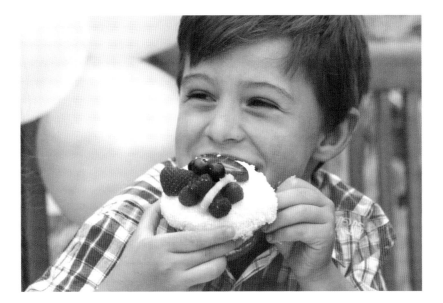

MY GOODNESS

All you need to know about children's health and nutrition

Written by Lisa Guy, ND

JCP

First published by Jane Curry Publishing 2010
(Wentworth Concepts Pty Ltd)
PO Box 780 Edgecliff NSW 2021

www.janecurrypublishing.com.au

National Library of Australia
cataloguing-in-publication data:

Lisa Guy   ISBN 978-0-9804758-9-0

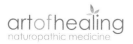

www.artofhealing.com.au
lisa@artofhealing.com.au

Edited by Kelli Wells.
Photographs by Lyndon Hawkins and Peter Logan.

Graphic design by Pauline Armour.

Cover: Harry Adkins, Skye George, Giorgia Floyd and
Toby Adkins. Photographed by Lyndon Hawkins.
Printed in China by Bookbuilders

Recipe Abbreviations
LF: Lactose-free   GF: Gluten-free

For Pete and my beautiful daughter Lily, who inspire me daily.

Acknowledgments

My deepest appreciation to my wonderful parents and partner for all their love, support and encouragement throughout this journey.

A special thank you to my dear friend Kelli Wells for editing my book, Libby Albert for all her help organising the photo shoots and Pauline Armour for designing this book so beautifully.

A big thank you to Lyndon Hawkins for bringing my book alive with his lovely photographs.

To all the gorgeous models photographed in this book, Lucy and Archie Benuska, Mia Clark and Harry Adkins, Toby Adkins, Skye George, Giorgia Floyd, Simon Anderson, Domenic Morocco, Mitch Walker, Henry Major, Taymon Cheal, Tylah Hutchinson, Jak Hall, Steve Pain and Rosie, a big thank you to you and your parents.

Thanks to Ben Hughes for letting me photograph Rosie (the VW combi van).

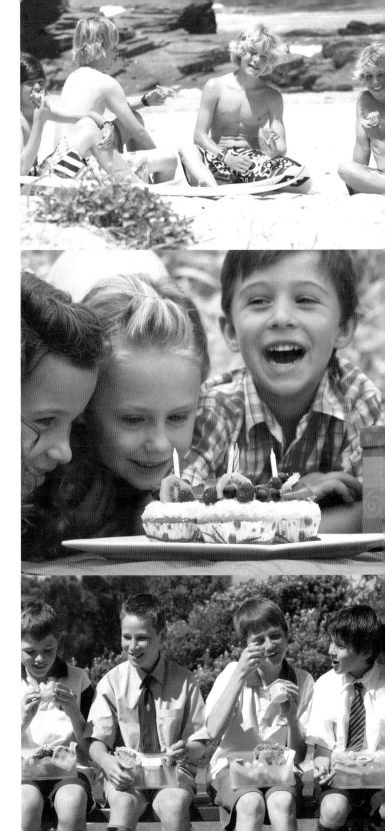

Contents

Introduction   7

Chapter 1: Back to basics   11

Going organic   12
Healthy cooking   15
Water   17
Enzyme-rich raw foods   18
Phytochemicals   19
Fibre   21
Glycaemic Index   26

Chapter 2: Essential nutrients   31

Macro-nutrients   32
Carbohydrates   32
Protein   34
Fats   36

Micro-nutrients   40
Calcium   41
Iron   44
Zinc   46
Vitamin C   48
Vitamin A & Beta-carotene   50
Vitamin E   52
B vitamins   54

Chapter 3: The five food groups   55

Wholegrain cereals   57
Fruit   60
Vegetables & legumes   64
Dairy foods   68
Meat, poultry, fish   73

Chapter 4: Extra foods   77

Refined sugars   79
Artificial sweeteners   84
Soft drink   85
Caffeine   88
Salt   89
Saturated & trans-fats   93

Chapter 5: Super foods   99

Berries   100
Fish   101
Garlic   102
Yoghurt   104

Chapter 6: Building healthy bones   105

Chapter 7: Vegetarian kids   109

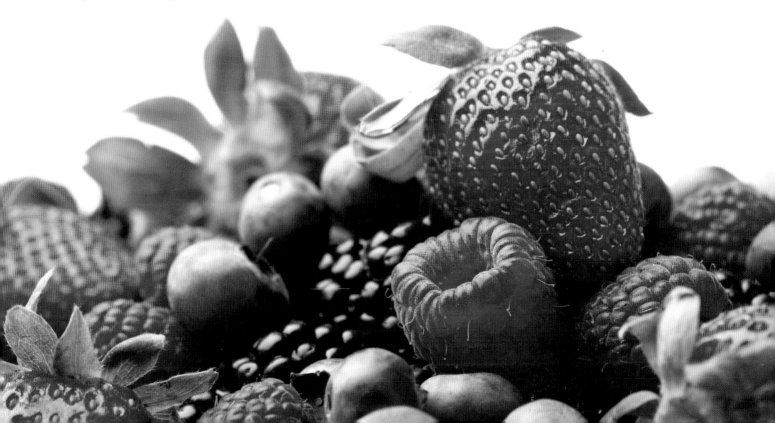

Chapter 8: Allergies & intolerances   115

Food Allergies   116
Milk allergy   117
Egg allergy   120
Peanut allergy   121
Food intolerances   122

Chapter 9: Kids with special needs   129

Childhood obesity   130
Children with diabetes   135
Kids with ADHD   139

Chapter 10: Packing a safe lunch box   141

Cooking with your kids   143

Recipes   145

Breakfast   147
Dips, sauces, salad dressings & chutneys   160
Salads   175
Winter soups   188
Baked goods & party treats   196
Lunch & dinner   215
Dessert   249
Beverages   258
Healthy party food   262
Sandwich & lunch box ideas   267
Cooking grains & legumes   271

References   274

Index   286

Introduction

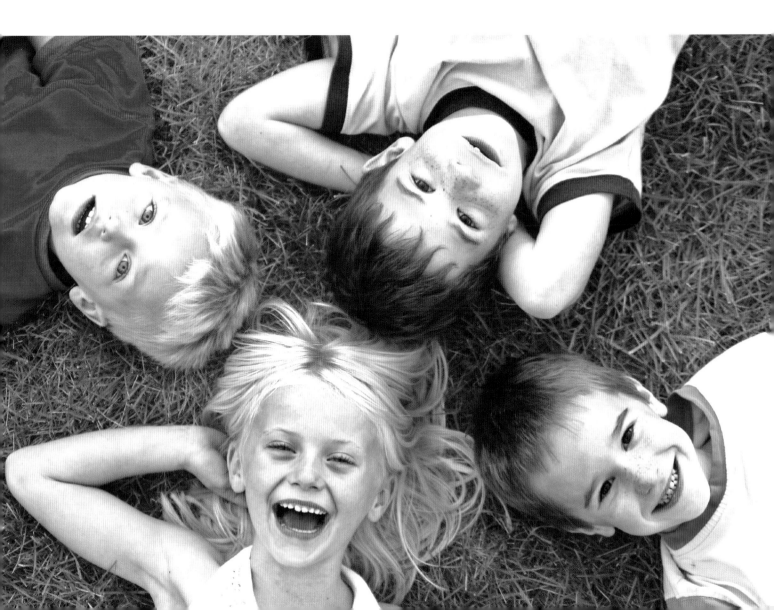

Obesity has become one of the most significant threats to the health of Australian kids. Over the last 20 years obesity rates in children have risen at an alarming rate in Australia and in many countries around the world.[1-3] In their most recent review of children's health, the NSW Centre for Overweight and Obesity exposed many 'questionable' eating habits in Australian children and reported a rapidly increasing prevalence of childhood obesity. According to the study, almost a quarter of Australian children aged between 5 to 16 years old are now overweight or obese.[4]

Equally concerning is that diseases such as type-2 diabetes, once seen only in adults, are now being seen in growing numbers in children. A significant number of these children are already showing signs of health problems caused by being overweight and having a poor diet. Precursors to cardiovascular and liver disease, elevated cholesterol, high blood pressure, high insulin levels and fatty liver deposits have been detected in an increasing number of children.

A major cause of childhood obesity and declining children's health in Australia is dietary-related.

Australian children are getting bigger and unhealthier as a result of their growing reliance on energy-dense junk foods that invariably include soft drinks, fast foods and processed snacks. These all tend to be high in saturated fats, sugars, salt and low in fibre.[5]

It is imperative that the current trend in Australian children's eating habits is corrected as soon as possible. If not, the not-so-long-term implications for Australians and Australian society are shocking: spiralling individual and public health costs; increasing morbidity rates, and a very real erosion of our kids' future quality of life.

In one sense, bucking the current trend can be as simple as steering children away from a diet dominated by these unhealthy, energy-dense junk foods. However, children are subjected to several influences that affect their food choices and preferences: family, friends, and the media, among others. Television commercials in particular have a powerful effect on the types of foods commonly desired, bought and consumed by children.[6] Children are constantly being bombarded with advertisements portraying unhealthy food and soft drinks as positive desirable choices, reinforcing children's bad dietary habits. The majority of these advertisements targeting children are for food products containing high amounts of saturated fats, sugars, and salt and foods that are low in dietary fibre.[7,8] Parents' efforts to encourage healthy eating are being undermined by unhealthy food advertising. Parents need to protect their children by helping them become educated young consumers making healthy dietary choices.

We are at the stage now where it is crucial that something is done to improve our children's health and eating habits. If we continue down this path the future implications for the health of our children will be frightening.

Prevention is the best cure. The best place to start addressing this problem is at home, with education and guidance from parents. It's while we're young that we are most susceptible to acquiring and learning attitudes towards food, diet and nutrition. Parents play a principal role helping their children develop positive attitudes towards food and healthy eating habits early on in their lives. There is evidence that establishing healthy eating patterns as a child will increase the likelihood of these patterns continuing throughout their lives.

To do this, parents need to learn about what foods their children should and shouldn't be eating. This book is a wonderful resource guide for parents, detailing everything they need to know about childhood nutrition.

When children start school they experience a new found independence when it comes to selecting and consuming food. School canteens and pocket money offer children the opportunity to choose their own foods, without the supervision of parents. With an increasing number of meals bought and eaten outside the home, school children are often eating at least one to two meals, plus snacks away from home each day. These new eating experiences benefit the development of children, exposing them to new foods, but can also pose a challenge to parents.

Parents and caregivers have the special responsibility to ensure their child receives nutritious, well balanced meals and snacks that meet all their nutritional needs. Childhood is an extremely important time for growth and development. If there is a period of poor nutrition during childhood your child will experience delayed growth. Poor nutrition during childhood will not only effect their growth and development, but can negatively affect their health for the rest of their lives.

Parents are one of the strongest influences and are role models for children. Parents need to be aware that their own food preferences and approaches to buying, cooking and eating foods have a big impact on their child's attitudes towards food.[9] It's important that children see food and mealtimes as fun and enjoyable. They will be encouraged to eat healthy foods if they see a positive association between meal time, healthy food and family.

One of the biggest concerns for all parents is whether their child is getting a balance of all the right nutrients through their diet. Children have special health needs and distinct nutritional requirements as they go through specific growth and development changes. Your child's growth, from the age of five to the onset of puberty is slow and steady. Their nutritional needs should be met by the continued consumption of a wide variety of food, increasing gradually as they get older, to meet their increased energy needs. Your child's

diet should consist of a nutritious breakfast, mid-morning snack, lunch, afternoon snack and dinner. This will ensure that your child has plenty of energy to sustain them throughout the day.

Not only are children's bodies steadily growing during this time, so are their brains. It's especially important that your children get all the necessary nutrients, such as omega-3 fats, to feed their growing brains. The growth and development of a child's brain continues right through until 16 years of age, and their intelligence, ability to concentrate and their school performance are all dependent on them receiving the right foods and nutrients every day from a young age.

Good nutrition is also essential for the healthy functioning of your child's immune system. Specific nutrients are needed for the production of protective immune cells, such as white blood cells, immunoglobulin and antibodies that fight infections and disease. Childhood is a very important time for the provision of protein, iron, zinc and vitamin C, which are all required daily to strengthen your child's immunity. Children who are lacking in any of these nutrients will be more prone to colds and viral infections and common childhood illnesses such as earaches and gastroenteritis.

Like the rest of their bodies, children's teeth will also benefit from a healthy balanced diet. Teeth are one of your child's most important possessions and how you help your child look after them will make a big difference to their health. This means not only how they clean them but also focusing on cutting down on sugary foods and drinks that are known causes of tooth decay.

Many adult health problems such as obesity, high blood pressure, heart disease, osteoporosis, type-2 diabetes and certain cancers can be prevented by good nutrition in childhood. Childhood symptoms to look out for, that may suggest that your child is not eating the right foods, include being over or under weight, poor growth and development for their age, chronic constipation, raised blood fats, dental cavities and unhealthy gums, constant tiredness, irritability, inability to concentrate and learning difficulties, as well as recurring infections and illness.

Only with appropriate guidance and education, and with reinforcement of positive attitudes to proper diet in the home, can we improve our children's health and curb this childhood obesity epidemic. The role of parents is critical. For parents to spread the healthy food gospel with the zeal that is truly required they must be empowered through 're-education' and awareness. They must learn the real meaning of healthy foods in the modern world. What we once knew as 'healthy' has become blurred in the face of the changing nutritional value of fresh produce, greater use of pesticides in agriculture, burgeoning preservative technologies in food, greater choices of packaged and processed products and, of course, the constantly evolving scientific view of what 'healthy' and proper dieting entails. Parents need to be mindful of this in the context of how the alternative – the modern energy-dense, junk food diet - deprives kids by way of their lifelong potential, and how the choices they make and provide in the home can influence lifetime eating behaviours.

This is why I have written this book - to equip parents with the tools necessary to ensure their children do not head down the path to overweight, obesity and poor health. It's my belief that parental education and guidance is the greatest weapon in fighting childhood obesity.

This book is a valuable resource and guide for parents, detailing everything they need to know about childhood nutrition and showing them how healthy foods can be prepared, combined and served in a way that your children will love.

In the subsequent pages you will find a number of delightful recipes that are presented in a way that does their true 'scrumptiousness' justice. I have taken great care to ensure all the recipes are fun, tasty and attractive to kids and parents alike. However, the fundamental appeal of all of my recipes is that they are healthy in every sense of the word, they meet all of the key issues and requirements for kids growth and development and give them the best chance of a healthy future.

Please enjoy learning about and implementing healthy nutrition for you and your kids. Thanks for your efforts for their goodness' sake. Good health and bon appétit.

"Parents play a principle role helping their children develop positive attitudes towards food and healthy eating habits early on in their lives."

Chapter 1:
Back to basics

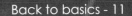

Going organic
your child deserves it

It's important to give children the very best start in life and that involves giving them the best quality, nutrient-dense food you can. Children need the best possible nutrition if they are to fulfil their potential both physically and emotionally. Natural, fresh foods, free from chemicals, preservatives and additives should make up the majority of your child's diet.

Organic produce is grown without the use of synthetic fertilizers, pesticides or herbicides. All of these have questionable effects on human health if they remain in the foods we ultimately eat. Therefore, organic manufacturers take their nutritional responsibilities very seriously, having strict standards at all levels of production and supply. The producers of organic products have a special consideration for the environment, caring for the soil, and work in harmony with nature to deliver a natural product that is free from chemicals. Organic products must be free from any artificial additives, flavourings, colourings, preservatives, hydrogenated fats or genetically modified ingredients.

Artificial additives

Many processed or commercial foods contain a vast number of additives in the form of chemical preservatives, antioxidants, stabilisers, thickeners, flavour enhancers and colourings. A UK Food Commission survey showed that 38% of children's food contained additives in products that were likely to form a large part of their diets (not including soft drinks, confectionery, chocolate and crisps).[1] In Australia there are hundreds of artificial additives added to processed foods.[2] As

has been the modern trend, children's consumption of processed and fast food has gathered pace and therefore so too has their intake of chemical additives.

Herbicides and pesticides

Over 170 pesticides, herbicides and fertilizers are routinely sprayed on commercially grown crops. Their toxic residues can be found in a variety of the foods children frequently consume. Some of these foods have been found to contain up to 14 different pesticide residues.[3] Several kinds of fertilizers also contain toxic heavy metals (mercury, lead, aluminium) that enter the soil and are absorbed and retained by these plant crops.[4]

There is a substantial body of evidence that suggests residues left in food by pesticides and other chemicals can be harmful to humans. Research has demonstrated that reduced immune resistance and reproductive function is associated with consumption of commercially versus organically grown produce.[5-8]

The literature also shows that excessive exposure to pesticide residues and the like can potentially disrupt the growth and development of your child's developing nervous and reproductive systems. As these continue to develop, until around 18 years of age, this has obvious implications for our kids and the diets they should be consuming.

Antibiotics

Also of relevance to children's health is the issue of antibiotic usage in livestock farming. Most non-organic livestock are given antibiotics and other drugs on a regular basis to maximize meat and egg production. There is growing evidence to suggest the long-term consumption of low levels of antibiotics has a detrimental effect on the development of children's immune function.

By choosing certified organic meats, poultry and eggs you can feel reassured that they will be free from antibiotics and their feed was free from pesticides, herbicides and genetic modification.

Higher nutrient levels

Much of the soil in Australia and other countries around the world is increasingly 'nutrient-poor' due to non-sustainable farming practises and the use of non-organic fertilizers. Perpetual farming of land can lead to soil de-nutrification. Manganese, zinc, iron, chromium, cobalt, magnesium, molybdenum and calcium, to name a few, which the growing plant takes from the soil, are never replaced. Subsequent crops draw from lowering levels of essential nutrients in the soil and, are themselves compromised in the same way.

There is little doubt that through the ages of commercial farming practice, mineral depletion of soils has occurred to a significant extent and that food crops today contains fewer nutrients than in the past. Reputable British and American studies have shown a decline in the vitamin and mineral content of commercially grown fruits and vegetables over the last 60 years.[9]

Sustainable (organic) farming techniques, however, such as manuring, composting, companion planting and crop rotation ensures that the soil is healthy and has an adequate supply of nutrients from which crops can grow.

There are more than 30 studies comparing the nutrient content of organic crops to those grown conventionally. The majority of these show that organic crops are nutritionally superior, having higher levels of vitamins and minerals.[10] Organic crops are also distinguishable by their superior taste.

Research by the Organic Advisory Service of the Organic Retailers & Growers Association of Australia (ORGAA) compared nutrient content of organic and conventionally grown vegetables. This study found that there were significantly higher mineral levels in organic produce by comparison to conventional produce. Calcium levels in some organic produce was superior to its levels in conventionally grown counterparts by eight times; potassium by ten times; magnesium by seven times; and zinc by five.[11] Organically grown produce has also been found to be superior to commercially grown crops in protein quality.[12]

Fruit and vegetables grown organically contain significantly higher levels of phytochemicals (antioxidants) than conventionally grown foods.[13,14,15] Phytochemicals are a part of a plant's natural defence system and also act as powerful antioxidants in humans. They help prevent cancers and other chronic diseases. Researchers have identified some pesticides and herbicides that actually inhibit the production of phytochemicals in plants.

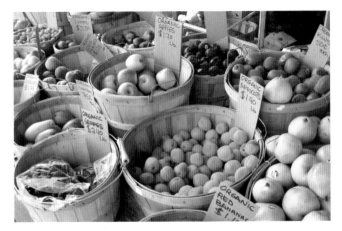

Keep chemicals out of your child's diet

The best way to remove toxins from your child's plate is to provide organic foods whenever possible. However, when consuming commercially grown products there are ways you can reduce pesticide residue:

1. Thoroughly wash all non-organic fruit and vegetables.

2. Peel all non-organic fruit and vegetables with skins such as carrots, potatoes, pumpkin, pears and peaches.

3. Peel foods such as cucumbers and apples that have a wax coating (wax prolongs their shelf life but also seals in harmful pesticide residues).

4. Rinse non-organic rice, grains and legumes well before cooking and use fresh water to cook with.

5. Choose organically farmed meats, chickens and eggs where possible. If you buy non-organic meat make sure you trim all visible fat, as toxins tend to accumulate in the fat of animals.

Genetically modified foods

One of the most important issues facing consumers today is the advent of genetic engineering of foodstuffs. Genetically modified (GM) foods have ingredients in them that have been modified by gene technology. This technology makes it possible to transfer genes between organisms to produce crops that are more resistant to herbicides and pesticides, and have a longer shelf-life. It is a complex and controversial issue involving our health and the environment.

Molecular biology has advanced so quickly that genetic modification of organisms today is dramatically different from cross-breeding first seen a century ago. Genetic engineering now crosses the natural boundaries between species, crossing plants with animals and micro-organisms.

There is a growing concern that introducing foreign genes into food plants may have an unexpected and negative impact on human health, including allergic responses. There remains a possibility that introducing a gene into a plant may create a new allergen or cause an allergic reaction in susceptible individuals. There has been insufficient research into the long-term effects of these gene altered foods on humans. It is suspected however that genetically modified foods are potentially harmful and may have a significant impact on children.[15]

Indeed, the potential health dangers in consuming GM foods are numerous. For example, GM foods might contain resistant bacteria or viruses and unlabelled allergic proteins. These may adversely affect immune function and of course, allergic sensitivity when consumed. Moreover, the extent of these changes can only be speculated upon as there is, by much estimation, insufficient understanding of the dynamic changes that take place in GM plants and little knowledge of what second and third-generation plants will produce. Certainly, the risk to children's health must surely be considerable when the possibility of immune-function type effects are considered.

Crops that are commonly modified in some countries include soy beans, canola (rape seed), corn and potato. Everyday products containing GM foods include breakfast cereals, soy products and vegetable oils. Australia requires mandatory labelling of all GM foods and products containing GM ingredients. However, in some countries like America, which produces the majority of GM foods, it is not mandatory to label GM foods or products containing them.

It is my sincere recommendation that, by virtue of the uncertainty surrounding GM foods and children's health, all food labels should be read carefully and products containing genetically modified foods should be avoided. The way that food is cooked has a significant effect on the amount of

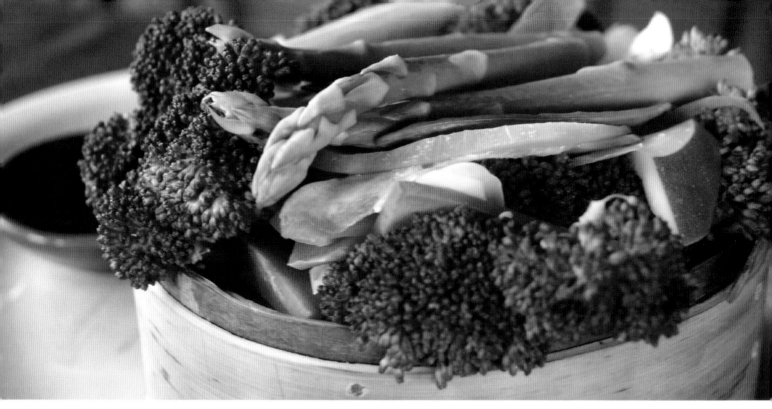

Healthy cooking
for healthy kids

nutrients that ultimately wind-up on the dinner plate. To ensure your children are getting the most out of the foods they eat, prefer cooking methods that preserve nutritional value (eg steaming vs boiling vegetables) and steer clear of adding harmful fats in the cooking process.

Keep 'off the boil'

Recent studies have confirmed that several nutrients and beneficial phytochemicals (antioxidants) in plant foods are damaged by particular cooking methods. Conventional boiling of vegetables can lead to a 66% loss of certain antioxidants compared to fresh vegetables, while microwaving vegetables can lead to a 97% loss of antioxidants.[1,2] Most nutrients are water-soluble and during boiling, a high percentage of nutrients are leached out of vegetables into the cooking water.

Thus, it is recommended that vegetables be cooked in a minimal amount of water in order to retain their nutritional value. Indeed, lightly steaming vegetables is the best way to retain their goodness and flavour as steaming leads to only minimal antioxidant loss. If you must boil vegetables only use a small amount of water and preserve lost nutrients by using the water as nutrient-rich 'stock' for soups or sauces.
In some cases, the availability of a nutrient might actually be enhanced by the cooking process.

Lightly stir-frying vegetables in a small amount of olive oil actually improves our ability to absorb fat-soluble vitamins (A and E) and other fat-soluble compounds (eg, carotenoids or phytochemicals) found in carrots, sweet potato and tomatoes.[3] Lightly steaming vegetables that contain carotenoids also improves our uptake of these compounds.[4]

When all is said and done children and adults alike should eat a combination of cooked and raw vegetables. Healthy stir-frying with a little olive oil, lightly steaming and oven baking remain the most effective methods of cooking vegetables to retain their nutritional value.

Oils aint oils

The most appropriate cooking oils for both children's and adult health are those that are low in saturated fat and high in monounsaturated fat. Olive oil is one example. Olive oil has a higher smoke point than other oils which means it does not 'oxidize' or degrade as quickly with repeated heating. Olive oil is a highly monounsaturated oil and therefore more resistant to hydrogenation and the formation of harmful trans-fats which play a significant role in cardiovascular disease. Studies have shown oxidation and hydrogenation occurs to a lesser degree in olive oil than in other oils. Avoid heating olive oil to very high temperatures. Moderate heat cooking is recommended.

Olive oil is a versatile and healthy choice for cooking. Cold pressed virgin or extra virgin olive oils are particularly preferable for stir-frying and oven baking. They can also be used in cakes and other baked goods, as in all my recipes, instead of butter.

Let your children enjoy the fresh, clean taste of foods without cooking them in unhealthy saturated fats such as vegetable oils and butter. Avoid deep frying meats, fish and chicken and instead use healthier cooking methods such as baking, grilling or healthy stir-frying with a little olive oil.

Finally, there is a growing body of research that suggests that burnt, overcooked, or charred meat, poultry and fish contain cancer causing compounds.[5]

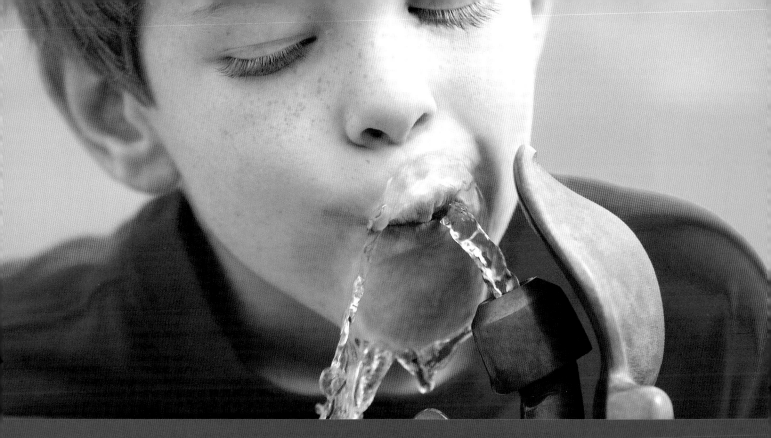

Water your child regularly

Water is an essential nutrient for life, making up around 60% of the human body. All biochemical reactions in the body occur in water that fills the spaces between all of our cells. Water is required for digestion, absorption and transportation of nutrients around the body, for the elimination of waste products and for temperature regulation.

Beverages are the main source of water in most people's diet, although water can also be obtained from a range of other foods, such as fruit and vegetables. Children should be encouraged to drink plenty of water throughout the day in preference to other fluids. Excessive consumption of soft drinks has obvious hazards, but too much fruit juice in the diet is not as healthy as it would seem. Both have high sugar content and can displace other dietary nutrients. High sugar intake may contribute to dental caries, weight gain and other nutritional deficiencies.

A balance between fluid intake and output is essential for efficient functioning of the body and for maintenance of good health. In the Australian climate, children, especially infants, are often at risk of dehydration. A child's fluid needs should be firstly met by water. Always pack a water bottle in their school bag. Pre-freezing is a good idea so it stays nice and cool over several hours. If, however, getting your children to drink more water is proving troublesome, mixing-in a little flavoursome fruit juice (eg apple and cranberry, tropical or pineapple) can work wonders (call it a healthy cordial).

Enzyme-rich raw foods

fruit, vegetables & sprouts

Scientific studies have confirmed the numerous health benefits obtained from eating enzyme-rich living foods. Fresh, raw sprouts (seeds, legumes and grains) are the best source of living enzymes. Other foods such as fresh, raw fruits and vegetables also provide living enzymes. Children can reap several positive health effects from a balanced diet rich in raw salad vegetables, sprouts and fruits and the plentiful enzymes that these provide.

Digestive enzymes are needed for all chemical reactions in the body associated with digestion. The body needs a regular supply of these enzymes to help break down proteins, carbohydrates and fats in foods, so the body can absorb and use them for energy, growth and development. Eating fresh raw foods containing living enzymes assists digestion, as these food enzymes can take the place of some of our body's digestive enzymes, sparing our body from having to make such concentrated digestive enzymes. This is beneficial not only for improving digestion but for the health of the whole body.

Unfortunately, most of the food children eat these days is enzyme-deficient. Processing and cooking of foods destroys many of these living enzymes. Therefore, a diet rich in processed foods places a greater demand on the body's energy and digestive enzyme supply.

Include enzyme-rich sprouted foods in your child's diet

1. Sprouting increases the nutritional value of legumes significantly. You can sprout most seeds, grains and legumes. Excess cooking will destroy valuable enzyme content and vitamin C and B - raw or lightly cooked is the healthiest way to eat sprouts.

2. Try combining sprouted grains into your kids' breakfast cereal (half sprouted half cooked grain). Add to cooked meals like stir-frys, soups or casseroles, rice and vegetable dishes and in salads. One tablespoon added to meals is all kids need to reap the wonderful health benefits of sprouted foods. Add some alfalfa or sprouted mung beans to your children's sandwiches and wraps for that extra crunch.

3. Buy only fresh looking sprouts from a reputable store. Sprouts are fresh when they are crisp and their roots are moist and white. Avoid musty-smelling, dark or slimy-looking sprouts. Keep sprouts refrigerated and use them in a timely manner. Wash the sprouts thoroughly with water to remove any dirt.

4. Bean sprouts go well mixed through stir-fries, salads and on sandwiches, wraps and burgers. Add sprouts to the centre of omelettes or top rice cakes spread with hummus or low-fat cottage cheese and sliced tomato.

Protect your child with
Phytochemicals

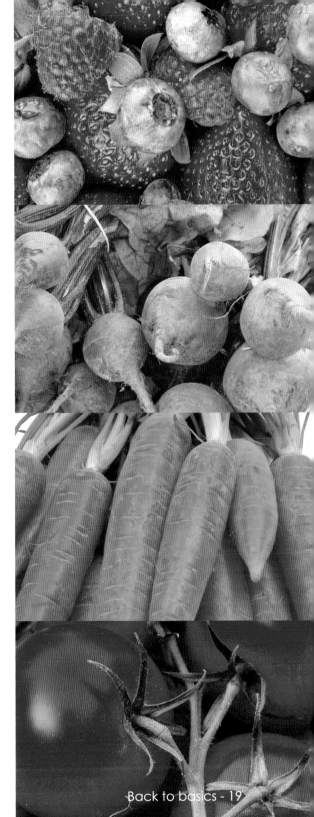

There are more than 1000 known phytochemicals derived from plant foods. Each of them works in a unique way to promote health. Plants produce these chemicals to protect themselves, but recent research demonstrates that many phytochemicals also protect humans and fortify against chronic disease. Wholegrain cereals, fruit, vegetables, legumes and herbs are all generally rich in phytochemicals.

Most phytochemicals have antioxidant activity that protects our cells against free radicals. Free radicals are highly reactive molecules that cause damage to cells in the body. By including antioxidants in the diet it reduces the risk of certain types of cancers and protects against cardiovascular disease.[1-3]

Carotenoids (beta-carotene and lycopene) and flavanoids (anthocyanins) are two of the better known phytochemicals found in the foods we eat.

Carotenoids

Carotenoids are found in red, yellow and orange fruits and vegetables such as carrots, sweet potato, pumpkin, mango, apricots and tomatoes. Like other phytochemicals they act as antioxidants, enhancing the performance of the immune system, protecting against certain cancers and playing a role in the prevention of heart disease and atherosclerosis.[4-7] Most carotenoids, namely beta-carotene, have pro-vitamin A activity, which means the body can convert them into an active form of vitamin A.

Lycopene is a carotenoid that gives the red colour to tomatoes, guava, watermelon and pink grapefruit. Lycopene is a powerful antioxidant which is particularly abundant in red tomatoes. Research shows that lycopene in tomatoes can be absorbed more efficiently by the body if processed into juice, sauce, and pastes. Epidemiological studies have shown that a high intake of lycopene containing vegetables is also protective against certain types of cancers, heart disease and other chronic diseases.[8, 9]

Flavanoids

Flavanoids are phytochemicals which are responsible for the yellow, red and purple colour in fruits and vegetables. They are found in apples, apricots, blueberries, beetroot, red cabbage, raspberries and strawberries. Flavanoids help protect blood vessels from rupturing and leaking and thus minimise bruising. Flavanoids enhance the power of vitamin C and have general antioxidant-enhancing activity which protects the cells from free radical damage and reduces inflammation throughout the body.

Anthocyanins are a major component of the flavanoid family and give berries, such as blueberries, their deep colour. Recent research shows that anthocyanins are powerful antioxidants that provide many potential health benefits, such as improving vision, balancing blood sugar levels, improving circulation and ultimately protecting against cancers and heart disease.[10] These flavanoids help promote healthy brain function, cardiovascular, urinary and skin health.[11]

Different phytochemicals have different health-promoting actions. It is important to give kids a variety of different fruits, vegetables, legumes and wholegrains in their diet to ensure they are exposed to the full gamut of protective phytochemicals.

"Include a variety of antioxidant-rich red, yellow and orange fruits and vegetables in your child's diet."

Fibre
your child's best friend

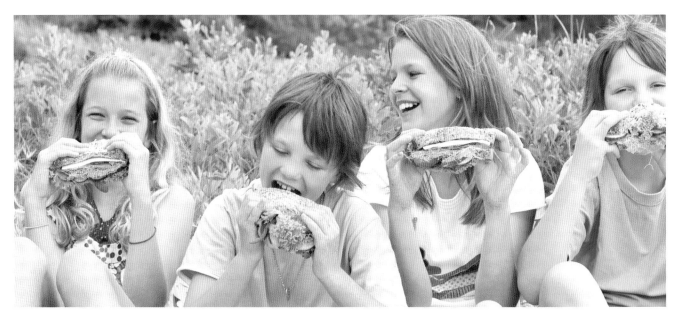

Dietary fibre is undoubtedly one of the most talked about nutrients for the promotion of health and prevention of disease. Fibre has many important health benefits and plays an essential role in children's health and wellbeing.

Dietary fibre is a type of indigestible carbohydrate derived from the edible parts of plants. Wholegrains, fruits, vegetables, legumes, nuts and seeds are all good sources of dietary fibre.

Maintaining a healthy colon and digestive system is crucial for your child's long-term health. Not only does the digestive system break down food to provide essential nutrients and energy, it is also a crucial component of a child's immune system in its own right. Beneficial bacteria found in the bowel, namely lactobacilli and bifidobacteria are needed for healthy immune function. There is also a high percentage (around 80%) of immune-producing cells found in the small intestine. In order to strengthen your child's immunity, you must start by supporting their digestive systems with appropriate nutrition. Dietary fibre should be included daily in your child's diet as it helps maintain the health of their colon and digestive system.

Previously it was generally thought that there were only two kinds of dietary fibre, soluble and insoluble. Over the last 20 years however, nutrition research has demonstrated the presence of a third kind called 'resistant starch'. All three kinds of fibre play specific roles in children's health.

Insoluble fibre

Insoluble fibre is found in the cell walls of plants, providing bulk and keeping kids 'regular'. It is found in wholegrain breads and cereals, unprocessed bran and wheat germ, nuts and seeds (flaxseed), and fruit and vegetables.

Constipation is strongly associated with colon cancer. If undigested food and waste products are not eliminated from the body they accumulate, putrefy, feed unfriendly bacteria and are reabsorbed back into the body. Over time these toxins can lead to chronic illness. Insoluble fibre helps maintain bowel regularity by increasing the bulk of the stool and speeding up the time it takes to travel through the intestines. This results in softer, larger stools and more frequent bowel actions. Diets rich in insoluble fibre are associated with a low prevalence of constipation and colon cancer.[1,2]

Soluble fibre

Soluble fibres are edible parts of plants that are resistant to digestion and absorption. They pass undigested through the small intestine. However, when they reach the large intestine they are fermented by bowel bacteria.

Soluble fibre helps protect the immune system and promotes intestinal health by acting as a 'prebiotic'. Prebiotics stimulate the growth and activity of beneficial bacteria in the large intestine.

Soluble fibre is found in many foods, including legumes (peas, beans and lentils), oats and oat bran, brown rice, fresh and dried fruit, vegetables and seeds.

When soluble fibre foods are eaten, they attract water in the gastrointestinal tract, forming a gel like substance. This gel delays the stomach emptying and slows digestion to help the body absorb vital nutrients from foods.

Soluble fibre has been scientifically proven to lower total and LDL 'bad' cholesterol, which helps reduce the risk of heart disease.[3] It helps to normalise blood glucose levels by slowing the rate at which food leaves the stomach, delaying the absorption of glucose from a meal. By slowing the rate at which food leaves the stomach, your child will be provided with a steady supply of energy to fuel their active minds and bodies throughout the day. This promotes a sense of satiety (fullness) after a meal which stops children from overeating and therefore gaining weight. Soluble fibre also increases insulin sensitivity and plays a role in the prevention and treatment of type-2 diabetes.[4] Insulin sensitivity is a critical factor in maintaining healthy blood sugar levels.

Resistant starch

The large intestine is composed mainly of colon where additional nutrients are absorbed through a process called fermentation. Beneficial bacteria, present in the colon, are responsible for the fermentation process that produces gases and short-chain fatty acids. It is these short-chain fatty acids that have significant health properties.

Resistant starch provides some of the health benefits of both soluble and insoluble fibre, plus some unique advantages of its own. Resistant starch escapes digestion and is then fermented in the colon where a range of beneficial short-chain fatty acids, namely butyrate, are produced.

Butyrate supports the health and integrity of the colon and immune system by maintaining healthy populations of 'friendly' bowel bacteria, bifidobacteria and lactobacilli. Acting as a prebiotic, butyrate stimulates the growth and activity of these beneficial bacteria and discourages the growth of pathogenic (harmful) bacteria.[5,6] Butyrate also stimulates the production of T helper cells, antibodies, leukocytes and other components that play crucial roles in immune protection. Researchers have found that butyrate has anti-cancerous properties, helping to reduce the risk of colorectal cancer.[7-9]

Resistant starch and soluble fibres are called fermentable fibres however, the fermentation of resistant starch produces more butyrate than that of soluble dietary fibre. Researchers have found that consuming resistant starch is an ideal way of adding more fibre to a wide range of products. Due to its slow fermentation characteristic resistant starch can be consumed in significantly higher quantities without the digestive side effects that can occur with larger amounts of soluble fibre.

Resistant starch improves digestive health and the overall health of the bowel by promoting regularity with a mild laxative effect. Resistant starch also has a stabilising effect on blood sugar levels by reducing the glycaemic response of foods. This slows the release of glucose into the bloodstream.[10] Like soluble fibre, foods rich in resistant starch have been shown to be protective against diabetes.[11]

Resistant starch is found naturally in seeds, legumes, unprocessed grains, potato, green bananas, rice and corn. Legumes and unprocessed cereal grains (particularly barley and corn) contain a substantially higher percentage of resistant starch. Heavily processed flours and processed grain-based products do not contain as much natural resistant starch as wholegrain varieties.

In Australia, resistant starch is now added to a variety of commercially made products such as breads, cakes, pasta, cereals, snacks and other baked goods in the form of corn (maize). While 'resistant starch' is not generally listed on ingredient panels, look out for terms such as 'fibre', 'starch', 'corn starch' or 'maltodextrin'.

"Maintain a healthy colon and digestive system with a daily dose of fibre."

How much fibre should children eat?

Giving children a variety of different wholegrain cereals, fruits, vegetables, legumes, nuts and seeds will provide them with all of the dietary fibre they need as well as a variety of soluble fibre, insoluble fibre and resistant starch.

Recommended daily fibre intake for children (AI*) [12]

- All children 4–8 years should eat 18 g of fibre a day.
- Boys aged 9–13 years should eat 24 g of fibre a day and boys aged 14–18 years should eat 28 g of fibre a day.
- Girls aged 9–13 years should eat 20 g of fibre a day and girls aged 14-18 years should eat 22 g of fibre a day.

* Adequate intake

Improve your fibre intake

1. Choose wholegrain breakfast cereals. A good kid's breakfast cereal should have more than 5% fibre, or more than 5g of fibre per 100g.

2. Choose wholegrain breads and crackers.

3. Bake with wholegrain flour instead of white flour.

4. Increase your child's fruit and vegetable intake. Skin of fruits and vegetables, like apples and potatoes, contain good amounts of fibre, so when buying organic produce leave the skins on.

5. Give your child whole fruit over fruit juice. If making fresh juices, make sure you add the pulp.

6. Increase legumes (beans, lentils, peas) in your child's diet. Add to soups, salads, stir-fries, make some hummus, dahl or baked beans. Mash some broad beans or white kidney beans through mashed potato. Make oven baked falafels.

7. Choose brown rice over white. Accustom your child to brown rice by cooking a mix of both brown and white. Brown rice takes around 45-50 minutes to cook, but for the extra fibre it delivers, it's worth the wait. If you soak brown rice for 30 minutes before cooking, it will cook quicker and have a softer texture.

8. Include raw and unsalted nuts and seeds in cooking, (stir-fries, biscuits and muffins) and sprinkled on breakfast cereals and salads.

9. Gradually increase your child's fibre intake to avoid gastrointestinal discomfort and increase their fluid intake at the same time to prevent constipation.

Fibre content of commonly eaten foods:

Food	Serving size	Total dietary fibre (g)
Shredded wheat biscuit	2	4.4
Whole oats	30g (1 medium bowl)	3.2
Wholemeal bread	1 slice	2.1
White bread	1 slice	0.5
Rye crispbread	4 crispbreads (36g)	4.2
Wholewheat pasta	230g	8.1
White pasta	230g	2.8
Brown rice	180g	1.4
White rice	180g	0.2
Dried apricots	6	3
Orange	1	2.7
Apple	1	1.8
Avocado	1/2 small	3.4
Baked beans	1 small can (200g)	7.4
Jacket potato	1 medium (180g)	4.9
Green peas	3 tbsp (90g)	4.6
Red Lentils	3 tbsp (90g)	1.7
Broccoli	85g	2
Carrots	60g	1.5
Sweet corn	3 tbsp (90g)	1.3

What is the
Glycaemic Index?

Most people will be familiar with the terms 'high GI' and 'low GI' that are commonly seen on the packaging of food products containing carbohydrates. However, what these terms mean and how they affect our health and the health of our children is not generally known.

Not all carbohydrate foods are created equal, in fact they behave quite differently in our bodies. The Glycaemic Index (GI) is a ranking of carbohydrate foods based on the effect they have on blood glucose levels. Foods high in fat or protein do not cause a significant rise in blood sugar levels so they are not included in the GI list. Foods containing carbohydrates are compared against glucose, which is the most quickly absorbed type of carbohydrate and has a (top) rating of 100%. High GI foods have a GI of 70 or higher, moderate GI foods have a GI of 56-69, and low GI foods have a GI of 55 or less. The speed at which these carbohydrates enter the bloodstream has an effect on how much insulin is released into the blood.

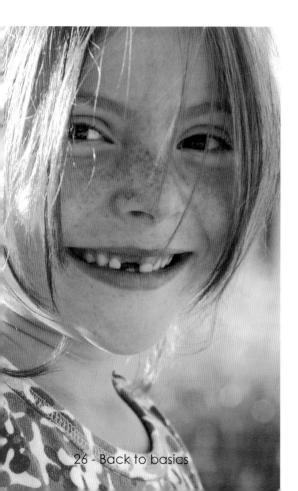

Parents can use the GI as a tool to prepare healthy meals. It helps to maintain an optimal level of blood glucose which is especially important for children with diabetes. Children who are overweight or obese will also stand to benefit from following a diet based on the GI.

High GI foods

Foods that contain carbohydrates that are broken down quickly during digestion and rapidly absorbed quickly into the bloodstream have the highest GIs. The consumption of high GI foods causes blood sugar levels to surge quickly which then triggers the release of insulin into the blood stream. A 'rush' of blood-insulin causes a rebound effect whereby blood sugar levels then begin to plummet. Low blood sugar levels are associated with tiredness, poor concentration, crankiness, irritability, and 'sugar cravings'. This is also a signal for the body to store fat.

The typical western diet, based on potato, bread and processed cereal products, is digested and absorbed rapidly, resulting in a high glycaemic load and a high demand for insulin secretion.[1] Studies have shown that a high glycaemic diet is associated with weight gain and obesity.[2] The consumption of high GI foods promotes a rapid return to hunger and increases food and energy intake, leading to overeating and weight gain.[3,4] Epidemiologic data suggests that a high dietary glycaemic load from refined carbohydrates increases the risk of coronary heart disease.[5]

The long-term consequences of an imbalance of insulin and blood sugar levels can result in the development of chronic diseases such as cardiovascular disease and type-2 diabetes.[6]

Low GI foods

Low GI foods contain carbohydrates that breakdown slowly and are associated with a gradual release of glucose into the bloodstream. These foods release their total energy slowly over a period of time. By eating foods with a low GI, the rate of glucose absorption and the amount of insulin secreted are tightly regulated. Low GI foods provide a steady supply of glucose which can sustain children's energy requirements longer, avoiding drops in blood glucose levels and helping to reduce energy slumps and mood swings - the brain receives a steady supply of glucose which allows children to concentrate and 'learn' at a more optimal level.

Low GI foods also promote a sense of satiety (fullness) that will help reduce hunger and overeating of unhealthy food.[7] The slower digestion of low GI foods is associated with minimal insulin secretion which can help prevent excess weight gain.[8,9] Studies have shown that, by comparison with high GI meals, low GI meals are usually followed by less energy (calorie) intake at subsequent meals.[10]

Researchers have found that giving children a diet containing medium to low GI carbohydrate foods will reduce their risk of chronic diseases (heart disease and diabetes).[11] A lower GI diet will improve insulin sensitivity and help maintain both healthy cholesterol levels and body weight.

Factors affecting the GI of foods

Wholegrain foods are rich in fibre and have lower GI's than many of the processed grain products such as white breads, white rice and commercial breakfast cereals. Wholegrain is not the same as 'wholemeal'. Even though the whole of the grain is included, it has been ground-up instead of left whole. For example, some mixed grain breads that include wholegrains have a lower GI than either wholemeal or white bread. Fruit and vegetables are also rich sources of fibre and are therefore low GI foods that should be freely included in the diet.

The presence of fat and protein in a food slows down the absorption of carbohydrates. Milk and other dairy products have a low GI because of their high protein and fat content. Legumes, nuts and seeds are also all low GI foods as they contain protein and unsaturated fats. Not all low GI foods are healthy choices however. For example, chocolate has a medium GI and potato chips have a lower GI than potatoes, due to their high fat content. For this reason it's important to use the GI only as a guide and not to rely exclusively on it for healthy food choices.

While a balanced consumption of low GI foods in the diet is clearly beneficial for health, high GI foods need not be avoided altogether. There are a number of healthy choice high GI foods that should be included in your child's diet. The glycaemic load of a given meal or snack can be balanced by combining high and low GI carbohydrate sources. For example, a puffed rice cake, which is a healthy cracker choice but with a high GI, can be balanced by spreading it with low GI hummus, cottage cheese or avocado. Healthy natural corn flakes or puffed brown rice (with no added sugar) have a high GI which can be balanced with the addition of milk or yoghurt, some fresh fruit and a sprinkling of nuts (all low GI foods). With white rice meals, low GI stir-fries containing lots of vegetables, legumes or tofu will balance-up the GI load. Likewise, dried fruits have high GIs however, if eaten in small quantities and combined with low GI nuts and seeds, can be consumed in a perfectly healthy manner.

Lowering the glycaemic load for kids

1. Choose wholegrain breakfast cereals over highly processed cereals. For example, give your child slow cooking whole oats instead of instant oats. Adding milk, yoghurt or fresh fruit to higher GI cereals like puffed brown rice or natural cornflakes will lower the total glycaemic load.

2. Choose wholegrain breads over white or wholemeal. Serve higher GI breads such as Lebanese breads with low GI dips (hummus, baba ghanoush) or serve as a wrap with lots of salad and some form of protein (lean meat, fish, chicken, egg, low fat cheese, falafel, tofu pattie).

3. Include plenty of whole fruit, vegetables and legumes in your child's diet.

4. Combine lower GI foods with higher GI foods in the same meal to lower the total glycaemic load of the meal.

5. Including fibre, protein or good fats in a meal will lower the meals total glycaemic load.

6. Use wholegrain flours instead of plain flour to bake muffins, cakes and cookies.

7. Include plenty of salad vegetables in your child's diet.

8. Include wholemeal pasta and noodles in your child's diet. Serve with plenty of fresh vegetables and some type of protein (lean meat, fish and chicken) to lower the total glycaemic load.

9. Choose brown rice over white rice.

10. Rice cakes, rye crackers and crisp breads are healthy snacks and should be included in your child's diet. Spreading crackers with low GI spreads such as hummus, baba ghanoush, low fat cheese or avocado will reduce the total glycaemic load.

11. Limit high GI foods like processed, sugary breakfast cereals and snacks.

12. Limit dried fruit to small servings and combine with some nuts, seeds and protein to help lower the total glycaemic load.

Glycaemic Index of carbohydrate foods[12]

Food	Glycaemic Index
COMMERCIAL BAKED GOODS:	
Lamingtons	87
Doughnuts	76
Crumpet	69
Croissant	67
Pancake, packet mix	67
Banana cake	47
Apple muffin	44
BREADS:	
Middle Eastern flat bread	97
Turkish bread, white	87
Lebanese bread, white	75
White bread	70
Wholemeal spelt	63
Rice bread	61
Pita bread, white	57
Wholegrain bread	51
Pumpernickel (rye) bread	50
Mixed grain bread	49
Fruit loaf	44
BREAKFAST CEREALS:	
Rice bubbles	95
Corn flakes	81
Coco pops	77
Sultana bran	73
Weet-Bix	69
Porridge, instant oats	66
Porridge, rolled oats	58
Porridge, whole oats	55
Special K	54
Muesli, natural	49
All bran	42
Muesli, gluten-free	39

Food	Glycaemic Index
BISCUITS:	
Puffed crisp breads	81
Puffed rice crackers	78
Water crackers	71
Rye crisp breads	64
PASTA & NOODLES:	
Gnocchi	68
Udon noodles	62
Rice noodles, dried	61
Rice vermicelli	58
Macaroni	47
Linguine, durum wheat	46
Spaghetti, white	42
Fettuccine, egg	40
Rice noodles, fresh	40
Spaghetti, wholemeal	37
Mung bean noodles	33

Food	Glycaemic Index
CEREAL GRAINS:	
Amaranth, puffed	97
Instant white rice	87
Millet, boiled	71
Cornmeal	69
Couscous	65
White rice, boiled	64
Basmati white rice, boiled	58
Long-grain white rice, boiled	56
Semolina	55
Brown rice	55
Buckwheat	54
Bulgur, cracked wheat	48
Wheat, whole kernel	41
Rye, whole kernel	34
Barley, pearl	25

Glycaemic Index of carbohydrate foods

Food	Glycaemic Index
VEGETABLES:	
Potato, peeled, boiled	87
Pumpkin	75
Beetroot	64
Sweet potato (kumera)	61
Potato, with skin, baked	60
Sweet corn	54
Carrots	47
Other vegetables	30
FRUIT:	
Dates, dried	103
Watermelon	72
Figs, dried	61
Pineapple	59
Sultana	56
Banana	52
Kiwi fruit	53
Mango	51
Grapes	46
Orange	42
Peach	42
Strawberry	40
Pear	38
Apple	38
Apricot, dried	31
Other fruit	30

Food	Glycaemic Index
DAIRY PRODUCTS:	
Ice cream	61
Custard	38
Whole milk	27
Yoghurt, reduced fat	27
SNACK FOODS & CONFECTIONARY:	
Jelly beans	78
Popcorn	72
Corn chips	63
Muesli bar	61
Milk chocolate, plain	43
SUGARS:	
Glucose	100
Sucrose	68
Honey	55
Fructose	19

"Parents can use the Glycaemic Index as a tool to prepare healthy meals."

Chapter 2:
Essential nutrients

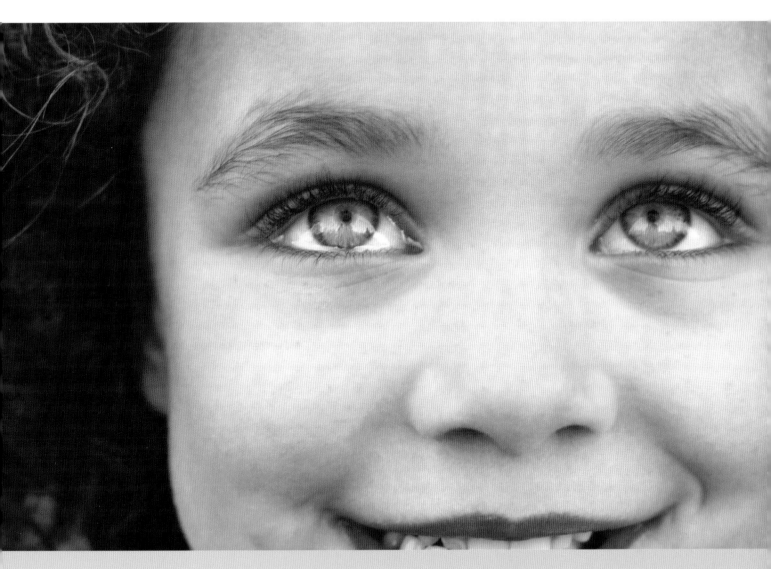

What children eat provides them with the raw materials needed for growth, development and the functioning of every cell in their body. There are two basic groups of nutrients that must be obtained through the diet - macro-nutrients and micro-nutrients. Macro-nutrients comprise proteins, carbohydrates and unsaturated fats while vitamins and minerals make-up micro-nutrients. All nutrients play different but vital roles in children's health and wellbeing.

Mighty
Macro-nutrients

Carbohydrates

Carbohydrates are the main energy-providing macro-nutrient. They can be easily converted into glucose by digestion and either used directly to provide energy for the body or stored in the liver for future use. A portion of carbohydrates may also be stored as body fat after a person has consumed more calories than have been burnt.

Glucose is the main fuel for brain and bodily energy requirements. It is required by the body for all metabolic processes, to power all muscle action (including heart function), for maintenance of body temperature, and the growth and production of new tissues.

Carbohydrates are found almost exclusively in plant foods such as grains, fruits, vegetables and legumes. Milk and milk products are the only foods derived from animals that contain a significant amount of carbohydrates.

There are two basic types of carbohydrates: simple and complex. Simple carbohydrates (or simple sugars) include fructose (fruit sugar), sucrose (table sugar), lactose (milk sugar) and glucose, as well as other compounds like honey. Simple sugars are easily identified by their sweet taste and are broken down quickly in the body to release energy.

Fruit and milk, containing natural simple sugars fructose and lactose, should be consumed daily as part of a well balanced diet. Fruits are the richest natural source of the simple carbohydrate fructose. When fruit is eaten whole, the fibre present in fruit slows the absorption of sugars, reducing the possibility of a surge in insulin and blood sugar levels. Milk is an excellent source of calcium and protein for children. Due to its high protein content, milk has a low GI and will not cause imbalances in blood sugar levels.

On the other hand, processed foods contain mainly only refined, simple sugars such as sucrose (table sugar) and fructose syrup. These should be reduced in the diet. High simple sugar foods include cakes, biscuits, other baked goods, lollies, chocolates, soft drinks, sugary breakfast cereals and muesli bars. If eaten to excess, especially over a period of many years, the large amounts of simple carbohydrates found in refined foods can lead to a number of disorders, including diabetes and obesity.

Honey is a natural alternative to white sugar. Produced by honeybees, honey is considered a simple sugar as it is composed of numerous types of simple sugars like glucose and fructose. A good quality raw, organic honey is a healthy addition to the diet. Raw honey has a lower GI than sucrose and contains beneficial nutrients and antioxidants. However, as with all sugars, honey should still be consumed in moderation as it can promote tooth decay and obesity if eaten in excessive amounts. Particular care should be taken however, with snacks like so called, 'health bars', that list honey as one of the main ingredients. Even though these products contain healthy elements such as oats, nuts and seeds, they are usually very high in sugars and fats.

Complex carbohydrates (starches) on the other hand are made up of long chains of simple sugar units bonded together (polysaccharides). Digestive enzymes have to work much harder to break these chains into individual sugars for absorption through the intestines. For this reason, digestion of complex carbohydrates takes longer. The slow absorption of sugars provides children and adults alike with a steady supply of energy.

Foods rich in complex carbohydrates include wholegrain cereals (breads, pasta, noodles, rice and crisp bread), vegetables (especially starchy root vegetables like potatoes, sweet potatoes, pumpkin and corn) and legumes.

As with foods containing simple sugars, some complex carbohydrate foods make for better healthy eating than others. Unrefined carbohydrate-rich foods should always be preferred as these are jam-packed with fibre and retain all of their vitamins and minerals. Throughout the processing stages, refined grains such as white flour and white rice lose the bulk of their valuable nutrient and fibre content.

	Simple carbohydrates	Complex carbohydrates
Should be included in diet	Fruit Milk & milk products Organic raw honey (small servings)	Wholegrain cereals (bread, breakfast cereals, pasta, rice, crisp breads) Vegetables (potato, sweet potato, pumpkin, corn) & legumes
Should be limited in diet	Table sugar Refined foods containing high levels of sucrose, fructose, glucose or honey – chocolate, lollies, soft drinks, flavoured milk drinks, breakfast cereals and bars, cakes, jams, desserts.	Refined cereal products that are low in fibre such as white flours and white breads.

Recommended carbohydrate intake for children

Complex carbohydrate foods should make up around 50% of children's diets with only 10% or less being made up of simple carbohydrates such as sugars, glucose, fructose and honey.

Protein

Proteins are highly complex molecules comprised of linked amino acids. They are broken down into constituent amino acids during digestion that are then absorbed and used to make new proteins in the body. Twenty-three different amino acids are used to construct proteins. Of these, eight are classified as essential amino acids as they must be supplied from the food we eat.

Protein is vital for the growth and repair of all cells and is the major source of building materials for muscles, blood, skin, hair, nails and internal organs. It is needed for the production of hormones and for the healthy functioning of the immune system. Protein is also needed for proper digestion, the formation of enzymes, the transporting of fats, vitamins and minerals and for carrying oxygen around the body.

Proportionately, children need more protein than adults as they are still growing and have greater demand for the formation of new cells. An adequate intake of protein foods, containing all essential amino acids, is thus crucial for optimal growth and development of all kids.

Proteins derived from animal sources are usually called 'complete proteins', which means they provide all the essential amino acids in the right amounts required by the body. Proteins from plant sources however, tend to be lacking in one or more essential amino acids. They are referred to as 'incomplete proteins'. These deficiencies can be overcome by combining different plant based proteins to achieve a better amino acid balance. Thus, when two different foods are combined, the amino acids of one protein compensates for those the other one lacks. This is called 'protein complementation'. Combining wholegrain cereals with legumes results in a high-quality protein, comparable to that of animal protein and is a good

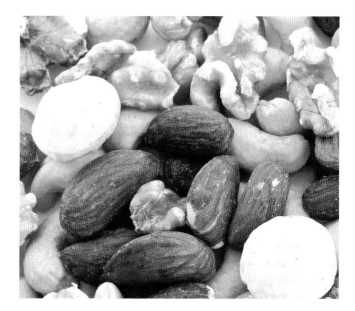

example of dietary protein complementation. (For more information on protein complementation go to the vegetarian chapter.)

Eating protein-rich foods also helps to stabilise children's blood glucose levels, which will in turn help curb sugar cravings and stabilise energy levels and mood. Protein creates a feeling of satiety (fullness), making protein an important part of any weight loss program for obese or overweight children.

Protein-rich animal sources include lean meat, fish, poultry, eggs and dairy products (cheese, milk and yoghurt).

Protein-rich vegetable sources include nuts and seeds (nut butters, tahini, ground nuts and seeds - LSA), legumes (beans, peas and lentils), hummus and patties made from legumes and seaweeds (kelp and nori).

Children should be eating around 25% of their daily calories from protein. A serving size for a piece of lean meat, fish or chicken should be roughly the width and thickness of your child's palm.

Protein content of commonly eaten protein-rich foods [1]

Food	Serving size	Total protein (g)
Lentils, raw	100g	25.8
Red kidney beans, raw	100g	22.5
Chickpeas, raw	100g	19.3
Chicken breast, roasted	80g	24.8
Lean lamb, roasted	80g	19.6
Tuna, canned	80g	20.4
Salmon, canned, bones	80g	18.5
Egg, hard boiled	1 egg	12.5
Pumpkin seeds	30g	7.4
Walnuts	30g	7.3
Almonds	30g	6.4
Flaxseeds	30g	5.9
Mozzarella, low fat	40g	9.7
Cottage cheese, low fat	40g	5.0

Recommended daily protein intake for children (RDI*) [2]

- All children aged 4–8 years should eat 20 g of protein a day.
- Boys aged 9–13 years should eat 40 g of protein a day; and boys aged 14–18 years should eat 65 g a day.
- Girls aged 9–13 years should eat 35 g of protein a day and girls aged 14-18 years should eat 45 g a day.

* Recommended dietary intake

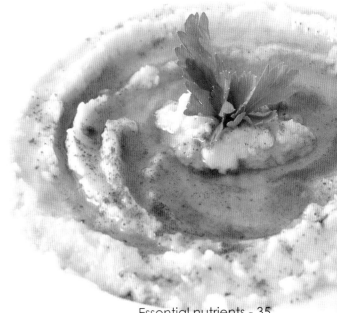

Unsaturated fats
the 'good fats'

Fats are a necessary and important part of every child's diet. However, they must be the right kind of fat. Children commonly eat too many saturated fatty foods in the modern diet. These are void of important essential fatty acids (EFAs) that are found in unsaturated fats or 'good fats'. The lack of EFAs in children's diets could play a significant role in the development of chronic degenerative diseases later in life. Eaten to excess, saturated fats are associated with elevated cholesterol, obesity, heart disease and increased risk of cancer.

Unsaturated fats eaten in moderation are needed for the absorption of fat-soluble vitamins A, D, E and K and are a concentrated form of energy.

If children do not obtain enough EFAs through dietary sources of unsaturated fats, numerous health problems can arise: eczema-like skin eruptions, susceptibility to infections and allergies, growth retardation, vision and learning problems and ADHD. EFA deficiency is also linked to conditions commonly seen in adults such as heart disease, cancer, insulin resistance and diabetes, asthma, depression, accelerated aging, stroke, obesity, arthritis and Alzheimer's disease.

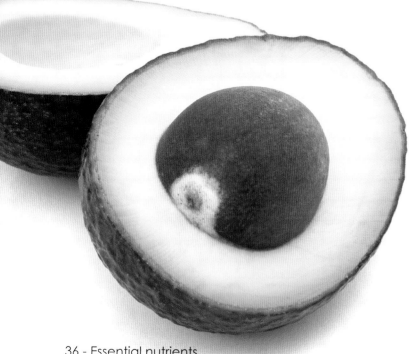

There are two main types of healthy unsaturated fats, the monounsaturated fats and polyunsaturated fats.

Monounsaturated fats

Monounsaturated fats are found in olive oil, canola oil, nuts (hazelnuts, almonds, cashews), almond oil, avocado, avocado oil, sesame seeds, sesame oil and pumpkin seeds. These fats are liquid at room temperature and are the most stable of the unsaturated fats. For this reason they are the best type of oils to cook with. Indeed, olive oil is one of the healthiest oils to cook with as it has a higher oxidation threshold than most other monounsaturated oils. Olive oil remains stable at higher cooking temperatures making it more resistant to hydrogenation and the formation of trans-fats, which are widely regarded as the worst type of fat.

Scientific studies have shown monounsaturated fats have a lowering effect on total cholesterol and LDL 'bad' cholesterol levels, as well as reducing triglyceride levels (blood fats) and blood pressure.[1,2] Diets containing monounsaturated fats are associated with a reduced risk of heart disease and cancer. These findings are consistent with the low incidence of heart disease and cancer in Mediterranean areas, where olive oil is the dietary fat of popular choice.

Monounsaturated fats have also been found to have beneficial effects on blood glucose levels, making them helpful in prevention and management of diabetes.[3,4] Moderate consumption of monounsaturated fats as part of a well balanced, low saturated fat diet, will help children maintain a healthy weight or assist in weight loss for the obese or overweight.[5]

Monounsaturated fats are typically high in phytochemicals and vitamin E, the antioxidant vitamin that is usually in short supply in many Western diets. In fact, it is likely that the significant health benefits derived from consumption of olive oil may be due to the vast number of phytochemicals it contains. To get the highest levels of protective phytochemicals from olive oil, cold pressed, 'extra virgin' or 'virgin' olive oils should be preferred as these varieties have endured minimal 'processing'. Care should still be taken to maintain phytochemical content by buying olive oil in dark bottles and by keeping it away from light and heat.

Polyunsaturated fats

Polyunsaturated fats are vital for children's health as they contain essential fatty acids (EFAs). EFAs cannot be manufactured by the body and therefore must be obtained from foods. There are two groups of polyunsaturated fats, omega-3 fatty acids and omega-6 fatty acids. Regular consumption of these 'good' fats is essential for the healthy growth and development of children.

The Western diet is abundant in omega-6 fatty acids, mainly from the wide spread use of vegetable oils rich in omega-6 FAs. Studies have shown that the ratio of EFAs consumed by adults and children is out of balance and is affecting our health.[6] Humans evolved consuming a diet that contained about equal amount of omega-3 and omega-6 FAs. Today, Western diets contain excessive amounts of omega-6 FAs and are deficient in omega-3 fats, with a ratio of around 16:1.[7] The healthy, natural balance of omega-3 to omega-6 has been destroyed.

This imbalance is believed to be a significant factor in the increasing rate of chronic inflammatory diseases. It's important to maintain an appropriate balance of omega-3 and omega-6 FAs in your child's diet as these two substances work together to promote good health. An inappropriate balance of these EFAs contributes to the development of disease while a proper balance helps maintain and improve health.

"Oily fish such as salmon, tuna and sardines, and flaxseed oil are rich sources of beneficial omega-3 fats."

Omega-3 fatty acids

Three of the most important omega-3 FAs are alpha-linolenic acid (ALA), eicosapentaenoic acid (EPA) and docosahexaenoic acid (DHA). EPA and DHA are found primarily in oily fish (salmon, mackerel, herring, sardines, tuna and trout). ALA is highly concentrated in certain plant oils such as flaxseed oil and to a lesser extent, canola and walnut oils. ALA is also found in dark green vegetables, parsley, seaweeds, nuts, seeds (pumpkin, sesame seeds and tahini), legumes, hummus and wholegrain cereals. Once ingested, the body converts ALA to EPA and DHA, the two types of omega-3 FAs more readily used by the body. Importantly, flaxseed, soybean or walnut oils should not be used for cooking as these oils are unstable at high temperatures, can easily oxidize and are more prone to hydrogenation.

Omega-3 FAs have a number of health benefits, notably in relation to the development and function of the brain and cardiovascular system. Omega-3 FAs play an important role in the prevention of many chronic diseases such as cancer, type-2 diabetes, cardiovascular disease, hypertension and arthritis.[8-19] They have triglyceride-lowering effects, reduce blood pressure and blood clots, and protect against atherosclerotic plaques.[20]

DHA is present in particularly high concentrations in the brain and retina, and appears to be most important for cognitive and behavioural function, as well as learning ability in children.[21,22] Consumption of these omega-3 FAs has been shown to help children with behavioural problems and ADHD. A link between depression and omega-3 deficiency has also been reported.[23]

Omega-3 FAs are needed for the proper growth and development of the nervous system and for the production of hormones such as oestrogen and testosterone. They are also important nutrients for healthy immune function as they help regulate inflammation and encourage the body to fight infection. While a diet containing too much omega-6 FAs actually promotes inflammation in the body, one that has abundant quantities of omega-3 FAs helps to prevent or inhibits inflammation.[24]

Omega-6 fatty acids

Linoleic acid (LA) is an EFA belonging to the omega-6 family. Like the omega-3 FA, LA cannot be manufactured in the body, so it has to be supplied through the diet. However, this EFA is in ample supply in our children's diets, commonly supplied through vegetable oils (safflower, sunflower, corn and soybean oils) in cooking. LA is also contained in less commonly used oils, like walnut, wheat germ and evening primrose oils.

Omega-6 FAs should not be thought of as 'bad' for health. They remain essential for a variety of health reasons. However, the fact remains that they form a very common part of most diets and are generally over-consumed. Commonly used vegetable oils such as safflower oil, corn oil and soybean oil all comprise over 50% omega-6 FAs with minimal content of omega-3 FAs. These oils should be used sparingly as they are unstable and easily convert to harmful trans-fats when heated.

Excessive consumption of omega-6 FAs and a very high omega-6/omega-3 ratio, found commonly in most children's diets, promotes the development of many diseases, including cardiovascular disease, cancer, and inflammatory diseases such as asthma and arthritis.[25] Research suggests that the consumption of excessive omega-6 fats may also lead to lower bone density with the increased risk of osteoporosis, whereas increased levels of omega-3 fats and a low omega-6/omega-3 ratio promote suppressive effects and prevent disease.[26,27]

Include 'good fats' in your child's diet

1. Include fish in your child's diet 2-3 times a week, grilled, in stir-frys, pasta dishes, patties and salads.

2. Flaxseed oil is an easy way of supplying EFAs to kids. Make sure you buy unrefined, cold pressed flaxseed oil. This oil has a mild taste so kids won't even notice it. Mix 1 tablespoon with their favourite food daily. Drizzle flaxseed oil on toast instead of butter, use it in salad dressings, hummus and mashed potato. Buy it from any health food store and keep it in the fridge. Don't cook with flaxseed oil as the heat will destroy the beneficial EFAs.

3. Avocado makes a great butter alternative, and a yummy dip or spread on crackers, toast, savoury muffins, pancakes and scones. Add diced avocado to salads or mix through mashed potatoes.

4. You can add nuts and seeds to a variety of dishes such as muffins, cakes, muesli, muesli bars, porridge, fruit salad, yoghurt, over veges, in patties, pasta dishes and salads. Use whole nuts, crushed or ground nuts and seeds. LSA (ground almonds, sunflowers and almonds) is a great way of sneaking extra EFAs into your child's diet. You can even mix it through mashed potato or sauces. Grind your own mix of nuts and seeds to add to meals or buy it ground from your health food store or supermarket. EFAs from ground nuts and seeds will be easier to absorb.

5. Use all natural nut butters or tahini (sesame seed paste) in moderation, as an alternative to peanut butter or butter. Add 1 tablespoon to patties, salad dressings, over vegetables, in stir-fries, spread on muffins, toast or scones, in muesli bars, cookie mix or in mashed potato. Mix with some mashed banana and spread on toast. Raw, unhulled tahini is the most nutritionally packed type of tahini, made from whole sesame seeds. However, unhulled tahini will have a slightly more bitter taste compared to hulled. You can mix a little organic honey with tahini for a sweeter spread.

6. Use olive oil for cooking, as it's one of the most stable oils for cooking with. All the baking recipes (cakes, muffins, biscuits, quiche bases) in this book use olive oil instead of butter.

Recommended fat intake for children

- For children over the age of 5 and for adolescents, approximately 30 % of their energy intake should be from fat, with no more than 10 % coming from saturated fats.
- Aim to reduce your child's total and saturated fat intake, replacing saturated fats with polyunsaturated and monounsaturated fats.
- Beneficial omega-3 EFAs are lacking in children's diets today, with Australian children's intakes estimated at being considerably less than recommended levels.[28] It is recommended to reduce your child's omega-6 intake and increase omega-3 FAs.

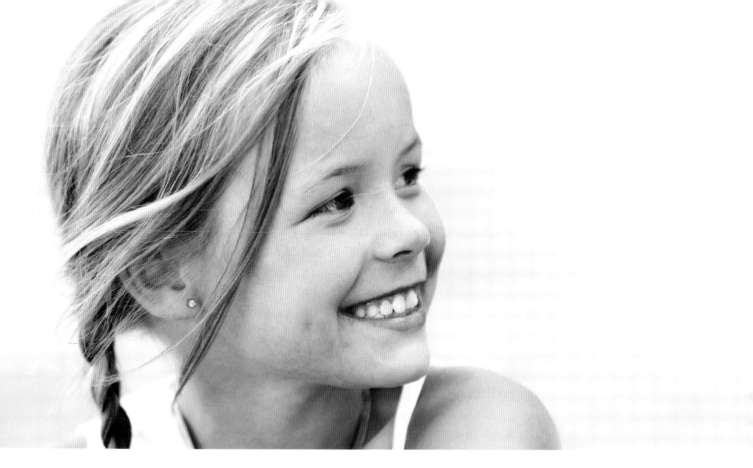

Micro-nutrients
essential vitamins & minerals

Although needed only in small amounts, micro-nutrients are essential for the proper functioning of every system in the body and are vital for children's growth and development. There are two classes of micro-nutrients, vitamins and minerals. Each vitamin and mineral has a specific role in bodily function. Our bodies cannot make these micro-nutrients, so they must be supplied through the diet. Different foods contain different levels of vitamins and minerals, so it's important that your child eats a wide variety of foods from the different food groups and a variety within each food group, to make sure they get an adequate supply of all the micro-nutrients they need.

There are certain vitamins and minerals that are especially important during childhood. These micro-nutrients are vitamin A, C, E, D and B group vitamins, as well as the minerals iron, calcium and zinc.

Calcium
for strong bones and teeth

Calcium is the most abundant mineral in the body and one of the most important for growth, reproduction and maintenance of the body. More than 99% of the body's calcium is stored in children's bones and teeth where it functions as structural support. The remaining 1 % is found throughout the body in blood, muscle and the fluid between cells.

It has long been known that calcium and calcium-rich foods are a 'must-have' in kids' diets. One of the most important functions of calcium during childhood is to build strong bones. This process is usually finished by the end of the teen years. Bone calcium begins to decrease in young adulthood and progressive loss of bone occurs with age, particularly in women. For this reason, children need to lay-down a strong bone foundation throughout 'the growing years'. Several retrospective studies suggest that higher calcium intakes throughout childhood are associated with greater bone mass in adulthood.[1-4] Children, especially girls, whose diets do not provide routine calcium in sufficient amounts are at greater risk of developing the bone disease osteoporosis in later life. Osteoporosis is associated with increased risk of bone fracture.

Calcium is needed to support proper functioning of nerves and muscles. Calcium is essential for muscle contraction, blood vessel contraction and expansion, normal heart beat, blood clotting, the secretion of hormones (for example insulin) and enzymes, and for nerve impulse transmission. If blood calcium levels are low (due to poor calcium intake), calcium is drawn from the bones in an attempt to maintain normal cell function. Thus, adequate dietary calcium is a critical factor in maintaining a healthy skeleton.

Although calcium is the nutrient consistently found to be most important for attaining peak bone mass and preventing osteoporosis, adequate vitamin D intake is also required for optimal calcium absorption. For this reason milk and a lot of soy milks are fortified with vitamin D. Calcium absorption is also reduced when there is excessive sodium and caffeine consumption in the diet. This results in an increased loss of calcium in the urine.

More than 85% of girls and 60% of boys aged 9 to 18 fail to get the recommended levels of calcium on a daily basis. Kids who drink soft drinks and other caffeinated beverages get even less calcium because those substances interfere with the body's ability to absorb and use calcium.

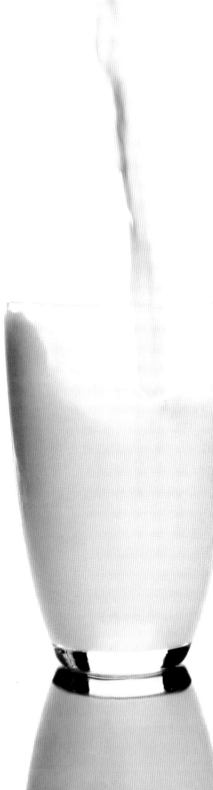

Increase your child's calcium intake

1. Including low-fat dairy foods in your child's diet is a great way to meet their daily requirements of calcium. Add milk to breakfast cereals, smoothies, sauces, quiches, scrambled eggs, mashed potato, cakes, muffins and desserts.

2. Pack a small tub of low-fat yoghurt in your child's lunchbox. Freeze yoghurts for a cool dessert. Add yoghurt to your child's porridge, quiches and dips. Use as a spread on pancakes and muffins. Yoghurt, used instead of milk, adds a lovely tang to muffins, cakes and pancakes. Serve yoghurt with nuts, seeds, muesli or fruit salad. Make your own sugar-free flavoured yoghurt by adding fruit puree and fruit pieces.

3. Low-fat buttermilk makes deliciously light, fluffy pancakes for after school treats or weekend breakfasts. Freeze leftovers and use them as lunchbox snacks.

4. Use low-fat cheese sprinkled over vegetables, homemade pizza and pasta dishes, in quiches, as a melt, in mashed potato and sauces, on rice crackers, or in wraps or sandwiches.

5. Nuts and seeds are extremely versatile. Use raw and unsalted, whole or ground (LSA – ground linseed, sunflower seeds and almonds) and add them to breakfast cereals, fruit salads, salads, sprinkled over quiches, stir-fries, desserts, patties, muffins, biscuits and cakes. This will add extra calcium, protein and EFA's to your child's meal.

6. Use almond butters and tahini (sesame seed paste) in dressings, cakes, muffins, biscuits, as a spread on toast, sandwiches, pancakes and crackers. Add tahini to homemade dips (hummus, babaghanoush) or mix through mashed banana and spread on toast. This will also supply extra protein and EFA's to these foods. You only need to use a small amount of these foods as they are energy-dense (high in calories).

7. Add canned salmon and include their soft bones, crushed up into patties, pasta dishes, quiches and through salads. Mix with some healthy homemade mayonnaise or salsa and add to a sandwich or wrap.

8. Include lots of green leafy vegetables in your child's diet. Add them to pasta dishes, soups, stir-fries, quiches, dips or just steamed on their own. Blending green leafy vegetables through pea soup is a great way of sneaking extra greens into their diet without them knowing.

Foods rich in calcium

Milk and other dairy products such as cheese and yoghurt are among the richest and most significant sources of calcium in children's diets. Milk is also a good source of phosphorus and magnesium that helps the body absorb and use calcium more effectively. Milk is fortified with vitamin D and is essential for the efficient utilization of calcium.

The saturated fat content of dairy products is a concern for children over the age of two. However, the fat content of milk can be easily reduced while maintaining calcium levels by preferring low-fat or skim milk dairy products. Calcium is not contained in the fat portion of milk, so removing the fat does not affect calcium levels.

For the lactose-intolerant child, daily calcium requirements must be met via the consumption of lactose-free dairy foods or non-dairy calcium-rich and calcium-fortified foods. When choosing an alternative to cow's milk you must consider the health benefits and nutritional balance of the milk. Soy, rice and almond milk contain little calcium so calcium fortified varieties are recommended. Rice and almond milks are normally not good sources of protein, however protein enriched varieties are now available. Children who do not drink cow's milk must also take care to obtain sufficient vitamin D in the diet. Non-dairy milks fortified with vitamin D are recommended.

In recent years there have been questions raised in regard to the safety of infants consuming soy formulas. Soybeans and soy products contain chemicals called isoflavones that exert a weak oestrogenic effect on the body. There are concerns that these isoflavones could potentially have a negative effect on children's growth and development if eaten to excess. To err on the side of caution limit your child's soy intake.

Other foods that contain good levels of calcium include nuts (especially almonds and almond butter), sunflower seeds, the bones of tinned fish (salmon and sardines) and tahini. Green leafy vegetables are also good sources of calcium. Several food products, such as breads and orange juice, are enriched with calcium making them a significant source of calcium too. However, it is difficult to eat adequate quantities of all of these types of foods to achieve optimal calcium intake. Care must be taken to ensure a wide variety of calcium-rich foods are consumed regularly.

Calcium content of commonly eaten foods [5]

Food	Serving size	Calcium (mg)
Cheddar cheese	40g	303
Milk	240ml	300
Yoghurt	240ml	300
Cabbage, cooked	1/2 cup	239
White beans, cooked	1/2 cup	113
Spinach, cooked	1/2 cup	115
Pinto beans, cooked	1/2 cup	45
Red beans, cooked	1/2 cup	41
Broccoli, cooked	1/2 cup	35

Recommended daily calcium intake for children (RDI*) [6]

- All children aged 4–8 years should have 700 mg of calcium a day.
- Boys aged 9–11 years should have 1,000 mg of calcium a day and boys aged 12–18 years should have 1,300 mg a day.
- Girls aged 9–11 years should have 1,000 mg of calcium a day and girls aged 12–18 years should have 1,300 mg a day.

* Recommended dietary intake

Iron
for healthy muscles and blood

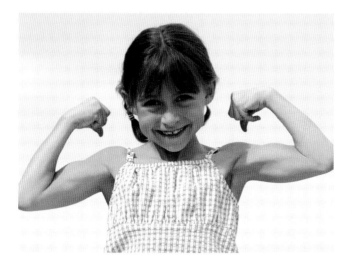

Iron is another extremely important mineral for your children's growth and development. It has a fundamental role in the functioning of many different body systems. Iron is necessary for the development of strong muscles and is required for the production of red blood cells. Red blood cells contain haemoglobin (Hb) a red, iron-rich protein that carries oxygen from the lungs to all of the body's muscles and organs.

Children need iron to build a healthy immune system and for the production of white blood cells and antibodies. Without sufficient iron, kids will be more likely to suffer from frequent colds and infections.

Iron is necessary for the production of energy from glucose, which is the main fuel for both the brain and the rest of the body. Iron is also essential for brain development and for the production of neurotransmitters required for normal brain function.

Iron deficiency

Iron deficiency is a common nutrient deficiency in children, with recent studies suggesting that a significant number of Australian children (up to 35%), may be iron deficient.[1] If iron deficiency is left untreated it can progress to anaemia, which is a condition characterized by low levels of red blood cells.

Children with iron deficiency and anaemia commonly appear to have pale skin, continual tiredness and have a decreased tolerance to strenuous activity or exercise. This condition is associated with decreased immune function (and thus a lowered resistance to infection), decreased muscular strength and poor physical growth. The relationship between anaemia and iron deficiency with brain development, kids' behaviour and performance issues, are well documented.[2-5] Iron is involved in the proper functioning of the brain and nervous system, both of which are sensitive to lowered iron levels long before anaemia is diagnosed. Low iron levels can impair a child's cognitive process (verbal learning and memory), as well as psychomotor development.

Foods rich in iron

Iron is found in a variety of animal and plant based foods. Haem-iron sources are animal based and are the best sources of iron. These include lean meat, chicken, fish and eggs.

Non-haem iron sources are plant based and include wholegrain breads and cereals, wheatgerm, legumes (beans, peas and lentils), baked beans, nuts (nut butters), seeds (tahini), green leafy vegetables and dried fruits. A wide range of iron-fortified food products including breakfast cereals and breads are also available.

Increasing iron absorption

Haem-iron sources have higher absorption rates (around 25%) compared to non-haem iron sources (around 15%). Therefore, even though some plant based foods contain iron, this is not usually absorbed as readily as the iron from animal based foods. Significantly, consumption of haem-iron in a meal containing both iron sources, can actually double the absorption rate of non-haem iron in that meal.

Adding foods rich in vitamin C to meals containing iron sources can greatly increase the absorption of iron from that meal.[6] For example, orange juice consumed simultaneously with food can increase iron absorption. Other ways of including vitamin C foods with meals include adding tomatoes or tomato sauce to wholegrain cereals like pasta or rice and adding fruit to breakfast cereals (oats), baked beans in tomato sauce on wholegrain bread, or adding vitamin C rich vegetables to dishes. This is particularly important for children who consume vegetarian diets or diets low in haem-iron sources.

Eating a variety of haem and non-haem iron sources will ensure that children receive adequate amounts of iron in their diet.

Iron content of commonly eaten foods [7]

Food	Serving size	Iron (mg)
Beef, cooked	85g	2.3
Tuna, light, canned	85g	1.3
Chicken, cooked	85g	1.1
Cashew nuts	30g	1.7
Prunes, dried	5 prunes (40g)	1.1
Raisins, seedless	40g box	0.9
Potato, with skin, baked	1 medium	3.8
Lentils	1/2 cup	3.3

Recommended daily iron intake for children (RDI*) [8]

- All children aged 4–8 years should be having 10 mg of iron a day.

- Boys aged 9–13 years should be having 8 mg of iron a day and boys aged 14–18 years should be having 11 mg a day.

- Girls aged 9–13 years should be having 8 mg of iron a day and girls aged 14-18 years should be having 15 mg a day.

* Recommended dietary intake

Zinc
for healthy immune function

Zinc contributes to the healthy functioning of every cell in the human body. It plays a vital role in growth and immunity and is a key factor in several metabolic pathways to energy production.

For kids in particular, zinc deficiency is highly problematic as it will lead to compromised growth and development. Research has shown that even mild zinc deficiency contributes to impaired physical and neuropsychological development and brain formation and function.[1]

Zinc is required for healthy functioning of the immune system needed for the production of white blood cells, which protects your child from colds and infections. Studies have found that children with inadequate zinc intakes have an increased susceptibility to infection.[2] Zinc also has antioxidant activity, helping to fight free radical damage in the body.

Several metabolic processes in the body are highly reliant on zinc. It is used in the synthesis and action of insulin – which helps balance blood sugar levels and assists in insulin function. Keeping blood sugar levels balanced helps to stabalise children's energy levels and moods.

Zinc is required to make new cells and is involved in over 300 enzyme systems in the body. It is needed to process carbohydrates, fats and protein in the food we eat, as well as being involved in the metabolism of EFAs. Zinc also plays a role in appetite-stimulation, and smell and taste sensitivity.

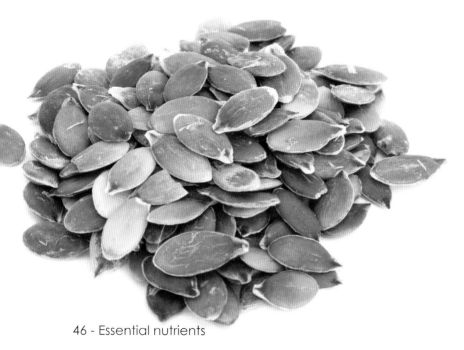

Food sources rich in zinc

The best food sources rich in zinc include lean meat, chicken, fish, milk and other dairy foods (cheese), brewers yeast, eggs (yolks), legumes (lima beans, lentils, peas), wholegrains (bread), sunflower seeds, pumpkin seeds and pecan nuts. A moderate amount of zinc is also found in vegetables. Zinc is lost during the refinement or processing of grains so wholegrain products should always be chosen over the refined equivalents, in order to maximize zinc intake.

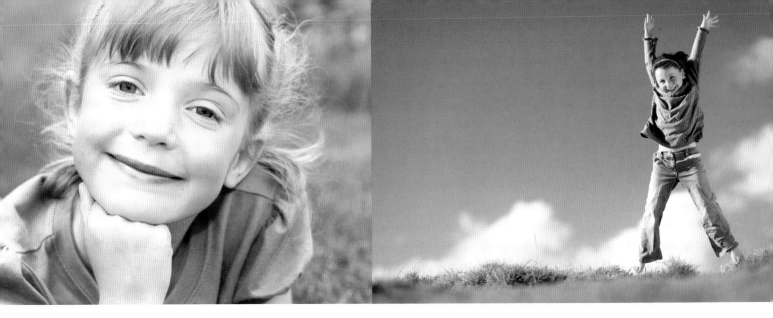

Zinc content of commonly eaten foods [3]

Food	Serving size	Zinc (mg)
Beef, cooked	85g	5.8
Pork, cooked	85g	2.2
Chicken, cooked	85g	2.4
Yoghurt, fruit	1 cup	1.8
Cheese, cheddar	30g	0.9
Milk	1 cup	1.0
Cashews	30g	1.6
Almonds	30g	1.0
Beans, baked	1/2 cup	1.8

Recommended daily zinc intake for children (RDI*) [4]

- All children aged 4–8 years should be having 4 mg of zinc a day.
- Boys aged 9–13 years should be having 6 mg of zinc a day and boys aged 14–18 years should be having 13 mg a day.
- Girls aged 9–13 years should be having 6 mg of zinc a day and girls aged 14-18 years should be having 7 mg a day.

* Recommended daily intake

Vitamin C

for healthy immune function and wound healing

Vitamin C, or ascorbic acid, acts as a highly effective antioxidant, protecting cells in the body from free radical damage. Research suggests that vitamin C is important for preventing cancer and cardiovascular disease.[1,2] Vitamin C also plays a significant role in the formation of collagen, which is a component of blood vessels, tendons, ligaments, bones, teeth and skin.

Vitamin C helps promote a healthy immune system to fight off colds and infections. It assists in wound healing and acts as a natural antihistamine that helps with the body's defence against allergies.

Vitamin C increases the absorption of non-haem iron and calcium and helps to convert folic acid into its active form for bodily use. Vitamin C also plays an important role in the synthesis of the neurotransmitter, norepinephrine. Neurotransmitters are critical to brain function and are known to effect mood.

Foods rich in vitamin C

Fruits such as citrus (oranges, mandarins, lemon), kiwi fruit and berries (strawberries, blueberries, raspberries) are excellent sources of vitamin C. Freshly squeezed orange juice and vitamin C fortified juices are also good sources of vitamin C. Ripe fruits have higher vitamin C content than unripe fruit. Vegetables such as red capsicums, broccoli, cabbage and parsley are also rich vitamin C sources.

Vitamin C is a very unstable vitamin and is destroyed by cooking. For children to reap the health benefits of vitamin C-rich foods, they should be fed a combination of fruits (in fruit salads, for example) and raw or lightly steamed vegetables. Sweet juicy berries are a delicious addition to fruit salads, smoothies, muesli, porridge, pancakes or desserts. Oranges should be cut or squeezed just before serving, as some of the vitamin C content can be destroyed if left sitting too long.

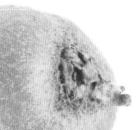

Vitamin C content of commonly eaten foods [3]

Food	Serving size	Vitamin C (mg)
Orange juice	¾ cup	75
Orange	1 medium	70
Grapefruit	½ medium	44
Strawberries	1 cup, whole	82
Tomato	1 medium	23
Sweet red pepper	½ cup, raw	141
Broccoli	½ cup, cooked	58
Potato	1 medium, baked	26

Recommended daily vitamin C intake for children (RDI*) [4]

- All children aged 4–8 years should be having 35 mg of vitamin C a day.
- Boys aged 9–18 years should be having 40 mg of vitamin C a day.
- Girls aged 9–18 years should be having 40 mg of vitamin C a day.

* Recommended dietary intake

Vitamin A & beta-carotene
for good eyesight and healthy gums

Vitamin A (retinol) is essential for maintaining mucosal membranes and skin. Vitamin A enhances the function of the protective mucous membranes of the respiratory and gastrointestinal tract that stops bacteria and viruses from entering the body. Vitamin A aids fat metabolism and is vital for good eyesight, healthy gums and bone development. Research has shown that even children who are only mildly deficient in vitamin A have a higher incidence of respiratory disease, diarrhoea, and infectious disease, than those who consume sufficient vitamin A.[1]

Vitamin A is commonly known as the anti-infective vitamin, because it is required for normal functioning of the immune system. The skin and mucosal cells (cells that line the airways, digestive tract, and urinary tract) function as a barrier to form the body's first line of defence against infection. Vitamin A is required to maintain the integrity and function of these cells and plays a central role in the development of white blood cells, such as lymphocytes. These are critical to all of the body's key immune responses. Vitamin A intake is also associated with reduced risk of certain cancers, allergies and recurrent infections. [2]

Red blood cells, like all blood cells, are derived from precursor cells called stem cells. These stem cells are dependent on vitamin A for normal differentiation into red blood cells. Additionally, vitamin A appears to facilitate the mobilization of iron from storage sites to the developing red blood cell for incorporation into haemoglobin, which carries oxygen around the body.

Foods rich in vitamin A

Vitamin A, in the form of retinol, can be found in animal based foods such as milk, cheese, egg yolk and fish liver oils. Vitamin A can also be produced in the body from beta-carotene (provitamin A). Beta-carotene is found in high levels in yellow and orange fruit and vegetables such as carrots, sweet potato, pumpkin, apricots and mangoes. Green vegetables like spinach also contain carotenoids, though the pigment is masked by the green pigment of chlorophyll.

Vitamin A content of commonly eaten foods [3]

Food	Serving size	Vitamin A (IU)
Cod liver oil	1 teaspoon	1,350
Fortified breakfast cereals	1 cup	180
Egg	1 large	909
Butter	1 tablespoon	97
Whole milk	1 cup	68
Nonfat milk (with vit A)	1 cup	150
Sweet potato	½ cup	959
Carrot, raw	½ cup	385
Spinach, cooked	½ cup	472
Squash, butternut	½ cup	572

Recommended daily intake vitamin A (retinol) for children [4]

- All children aged 4–8 years should be having 400 IU of vitamin A daily.
- Boys aged 9–13 years should be having 600 IU of vitamin A daily and boys 14–18 years should be having 900 IU a day.
- Girls aged 9–13 years should be having 600 IU of vitamin A daily and girls 14-18 years should be having 700 IU a day.

* Recommended dietary intake

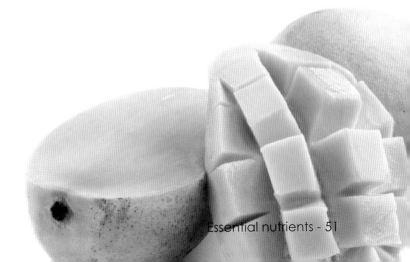

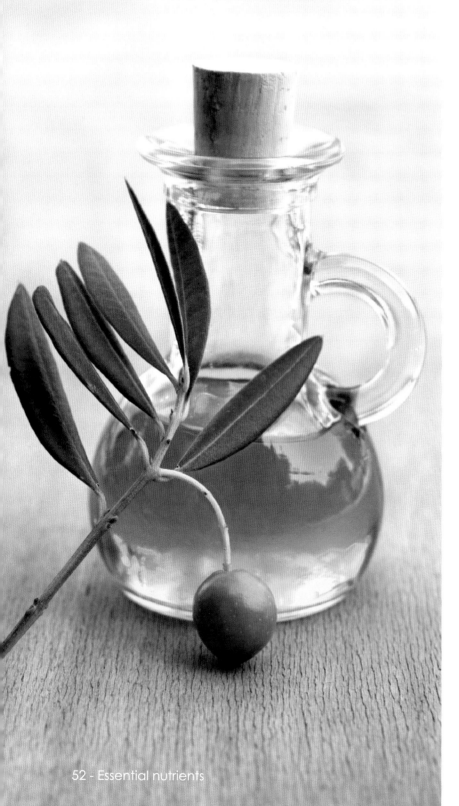

Vitamin E
a powerful antioxidant

Vitamin E is vital for the maintenance of all the cells in the body. The main function of vitamin E is that of an antioxidant, being one of the body's primary defenders against free radical damage. Free radicals are formed primarily in the body during normal metabolism and after exposure to environmental pollutants. Vitamin E maintains the health of the lungs by protecting lung cells from air pollution. Fats, which are an integral part of all cell membranes, are vulnerable to destruction through oxidation by free radicals. Vitamin E is uniquely suited to intercepting free radicals and preventing them from destroying cells, such as red blood cells, from oxidative damage.

Vitamin E has been shown to enhance immune function, help maintain healthy nerves and muscles, strengthen capillary walls, improve circulation, and promote healthy skin and hair. Vitamin E helps reduce scarring from wounds and is necessary for normal wound healing.

A diet rich in vitamin E is beneficial in the treatment and management of children's allergies such as asthma, hay fever and other allergic conditions. Studies suggest that vitamin E intake is associated with a decreased risk of heart disease and possibly some cancers.[1-4]

Food sources rich in vitamin E

Foods rich in vitamin E include cold pressed olive oil, sunflower oil, safflower oil, wheat germ, wholegrains, green leafy vegetables, avocado, fish, eggs and raw nuts and seeds.

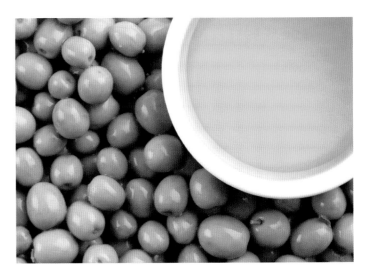

Vitamin E (α -tocopherol) content of commonly eaten foods [5]

Food	Serving size	Vitamin E (mg)
Olive oil	1 tablespoon	1.9
Corn oil	1 tablespoon	1.9
Canola oil	1 tablespoon	2.4
Safflower oil	1 tablespoon	4.6
Sunflower oil	1 tablespoon	5.6
Almonds	30g	7.3
Hazelnuts	30g	4.3
Spinach, raw	½ cup	1.8
Carrots, raw	½ cup	0.4
Avocado	1 medium	3.4

Recommended daily vitamin E (α -tocopherol) intake for children (AI*) [6]

- All children aged 4–8 years should be having 6 mg of vitamin E daily.
- Boys aged 9–13 years should be having 9 mg of vitamin E daily and boys 14–18 years should be having 10 mg a day.
- Girls aged 9–18 years should be having 8 mg of vitamin E a day.

* Adequate intake

B vitamins
for energy production and nervous system health

The B vitamins are a closely related group of vitamins that are needed to perform a wide variety of functions in the body. B vitamins play a crucial role in energy production, helping the body use carbohydrates, proteins and fats as fuel. Without adequate B vitamins children will lack energy. Brain function, metabolism, cell multiplication and the production of red blood cells all depend on the uptake of adequate amounts of B vitamins. Children also need B vitamins for healthy skin, eyes, liver and nervous system function.

Food sources providing B vitamins

Foods rich in B vitamins include wholegrain cereals and bread, wheat germ, nuts, seeds, legumes, meat, poultry, salmon, eggs, milk and green leafy vegetables (a good source of folate).

Different types of B vitamins

B1 (Thiamine) is essential for the metabolism of carbohydrates and keeps nerve and muscle tissues healthy.

B2 (Riboflavin) aids metabolism and growth and keeps the eyes, nails, skin and mucous membranes healthy.

B3 (Niacin) helps the body process food into energy, reduces cholesterol and keeps the nervous and digestive systems healthy.

B6 (pyridoxine) aids metabolism of fat and digestion and is important for nervous system function and red blood cell formation and function.

B_{12} is needed only in small amounts, yet it is vital to red blood cell production, cell growth and metabolism, and for a healthy nervous system. B_{12}, in conjunction with folate, plays a role in the synthesis of DNA. CSIRO research has demonstrated the importance of B_{12} in maintaining genetic stability and preventing chromosomal damage.[1,2] Low B_{12} status has been associated with impaired cognitive function in relation to being not able to assimilate and use new information.[3] Vitamin B_{12} is present in animal products such as meat, poultry, fish (including shellfish), and to a lesser extent dairy products (milk and yoghurt). Beneficial bowel bacteria can also synthesize vitamin B_{12}.

Folate (folic acid) is necessary for cell division and the production of haemoglobin (with B_{12}). Folic acid is the B vitamin that is particularly important during pregnancy, as it is vital to nerve development of the foetus, preventing neural tube defects including spina bifida. Particular emphasis is being focused at present on the importance of folate in reducing blood levels of the compound homocysteine, which is a possible risk factor for coronary heart disease.[4,5] A major source of dietary folate is green leafy vegetables.

Recommended daily vitamin B_{12} intake for children (RDI*) [6]

- All children aged 4–8 years should be having 1.2 µg of B_{12} daily.
- Boys aged 9–13 years should be having 1.8 µg of B_{12} daily and boys 14–18 years should be having 2.4 µg a day.
- Girls aged 9–13 years should be having 1.8 µg of B_{12} daily and girls 14-18 years should be having 2.4 µg a day.

* Recommended dietary intake

Chapter 3:
The five food groups
the key to a well balanced diet

1. Wholegrain cereals (breads, pasta, rice & noodles)

2. Fruit

3. Vegetables & legumes

4. Dairy products and calcium-rich alternatives

5. Meat, poultry, fish, eggs and protein-rich alternatives

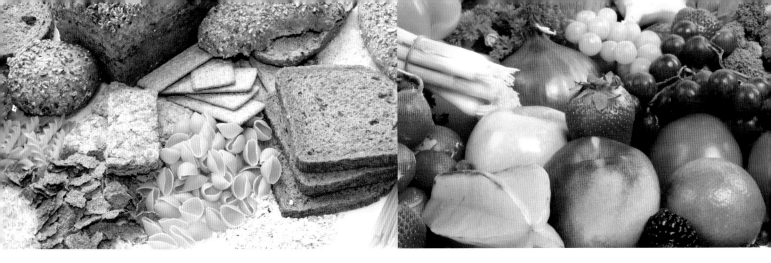

One of a parent's greatest concerns is whether their children are getting all the essential nutrients they need to grow and develop into healthy adults. The five food groups provide a simple system for helping parents create well balanced, nutritious meals for their children. All foods are grouped according to the main nutrient they contain.

There are two basic principles to a nutritionally sound diet, variety and wholesomeness. Your child's diet should be made up of a wide variety of different foods from the five food groups and the majority of their diet should contain natural, unprocessed foods made from wholegrains and foods rich in nutrients and phytochemicals (chemicals found in plants that protect us from chronic disease).

It is important to select a variety of foods from the five food groups, as different foods provide more of some nutrients than others. For example: dairy foods are rich in calcium, whereas fruits are rich in vitamin C.

It is also important to regularly introduce your child to new foods, adding a variety of flavours, textures and tastes to their diet. Variety is definitely the spice of life and a primary factor in the development of life long healthy eating habits. Start experimenting with different recipes and remember that meal time should be fun and enjoyable for the whole family.

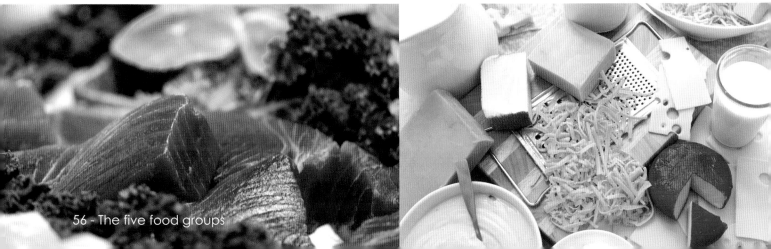

Wholesome
Wholegrain cereals
bread, pasta, rice & noodles

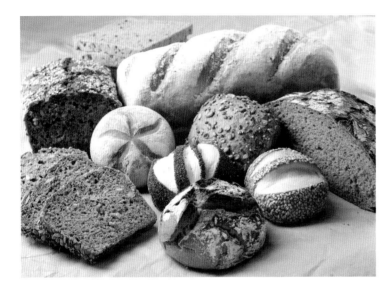

The 'wholegrain cereal' group consists of any foods made from wholegrains or partially processed grains such as breads, breakfast cereals, rice, pasta, noodles, crisp breads and products made from different types of flour and other plain cereal products such as polenta, semolina, burghul, oat bran and wheat bran.

It is recommended that wholegrain breads, breakfast cereals, rice, pasta and noodles form the basis of children's diets. Processed, cereal-based foods such as cakes, biscuits, pastries and breakfast cereals and bars, which usually have high levels of sugars and saturated fat, are not included in this group and should only be eaten occasionally.

Wholegrain vs. refined

Wholegrain cereals are recommended over refined cereals, as wholegrains contain all of the nutritious elements of the grain. When grains are milled or refined, the bran and germ elements of the grain are removed, taking away their fibre rich outer layer along with a lot of their phytochemical and nutritional value. Phytochemicals are natural substances found in plants that possess health-protective benefits – they help to prevent the development of chronic diseases such as heart disease, osteoporosis, some cancers, diabetes and hypertension. The active phytochemicals in grains are concentrated in the bran and the germ. Only when grains are eaten in their whole state can all of the health benefits of these nutrient-rich grains be realised.

Cereal grains are excellent sources of carbohydrate, which is especially important to meet the energy demands of active children. These grains are mostly low in fat and supply a good amount of folate and other B vitamins, vitamin E, iron, zinc, magnesium and phosphorus - essential for children's growth and development. Cereal grains are also an important source of protein, ranging from 8-16g per 100g. Two of the main cereal groups, breakfast cereals and breads are often fortified with vitamins and minerals such as iron, fibre, folate and omega-3 fats.

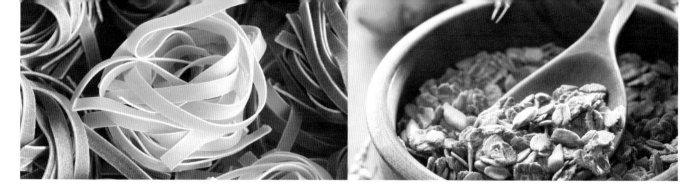

Wholegrain cereals are rich sources of fibre (soluble, insoluble and resistant starch) that are important for bowel health and regularity, promoting cardiovascular health, lowering cholesterol levels, maintaining healthy blood sugar levels and promoting a healthy body weight. A diet rich in high-fibre cereal is associated with a reduced risk of colorectal cancer, breast cancer, and other cancer such as prostate cancer.[1-5]

The National Heart Foundation of Australia along with many recent scientific reviews, support the beneficial effects of fibre-rich wholegrains in relation to decreased risk of coronary heart disease.[6-10] Consuming these fibre-rich foods will decrease children's risk of developing type-2 diabetes and obesity.[11-14]

Choose a variety of wholegrain cereals

Different cereals provide varying amounts and types of dietary fibre, as well as differing levels of nutrients and phytochemicals. The levels of some nutrients (such as selenium) in cereals vary considerably according to the region in which they are grown. It is important to eat a wide variety of cereal foods to maximize their nutritional benefits. Another reason why it's a good idea to offer kids a variety of cereals is to prevent the possibility of them developing sensitivities to certain foods, namely wheat. Western diets are dominated by wheat and some children can develop wheat-sensitivity if the majority of their diet is made up of wheat and wheat-containing products. Children therefore should be fed a variety of wheat and wheat-free grains like brown rice, whole oats, amaranth, buckwheat, millet and quinoa in breakfast cereals, salads, stir-fries, cakes and muffins.

Children's recommended daily intake for wholegrain cereal[15]

Wholegrain cereals should make up around 50% of your child's diet.

- Children aged 4 - 7 years should eat between 3-4 servings of wholegrain cereals a day.
- Children aged 8 - 11 years should eat between 4-6 servings of wholegrain cereals a day.
- Adolescents aged 12 - 18 years should eat between 4-11servings of wholegrain cereals a day (depending on energy requirements).

Example for 1 serving = 2 (60g) slices bread; 1 medium bread roll; 1 cup (155g) cooked rice, pasta or noodles; 1 cup (100 g) oats or 1 small wholemeal muffin.

Include more wholegrain cereals in your child's diet

1. Wholegrain breakfast cereals such as oats and muesli (unsweetened) make a wonderful start to your child's day, packed with fibre and nutrients.

2. Use wholegrain breads instead of white bread for your child's sandwiches and toast.

3. Keep it interesting and try different types of bread including flat breads (lavash, Lebanese bread, mountain bread, pocket/pita bread, tortillas) which are made from different types of grains including sourdough, wheat, oat, rye, soy and linseed, spelt, corn, barley, rice, fruit breads, sunflower and pumpkin seed and multigrain. Use flat breads for wraps, pizza bases, taco shells and toasted chips to serve with dips.

4. Use brown rice instead of white. If your child dislikes brown rice, try ½ brown, ½ white to get them use to it. Brown rice takes around 45-50 minutes to cook, but its wonderful nutty flavour and health benefits come from its fibrous husk, so it's worth the wait. Soak brown rice in water for 30 minutes before cooking, it will cook quicker and have a softer texture.

5. Add cooked wholegrains such as quinoa, millet, barley, buckwheat, burghul and couscous to soups, stir-fries and salads.

6. There are a wide variety of asian noodles available at your supermarket or local asian grocer. Usually made from wheat or rice, you can add them to stir-fries, laksas or salads. Choose from flat rice noodles, rice vermicelli, egg noodles, ramen, udon, soba, somen, hokkian, bean vermicelli and buckwheat noodles. Avoid buying instant noodles as most of them contain significant amounts of added salt and MSG and are high in saturated fat.

7. There is a wide range of Italian pastas to choose from, including spaghetti, fettuccine, macaroni, lasagne sheets, gnocchi and ravioli. Wholemeal pasta is preferred as it contains extra fibre. Pasta is usually made from wheat, but wheat-free pasta (usually made from rice) is also available from supermarkets and health food stores. Avoid buying pre-packaged flavoured pasta mixes as most of them contain significant amounts of salt and are high in saturated fat.

8. Use wholegrain flours for cooking instead of white flours. Make wholesome, homemade, wholegrain muffins, biscuits and cakes, ready for after school snacks or lunch box treats.

9. Make delicious desserts with brown rice, tapioca, oats and couscous.

10. Other healthy breakfast cereals include puffed cereals (brown rice, amaranth, buckwheat and corn), natural corn or spelt flakes and brown rice porridge. Puffed cereals and flakes make a lovely light addition to muesli.

Fruit

an apple a day keeps the doctor away

The bright, vibrant colours and delicious tastes and textures of fruit make this group one of the most stimulating food groups for children.

There is a huge variety of different types of fruit including citrus fruit (orange, lemon, lime, grapefruit, tangerine, mandarin), stone fruit (peaches, plums, apricots, nectarines), tropical fruit (pineapple, mango, banana, guava, papaya), berries (blueberries, blackberries, strawberries, raspberries, cranberries, gooseberries, boysenberries) and melons (rock melon, honey dew, watermelon) which are all highly nutritious. Avocados and tomatoes are also classified as fruit.

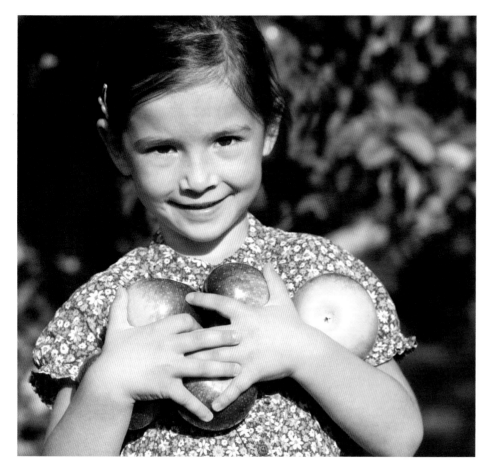

Fruit derive their sweetness from the natural sugar, fructose, which is a type of simple sugar carbohydrate, providing children with energy. Due to fruit's high fibre content, these natural sugars are digested and absorbed slowly, helping to keep children's blood sugar levels stable.

Fruit contains both soluble and insoluble fibre and are rich sources of vitamins C, A and beta-carotene, B vitamins (including folate), and minerals phosphorus, iron, magnesium, calcium and potassium.

Fruit is abundant in phytochemicals, called flavanoids, that are found mostly in richly coloured red, blue and purple fruit such as raspberries, blueberries, strawberries, plums and

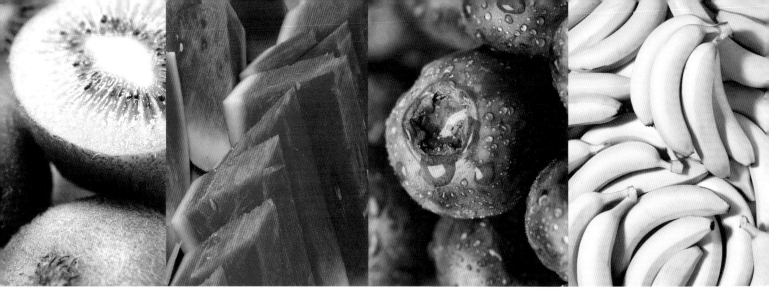

grapes. Flavanoids are known for their powerful antioxidant properties. They protect against many diseases marked by free radical damage such as heart disease, cancer, diabetes and neurological diseases.

There is substantial scientific evidence for the disease-preventing benefits of eating fruit (and vegetables) daily. Regular consumption of fruit (and vegetables) reduces the risk of many chronic diseases such as coronary heart disease, hypertension, stroke, obesity and type-2 diabetes.[1-11] The risk of bowel cancer and several other major cancers is also reduced by a diet rich in fruit (and vegetables).[12,13] Kids' bones will also benefit from consuming fruit (and vegetables), by increasing bone mineralization and reducing the risk of osteoporosis.[14]

Different fruit contains varying levels of nutrients and phytochemicals. It is important for children's diets to contain a variety of fruit and fruit of different colours.

Children's recommended daily intake for fruit [15]

- Children aged 4 - 11 years should consume at least 2 servings of fruit a day.
- Adolescents aged 12 - 18 years should consume 3-4 servings of fruit a day.

Example for 1 serving = 1 medium sized fruit (150g/5¼ oz), 1 cup (150 g/5¼ oz) diced pieces of fruit, ½ cup (125 ml/ 4 ½ fl oz) juice, 1 piece of large fruit (apple, orange, banana), 2 pieces of smaller fruit (plum, kiwi, apricot, passionfruit), ¼ cup (40 g/1¼ oz) grapes or berries.

"It is important for children's diets to contain a variety of fruit and fruit of different colours."

Include more fruit in your child's diet

1. Serve fruit to your children in a variety of different ways. Cut fruit up into fruit salads, yoghurt, breakfast cereals or heated up in porridges. Make fruit muffins, pancakes, fruit smoothies and ice blocks. Try making fruit fun by threading fruit chunks on skewers (melon balls, grapes, strawberries, banana, apple, kiwi) and serve with a small dish of yoghurt. Kids love biting into juicy watermelon slices (leave the skin on). Cut watermelon into rectangles and bananas in half and place a paddle pop stick down the centre of each, place in the freezer until ready to eat. Have fresh fruit pieces in the fridge, ready to go.

2. Canned fruit in natural juice without added sugars can also be a good alternative when you're unable to give your child fresh fruit. Avoid canned fruit packed in heavy syrups containing high amounts of sugar. Pack a small can of mixed fruit into your child's lunch box with a spoon.

3. Pureed fruit makes a wonderful, healthy alternative to sugary, commercially made syrups. Use it as a topping for ice cream, pancakes and other desserts or stir through yoghurt.

4. Make your own mango chutney to liven up sandwiches and meals.

5. Mash banana and some tahini or nut butter together for a tasty spread for toast, rice cakes, wholemeal crackers, pancakes or muffins.

6. Baked fruit makes a delicious dessert served with yoghurt or homemade ice cream. Place peach, nectarine, pear or fresh figs under the griller for 5 minutes, until golden brown, drizzle with a little honey and top with yoghurt, homemade ice cream or low-fat ricotta, sprinkle with flaked almonds. Place a banana in foil, cover with lemon juice and sprinkle with cinnamon, bake in 200*C oven for 10-15 minutes. Place peeled and cored apple halves in an oven proof dish, fill each core with raisins and sprinkle with cinnamon or mixed spice, bake covered for 30 minutes in 180*C oven.

7. Stewed fruit is a delicious accompaniment to muesli, porridge, yoghurt, homemade ice cream and custard, muffins and pancakes. Dice fresh fruit (apple, pear, apricot, figs), add a cinnamon stick and the zest of half a lemon, then add water (just enough to cover fruit). Simmer on low heat until fruit is stewed, then add 1 tablespoon of organic honey if desired.

8. Use avocado instead of butter on toast, sandwiches, or as a dip (guacamole) with rice crackers and vegie sticks. Cut avocado up into salads or salsa.

Dried fruit

Sun-dried fruit, in small amounts, can be a nutritious snack or addition to breakfast cereal (muesli and porridges), yoghurt, muffins, cookies and slices. Dried fruit however, is an energy dense food and could displace other more nutritious foods in your child's diet if eaten in excess. Dried fruit is a concentrated source of natural sugars; it can stick to the teeth and can contribute to tooth decay and the intake of excess calories. Dried fruit eaten in small amounts is a healthy addition to your child's diet. No more than one serving a day is recommended. A small box of sultanas or 4 apricots or apple pieces makes for a naturally sweet treat or a healthy alternative to chocolates and lollies.

One serving = 1 ½ tablespoons of small dried fruit (sultanas) or 4 larger pieces dried fruit (apricots, apples).

Popular examples of dried fruits are apricots, apples, sultanas, dates, bananas, figs and prunes. Other fruits that may be dried include plums, cranberries, mangoes, pawpaw, peaches, pineapples and pears.

Care must be taken when buying dried fruit that only sun-dried varieties are chosen. These are sulphur-free. Most commercially prepared dried fruit contains the preservative sulphur dioxide that can cause reactions in sensitive children, notably triggering asthma attacks. The drying process also destroys most of the fruit's vitamin C content.

Sulphur dioxide is used to prevent or reduce discoloration of light-coloured fruit. Look out for its other names such as sodium sulphite, sodium and potassium bisulphite, and sodium and potassium meta bisulphite which can also be found on food labels. When buying dried fruit, also check the label for added sugars and vegetable oil. Banana chips are usually fried in vegetable oil to make them crispy, so go for the healthier sun-dried variety instead.

Fruit juice vs. whole fruit

Although fruit juice can be a healthy part of kids' diet, it should not replace whole fruit. Fruit juice provides nutrients such as vitamin C and folate. Some commercially bought juices are also fortified with extra vitamin C and calcium. However, unless pulp is included, juice contains no fibre. Because of their lower fibre content, fruit juice is a high GI beverage.

Fruit juice is an energy-dense beverage that provides a great deal of calories from fruit sugars. Excessive consumption of fruit juice can displace other more nutritious food in the diet. This has the effect of reducing the nutrients that kids get over the day and can lead to nutritional deficiencies. One glass of juice can contain up to 4 pieces of fruit, so even a small juice can fill a child's small stomach and quickly replace meals.

Excessive consumption of fruit juice by children is associated with health problems such as obesity, dental erosion and dental caries.[16-18]

Fruit drinks are not nutritionally equivalent to fruit juice. Fruit juices contain 100% juice, while fruit drinks typically contain a much smaller proportion of juice, which is supplemented with water, sugar and other ingredients.

Children should be encouraged to eat whole fruit to meet their recommended daily fruit intake and limit fruit juice consumption to 1 serving (½ cup/125 ml/4½ fl oz) a day. Water is a far healthier choice of beverage for children and should be consumed liberally throughout the day.

If parents do serve fruit juice, care should be taken to ensure the juice is 100% natural, preferably freshly squeezed and with no added sugars. Fruit juice can make a healthy alternative to cordials when it is diluted with chilled water.

Squeezing your own fresh juice at home is the healthiest option. Try adding some vegies into the mix. Apple, pineapple and orange disguise the taste of carrot, celery and beetroot. Experiment with different combinations, adding only a small amount of vegetable to start with.

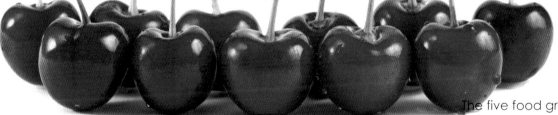

Vegetables & legumes

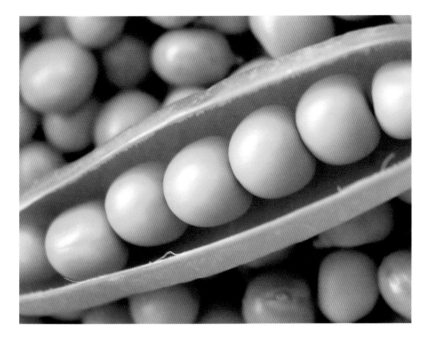

Regular consumption of foods from the 'vegetables and legumes' food group is one of the most important ways for your child to maintain good health and prevent disease.

Vegetables include all green leafy vegetables (spinach, lettuce, silver beet, bok choy), members of the crucifer family (broccoli, cauliflower, cabbage, brussel sprouts), all root and tuber vegetables (carrot, sweet potatoes, potatoes), edible plant stems (celery, asparagus), gourd vegetables (pumpkin, cucumber), allium vegetables (onion, garlic, shallots, leek) and corn.

Legumes refer to pulses and include all beans, peas and lentils - canned, fresh or dried. This group also includes any vegetarian product containing these foods such as hummus, falafels, baked beans, tofu, legume flours and patties. Commonly eaten legumes include split peas, green beans, snow peas, lentils, soya beans, chick peas (garbanzo), red kidney beans, broad beans, butter beans, lima beans, mung beans and navy (haricot) beans. Legumes are usually cooked, as it improves their nutritional value and digestibility.

Vegetables and legumes are rich sources of a large variety of vitamins, minerals, soluble and insoluble fibre and phytochemicals. It was more recently discovered that legumes are not only rich in soluble fibre but also in resistant starch. Both vegetables and legumes are good sources of complex carbohydrates for slow sustained energy as well. Legumes are also a valuable source of high quality protein (especially important for vegetarians).

Foods from this food group are excellent providers of vitamins A, C, E, beta-carotene, folate and other B vitamins; along with minerals zinc, selenium, phosphorus, magnesium, iron, potassium, manganese and calcium.

Phytochemicals

Vegetables and legumes are both good sources of cancer and heart-protective phytochemicals. Some of these include indoles (cruciferous vegetables - broccoli and cabbage), allium (garlic and onion) and lycopene (red pepper).

In Australia there is a preference for potato as the vegetable of choice among children. This is a concern as potatoes are not as rich in phytochemicals as many other vegetables. To make sure your child is getting the best protection against chronic disease, it is important for them to receive a wide variety of phytochemicals through their diet.

Different vegetables and legumes provide differing levels of vitamins, minerals and phytochemicals. It is important to give your child a wide variety of foods from this group to maximize their nutritional benefits. Giving your child a variety of different coloured vegetables is also important, as different colours represent different phytochemicals. Yellow and orange vegetables, like carrots and sweet potatoes are rich in carotenoids, whereas red vegetables, like red capsicums contain lycopene.

Disease prevention

Numerous scientific studies around the world conclude that regular consumption of vegetables and legumes reduces the risk of many chronic diseases including coronary heart disease, stroke, several major cancers and type-2 diabetes.[1-8] Allium vegetables (garlic and onion) in particular are recognised for their anti-cancerous properties.[9] Researchers have found that legumes can lower LDL 'bad' cholesterol levels, help control blood sugar levels and can assist in weight maintenance.[10-13] This makes legumes an extremely beneficial addition to children's diets, especially for children who are diabetic, overweight or obese.

Your child's bones can also benefit from consuming foods from this food group, by increasing bone mineralization and therefore reducing the risk of osteoporosis.[14]

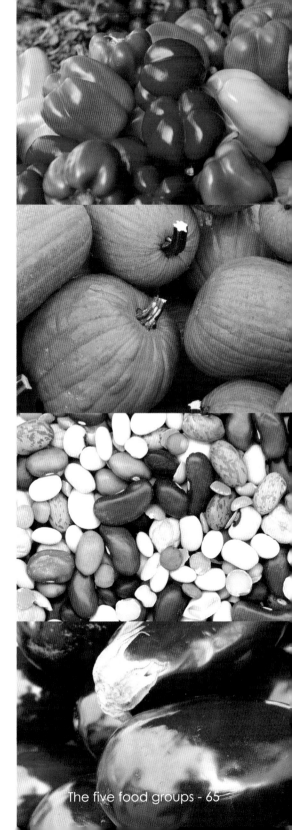

Frozen vs. fresh

Frozen vegetables can be convenient when you're a busy parent. Although it is recommended to eat fresh vegetables where you can, frozen vegetables can provide similar nutritional value to that of fresh vegetables. Freezing is a very effective method of preserving nutrients in many vegetables, with most nutrients keeping well.

Carotene (a compound that is converted to vitamin A in the body) may actually be better preserved in frozen produce because packaging keeps the vegetables away from light (which destroys carotene). While vitamin levels of vitamin C (25%), folate and thiamin (Vitamin B1) are lost during blanching. Blanching is the exposure of the vegetables to boiling water or steam for a brief period of time, a process which precedes commercial freezing. Other vitamins are generally fairly heat stable and are largely retained during the blanching process. Nutrients, other than vitamins, are not significantly affected by the freezing process.

Fresh, especially raw foods are highly nutritious because they still contain all of their vitamins, minerals and enzymes. Enzymes are important because they assist in the digestion and absorption of food. The human body requires a regular supply of these enzymes which are found in fresh vegetables (fruit and sprouted foods). Blanching of vegetables, as is done when commercially freezing, destroys valuable enzymes.

Children's recommended daily intake for vegetables and legumes[15]

- Children aged 4 - 7 years should consume at least 4 servings of vegetables and legumes a day.
- Children aged 8 - 11 years should consume 4-5 servings of vegetables and legumes a day.
- Adolescents aged 12-18 years should consume 3-4 servings of vegetables and legumes a day.

Example of 1 serving = ½ cup (75g/2¾ oz) cooked vegetables or legumes, 1cup (63 g/2¼ oz) salad vegetables, 1 small potato.

The most recent National Health Survey reported that only 15-25% of Australian children eat at least four serves of vegetables per day, most consuming only 2 serves a day.[16]

Include more vegetables and legumes in your child's diet

1. The best way to encourage your children to eat more vegetables is to make them more appealing to the taste buds by adding extra flavour, such as a little tamari to spinach and greens, melt a little cheese over broccoli and cauliflower; add some tomato and basil sauce to veges; add a creamy, cheesy or yoghurt sauce, or make a vege bake. Roast vegetables or make crispy chips and serve with a dip. Add a little honey to carrots and mint to peas. Lightly steam vegetables and add to a salad with a healthy dressing. Blend vegetables together to make a sauce for chicken, meat, casseroles or pasta dishes. Blend vegetables together to mae a soup or a spicy dip to serve with toasted pita bread.

2. Make delicious, crisp salads and top them with healthy, nutritious salad dressings.

3. Keep cut up vegie sticks such as carrots, celery and zucchini in the fridge with healthy dips, readily availably for kids to snack on.

4. Have healthy dips made from legumes and vegetables on hand such as hummus, babaghanoush, beetroot and spicy vege dips. Use these dips with vege sticks, crackers or toasted breads, or as a spread on sandwiches, burgers or wraps. Hummus is great served on wholegrain toast as a snack or for a quick breakfast.

5. Canned legumes and baked beans are very handy to have in the cupboard. Make sure you buy low-salt varieties. Add canned legumes to stir-fries, salads, soups, casseroles and patties. Make your own baked beans and hummus.

6. Legumes contain compounds that can sometimes be difficult to digest, often leading to flatulence (gas). Cooking beans with a strip of kombu (a type of seaweed) can help reduce this problem by partially breaking down these compounds and improving their digestion.

7. Make sure your child eats a variety of raw and cooked vegetables. Add grated vegetables (beetroot, carrot, zucchini) to salads and sandwiches. Roast vegetables and add them to sandwiches, wraps and pizzas. You could also make veggie skewers to cook under the grill or on the BBQ.

8. Make some beetroot chutney to liven up sandwiches or use as a side dish with BBQ meats and salads.

9. Make homemade, ovenbaked sweet potato chips, spray with a little olive oil and sprinkle with paprika. You could make half potato and half sweet potato.

10. Spice up boring mashed potato. Mash with green peas and some fresh mint; mash sweet potato; mash with some corn; add some garlic, a little miso paste, pesto, wholegrain mustard, grated low-fat cheese or other desired herbs and spices.

11. Dishes such as stir-fries, casseroles, soups, quiches, pasta dishes and patties are great to hide extra vegetables. Puree vegetables and make them into sauces for pasta dishes and casseroles (blend them with tomato based sauce). Grate vegetables into pattie or quiche mixes. Blend extra vegetables into soups.

12. Thicken stir-fries and casseroles by mixing mashed pumpkin or sweet pototo through it.

13. Blend vegetables of the same colour into soups eg. mix spinach, zucchini and broccoli into pea soup or carrots into pumpkin soup. Mix pale coloured vegetables, such as cauliflower, butter beans and chickpeas into mashed potato. Watch you don't overdo it and make sure there are no lumps or your kids will be suspicious.

14. Pureed legumes and peas make a delicious topping for other vegetables, fish, meat or chicken. Add roast garlic, fresh herbs or a little miso paste, pesto or tamari to puree.

15. Finely grate vegetables, such as carrots and zucchini, into patties. Mash legumes and sweet potato into patties. You can disguise vegetables by adding a little wholegrain mustard, tomato paste, pesto or cheese to patties.

16. You can even hide vegetables in muffins and cakes. Try a tasty carrot and zucchini cake, beetroot and carob cake or pumpkin and corn muffins from this book.

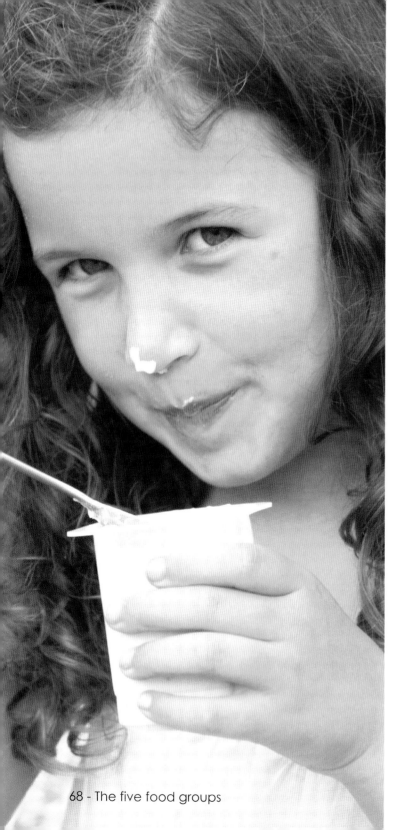

Dairy foods
& calcium-rich alternatives

Foods in the 'dairy foods and calcium-rich alternatives' food group are all excellent sources of calcium. Calcium is required for the normal development and maintenance of your child's bones and skeleton. Calcium is stored in teeth and bones, where it provides structure and strength.

Dairy foods are a major source of calcium in the Australian diet. Dairy foods contain high quality protein and are valuable sources of several nutrients including B vitamins (B2, B3, B6 and B12), vitamin A, magnesium, phosphorus and zinc. Dairy products also provide vitamin D through fortification.

This food group does not include dairy food that contain high levels of sugar, such as flavoured milk, ice cream, milk based desserts, sugary dessert type yoghurts or highly processed cheese.

Children's bones are in a phase of steady growth throughout childhood. Calcium seems to be the most important nutritive factor determining peak bone mass in young adults.[1,2] High peak bone density reduces the risk of osteoporosis later in life. Osteoporosis, a condition of low bone mass, can lead to bone fragility and increased risk of fractures. A number of studies have shown that milk consumption in childhood has positive effects on adult bone mass density.[3-5] Your child taking part in regular weight-bearing physical activity such as running, walking, dancing and ball sports also helps to maximize bone strength and bone mineral density, which are both important predictors of osteoporosis.

Should children have low-fat dairy foods?

Milk and other dairy foods, such as cheese, are a major source of saturated fats, providing around a third of the saturated fat in a child's diet. For this reason, low-fat varieties are recommended (except for children less than 2 years old). After the age of 2, children do not necessarily require whole fat milk, with the exception of children who are not gaining weight adequately.

Low-fat milks, cheeses and yoghurts are readily available and usually contain 75% less fat and the same amount of calcium as the equivalent full fat product. Regular full-fat milk contains around 115mg of calcium per 100mL, and low-fat varieties usually contain even more. However, low-fat soft cheeses, such as cottage cheese and ricotta, have lower calcium contents, therefore cannot be counted as a full serving.

Cheese

The calcium content of different types of cheese is largely influenced by how it's manufactured. A portion of calcium is removed during the manufacturing process. Sodium content is also variable as it is an optional added ingredient. One small 21 g slice of cheese can provide over 20% of the upper level of daily sodium intake acceptable for an 8 year old. Highly processed cheeses are traditionally made with a lot of added salt, preservatives and food colourings and should be avoided. Cheese, in general, is usually high in saturated fat and salt, so check labels carefully and buy cheese with higher calcium and lower fat and salt content.

There are many different varieties of cheeses. Harder cheeses such as parmesan, mozzarella, cheddar, Swiss and edam have the highest calcium levels. Softer cheeses such as cottage, goats, fetta and ricotta have lower calcium levels but still make a healthy addition to a child's diet.

"Dairy foods are rich sources of calcium needed for strong, healthy bones and teeth."

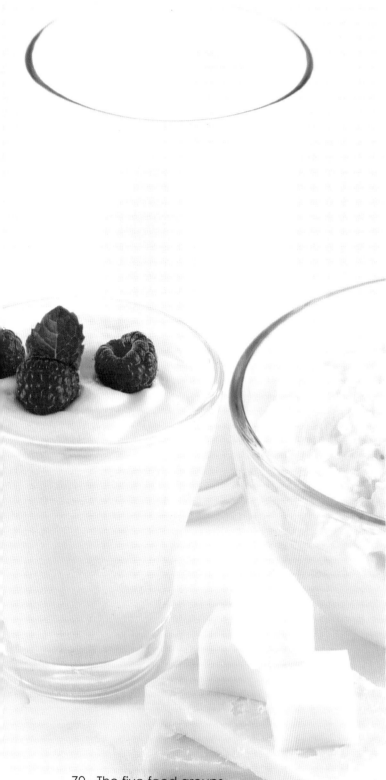

Yoghurt

Yoghurt is a wonderful addition to any child's diet. Yoghurt contains beneficial bacteria that help to promote a healthy balance of bowel bacteria. Beneficial bowel bacteria are an important part of your child's immune system needed to produce vitamins B_{12} and K and for proper digestion. Lactose-free yoghurts are available for lactose intolerant children however, dairy based yoghurts are usually well tolerated, as they have already been partially broken down by bacteria. A lot of low-fat yoghurts are surprisingly high in added sugars, with manufacturers adding up to five or more teaspoons of sugar to many flavoured yoghurts on the market. Make sure you buy good quality yoghurt without added sugars, artificial sweeteners or flavourings. Watch out for sugar listed in the top few ingredients on the ingredient panel.

Non-dairy alternatives

If your child does not eat dairy products because they are lactose intolerant, vegan or some other reason, it's important to ensure that their calcium and vitamin D requirements are being met. Calcium and vitamin D fortified soy, rice and almond milks are available. Rice milk is not a good source of protein and should not be thought of as a nutritional replacement for cow's milk. In this case additional protein rich foods should be included in the diet.

In recent years there has been questions raised in regards to the safety of infants consuming soy formulas. Soybeans and soy products contain chemicals called isoflavones that exert a weak oestrogenic effect on the body. There are concerns that these isoflavones could potentially have a negative effect on children's growth and development if eaten to excess. Organic soy milk and soy products can still be consumed by children in moderation as part of a well balanced diet. If your child is lactose-intolerant give them a variety of milk so their diet is not dominated by soy.

Calcium can also be found in wholegrain cereals, nuts (especially almonds, nut butters), seeds (tahini, LSA), green leafy vegetables, legumes and sardines and salmon with their bones.

Lactose-free milks, cheeses and yoghurts are now available so children with lactose intolerance can also enjoy dairy products and increase their calcium intakes.

Ca-rich dairy foods	Ca-rich non-dairy alternatives
Low-fat milk	Ca fortified rice, almond and soy milk
Low-fat yoghurt	Legumes
Low-fat cheese	Wholegrain cereals
Low-fat cottage cheese	Nuts (almonds and nut butters)
	Seeds (tahini and LSA)
	Green leafy vegetables
	Salmon and sardines with bones

Children's recommended daily intake for dairy or calcium-rich alternative foods [6]

Include a variety of dairy products and calcium-rich alternatives in your child's diet.

- Children aged 4-11 years should consume 2-3 servings of dairy foods or calcium-rich alternatives a day.
- Adolescents aged 12-18 years should consume 3-5 servings of dairy foods or calcium-rich alternatives a day.

Example of 1 serving = 1 cup (250 ml/9 fl oz)) of low-fat milk; 1 small tub (200g/7 oz) of yoghurt; 1 (40 cm) square of cheese or 2 slices; or ½ cup (60 g/2 oz) grated low-fat cheese; 5 sardines; ½ cup (85 g/3 oz)of pink salmon with bones.

Make sure you're not giving your child excessive quantities of milk. Due to its high protein content, it has a greater satiating (filling) effect than other drinks. Consuming too much milk during the day can diminish your child's appetite and displace other nutritious foods, which could lead to nutrient deficiencies.

Include more dairy foods or calcium-rich alternatives in your child's diet

1. Pack a small tub of yoghurt in your child's lunch box or keep them handy in the fridge for a healthy easy to grab snack.

2. You can always add extra flavour to natural yoghurts by adding fruit pieces, mashed banana, fruit puree (berries), grated apple or pear, or finely diced dried fruit. Put yoghurt on your cereal, in smoothies and on desserts instead of ice cream. Use yoghurt in quiches, salad dressings, dips, pancakes and muffins for a lovely fresh tangy flavour. Add natural yoghurt to mashed potatoes.

3. Make yoghurt cheese. Place some natural yoghurt into a piece of muslin cloth, tie it and let it drip into a pan overnight. You will end up with what looks like curd cheese. It can be used instead of sour cream on baked potato or add to salads or spread on sandwiches. Add desired herbs, spices or crushed roasted garlic for a little extra flavour.

4. Try to avoid sweetened milk drinks. Make healthy smoothies at home with fruit (strawberries, frozen raspberries and bananas). They taste better and don't contain all the added sugar and artificial colours and flavourings.

5. Low-fat cottage cheese is great served as a dip with crackers or spread on rice cakes. Low-fat creamed cheese or ricotta make a great spread for sandwiches and wraps.

6. Your child doesn't have to drink a glass of milk and eat slices of cheese to meet their daily calcium needs. Make it more interesting by adding milk to soups, casseroles and sauces; including cheese in dishes such as omelettes, quiches and vegetables, or as a melt. Milk and cheese can also be added to mashed potato.

7. Use almond nut spreads and tahini on sandwiches and wraps. Add them to dips, muffins, cookies, slices, sauces and salad dressings.

8. Sprinkle LSA (ground linseeds, sunflower seeds and almonds) on cereals. Add crushed nuts and seeds in cooking (cakes, muffins, biscuits, patties, rice and vegetables) or sprinkled over breakfast cereals (porridge and muesli) or on yoghurt.

9. Include the soft crushed bones of sardines and salmon when making fish patties, quiches and sandwiches.

Meat, poultry, fish
and protein-rich alternatives

The 'meat, poultry, fish and protein-rich alternatives' food group provide the richest sources of protein. Protein is essential for growth and repair of every cell in your child's body. Hormone and enzyme production as well as immune system health are all dependant on your child getting adequate amounts of protein through their diet.

This group also contains some of the highest levels of iron and zinc, needed for production of red blood cells, the transportation of oxygen around the body, healthy immune function and reproductive health. Other important nutrients this food group provides include B vitamins (thiamine, riboflavin, niacin and B_{12}) and omega-3 fats.

This food group includes all meats, poultry (chicken and turkey), fish and protein-rich alternatives such as eggs, legumes, legume products (hummus, chickpea and lentil patties), organic tofu and tempeh, nuts and seeds (including nut butters and tahini).

Some meat, fish and poultry products and dishes that are popular in Australia are usually of poor quality and contain significant amounts of saturated fat and sodium. Foods such as pies, sausage rolls, sausages, fish fingers, chicken nuggets, hamburgers, hot dogs and salami are not included in this food group and should only be eaten occasionally as part of a well balanced, nutritious diet. For example, one serving (125 g) of chicken nuggets typically only contains 55% chicken and 20 g of fat, more than three times the fat you would get from the same amount of BBQ chicken breast.

Red meat, pork & poultry

Red meat is a valuable source of dietary protein and the best source of bioavailable iron in the Australian diet. Pork and poultry also contain protein in equivalent amounts to those in red meats, about 20 g per 100 g. A substantial amount of iron, zinc and vitamin B_{12} are also found in these foods however, the content of these minerals in pork and poultry is substantially less than in red meat.

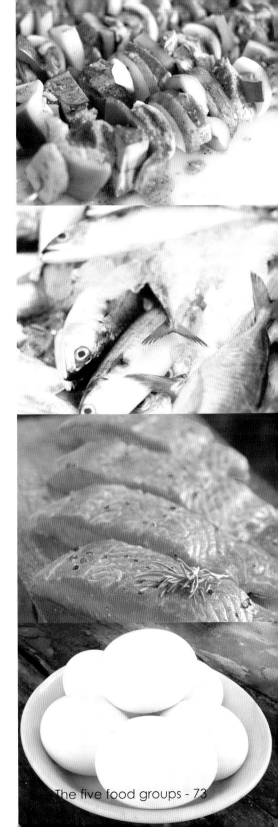

To lower your child's saturated fat intake, buy lean pieces of red meat and cut off any visible fat. The fat content of lean pork and skinless chicken is in the same range as that of lean meats. If buying sausages, choose quality, low-fat sausages. Avoid using deli meats that contain the carcinogenic preservative nitrate. Deli meats can also be high in saturated fats so choose low fat varieties.

It's a good idea to buy organic chickens where you can, as commercial farmers use antibiotics in their feed. Always take the skin off chickens, as the majority of toxins are stored in the animal's fat.

Fish

Fish contains high quality protein equivalent to that in red meat, pork and poultry. Fish also provides good levels of iron and zinc (in lower levels than red meats) and vitamin B_{12} (similar to that of red meat). Consuming fish will supply children with the important mineral, iodine. Iodine is vital for the growth and functioning of children's thyroid glands and is very important for brain growth and function. Iodine deficiencies in children can hamper the growth of their brain and can reduce their IQ, causing learning difficulties. Results from a recent study have confirmed that a majority of Australian children have inadequate iodine intakes and are borderline deficient.[1]

Fish, particularly oily fish, is the richest source of omega-3 polyunsaturated fats and is low in saturated fat. These omega-3 fats have been shown to provide specific health benefits, notably in relation to brain development and function and cardiovascular health. A well balanced diet that includes fish, can contribute greatly to your child's health, both mentally and physically.

Choose from a variety of cold water, oily fish like salmon, mackerel, herring, sardines, tuna and trout.

Tinned salmon, tuna and sardines can be used as an alternative to fresh fish. Keep a stock of tinned tuna and salmon in the pantry for sandwiches, fish patties and salads. Make sure you buy varieties without vegetable oils. Choose fish in spring water or olive oil. Including the soft crushed up bones of sardines and salmon with fish meals will provide your child with extra calcium.

It's recommended that children eat 2-3 fish meals (high in omega-3 fats) a week.

What about mercury levels in fish?

Some types of fish contain higher levels of mercury than others. Young children are more vulnerable to the effects of mercury, due to their smaller size and developing nervous system. Fish more likely to accumulate higher levels of mercury are larger, longer living species that are at the top of the food chain. Children should continue to consume a variety of fish as part of a healthy diet but limit their consumption of certain species.

There are a few types of fish that should be limited in children's (and adults') diets, due to their higher levels of mercury, PCBs and pesticides – these are billfish (swordfish/broadbill and marlin), shark/flake, orange roughy (also sold as sea perch) and catfish.

Fish that contain lower levels of mercury and can be consumed safely up to 3 times a week include fresh and canned salmon (Atlantic red salmon is a good choice), canned light tuna, trout, mackerel and sardines. Limit albacore 'white' tuna as it generally contains higher levels of mercury than canned light tuna. Choose wild salmon as farmed salmon has been found to contain more toxins such as PCB's. Most canned salmon is wild salmon. Trim all visible fat off fish, since PCB's are stored in the fat.

Protein-rich alternatives

A number of foods can provide some of the key nutrients found in meats, fish and poultry. These foods include eggs and plant based foods such as legumes (hummus), organic tofu and tempeh, nuts and seeds. These foods are generally good sources of protein but can have highly variable amounts of bioavailable iron, zinc and vitamin B_{12}.

Eggs are excellent sources of protein, having slightly lower protein content than red meat. Eggs are also a good source of B vitamins (thiamine, riboflavin, niacin, B_{12}) and provide substantial amounts of iron and zinc. Egg yolks also contain iodine.

Protein combining

Proteins derived from animal sources are usually called 'complete proteins', which means they provide all the essential amino acids in the right amounts required by the body. Proteins from plant sources however, tend to be lacking in one or more essential amino acids. They are referred to as 'incomplete proteins'. These deficiencies can be overcome by combining different plant based proteins to achieve a better amino acid balance. This means that when two different foods are combined, the amino acids of one protein can compensate for those the other one lacks. This is called 'protein complementation'. For example, combining wholegrain cereals with legumes results in a high-quality protein, comparable to that of animal protein. (For more information on protein complementation go to Chapter 7: Vegetarian kids).

Recommended intake for meat, chicken, fish and protein-rich alternatives for children[3]

- Children aged 4 - 7 years should consume ½ -1 serving a day of foods from the 'meat, poultry, fish and protein-rich alternative' food group.

- Children aged 8 - 11 years should consume 1-1 ½ servings a day of foods from the 'meat, poultry, fish and protein-rich alternative' food group.

- Adolescents aged 12 - 18 years should consume 1-2 servings a day of foods from the 'meat, poultry, fish and protein-rich alternative' food group.

1 serving = 65-100 g (2¼ - 3½ oz) cooked meat or chicken; ½ cup (85 g/3 oz) lean mince; 2 small chops; ½ cup (85 g/3 oz) tuna or salmon; ½ cup (110 g/4 oz) cooked legumes, lentils, chickpeas, split peas, or canned beans; 80-120 g (3 – 4¼ oz) cooked fish fillet; 2 small eggs; 1/3 cup (57 g/2 oz)almonds; 1 tablespoon nut butter; ¼ cup (40 g/1½ oz) sunflower or sesame seeds.

Include more protein-rich alternative foods in your child's diet

1. Although nuts and seeds have a relatively high fat content, most contain beneficial omega-3 polyunsaturated and monounsaturated fats. Nuts and seeds are extremely versatile and can be added to fruit and vegetable dishes, stir-fries, breakfast cereals and desserts.

2. A handful of raw unsalted nuts (almonds, cashew, Brazil, hazelnuts) and seeds (sunflower, pepitas) make a great snack. Check with your child's school before packing nuts in their lunch box. Most primary schools have a 'no nut policy'.

3. Add a couple of teaspoons of LSA (ground linseed, sunflower and almonds) or ground nuts to your child's yoghurt, breakfast cereal, fruit salad, vegie, mashed potato or salad. You will be also adding valuable omega-3 EFA's and protein to your child's meal without them even knowing.

4. Sprinkle whole nuts and seeds (linseeds, sesame, sunflower, pepitas) on cakes, muffins, muesli, porridges or salads.

5. Healthy nut butters and tahini (sesame paste) are also a great ways of supplying protein, EFA's and zinc into your child's diet. Spread a small amount on sandwiches, rice cakes, in dips or sauces, on pancakes, muffins or mixed through mashed potato.

6. Eggs are wonderfully versatile and can be eaten in many different ways. Make your child eggs on toast for breakfast (poached, scrambled or fried in a little olive oil), pack a boiled egg in their lunch box as a snack, or mash an egg up with some healthy homemade mayonnaise on a sandwich for school lunches. They also make great easy frittatas and quiches.

7. Legumes are another extremely versatile protein source. Hummus made from chickpeas and tahini is delicious with raw vegie sticks, on bread or with crackers. Add legumes to salads, stir-fries or vegie patties. Mash peas, cannelloni, broad beans or hummus through mashed potato. Add oven baked falaffels to salads and wraps with some taziki.

"Protein is essential for growth and repair of every cell in your child's body."

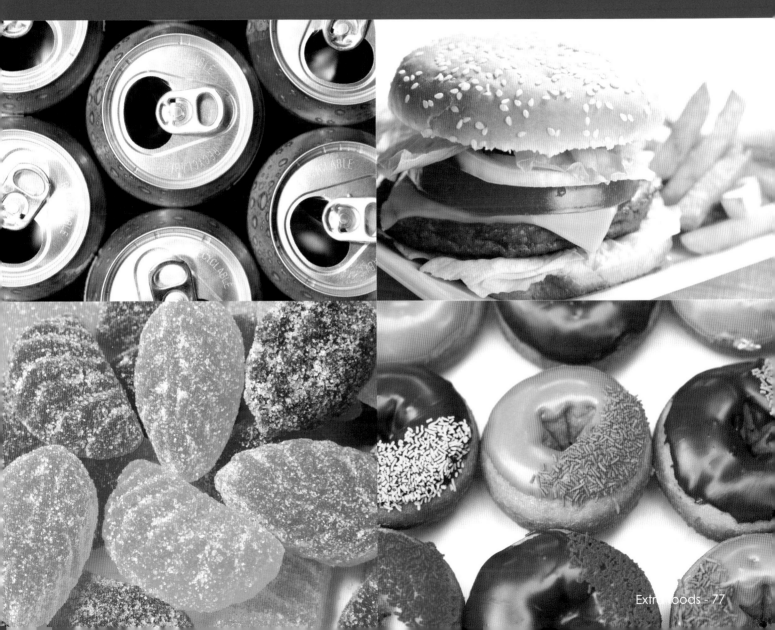

Chapter 4:
Extra foods
foods that should be avoided or limited in your child's diet

Foods that are included in the 'extras' food group are not sources of essential nutrients and give no nutritional benefit to your child's diet. This group includes foods containing high levels of added sugars, saturated and trans-fats, salt, artificial sweeteners, nitrates and caffeine. These ingredients are commonly found in large quantities in processed snack foods, take away foods and soft drinks, which have unfortunately become a large part of many children's diets. These processed foods will often have health claims and terms such as healthy, nutritious and low GI splashed across their packaging, in the hope to distract you from what makes up the majority of the product - usually sugar, saturated fats and salt. Make sure you read labels carefully and don't be fooled by trick marketing.

Kids will be kids and sometimes snack on chips, ice creams, chocolates and lollies on the way home from school, at parties or at their friend's houses. Being over controlling and totally restricting junk food from your child's diet tends to result in children craving and secretly over indulging in these forbidden foods. Eaten occasionally, these foods aren't going to be detrimental to your child's health.

"What's most important is what children eat most of the time. Make sure the majority of their diet is made up of nutritious foods from the five food groups."

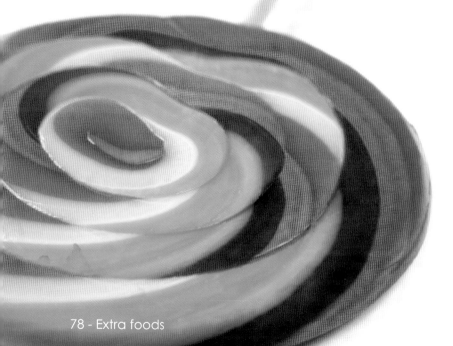

Refined sugars
should be limited in a child's diet

Changes in food processing over the past 30 years, particularly the addition of sugar to a wide variety of foods, has created an environment in which our foods are essentially addictive. In turn, this dooms some children to being overweight. The popular Western diet, full of sugary, high GI, energy-dense, low-fibre foods appears to be a major contributor to the increasing obesity epidemic.

This 'refined sugars' group includes all sugars and sugar-containing ingredients added during processing or food preparation as well as sugars eaten separately (like confectionary) or added at the table. This group does not include naturally occurring sugars found in fruit (fructose) or milk and dairy products (lactose).

Unfortunately sugar has become an integral part of most of our children's lives and is a significant source of energy in the Australian diet. Sugar is a hidden ingredient in many commercially prepared foods. Refined sugars such as sucrose (table sugar), glucose, dextrose (corn sugar) and high-fructose corn syrup are added during processing to increase food palatability and sometimes to add bulk.

Sugar is a crystalline carbohydrate extracted from sugar cane (and sugar beets and corn). During the manufacturing process, sugar cane is robbed of most of its natural and valuable constituents, destroying any enzymes, amino acids, fats and vitamins present. A diet high in refined sugars will rob the body of important micro-nutrients. When you consume processed foods containing refined sugars which lack vitamins and minerals, these nutrients will be leached from the body's stores, since they are still required for the metabolism of carbohydrates (sugar). Consequently, chromium is one of the nutrients removed during the refining process of processed foods, and chromium deficiency increases sugar cravings.

All your child's sugar needs are met when the body metabolises (breaks down) complex carbohydrate-containing foods such as wholegrains, legumes, fruit and vegetables. Children do not require refined sugars in their diet to meet their energy requirements.

Honey

Honey, 'nature's sweetener', is a natural alternative to white sugar. However, honey is considered a sugar as it's composed of numerous types of simple sugars like glucose and fructose. Raw honey is a natural and unrefined product that does not contain any harmful chemicals or additives. Honey contains small amounts of nutrients such as amino acids, magnesium, potassium, calcium, iron and B vitamins. Raw honey, especially darker shades of honey, possesses phytochemicals which act as antioxidants, having cancer-preventing and anti-tumour properties. However, when raw honey is processed and heated, the benefits of these phytochemicals are largely eliminated. Choose a raw, organic, 100% pure honey. Avoid commercial honey that has been heated to keep a clear, smooth consistency on the supermarket shelves.

Even though honey is natural it is still considered a sugar and should be eaten in moderation. A teaspoon of honey contains the same amount of calories as a teaspoon of table sugar, so don't go layering it on your children's sandwiches and toast or over their breakfast cereal. Honey can still cause tooth decay and obesity if eaten in excess. So beware of so called health bars that list honey as one of its top ingredients.

Foods high in refined sugars

Foods commonly known to contain large amounts of refined sugars include soft drinks, jams, cordials, ice cream, chocolate, lollies, frozen desserts, pastries, biscuits, breakfast cereals and bars, muesli bars and cakes. It also turns up in foods you might not expect, like salad dressings, tomato sauce, mayonnaise, peanut butter, savoury biscuits, bread, canned foods (baked beans, fruit), yoghurts and fruit juices. It can be quite surprising when you add up how much sugar your child consumes in a day, when one serving of tomato sauce can contain one teaspoon of sugar, one serving of baked beans can contain two and a half teaspoons, and one small tub of sweetened yoghurt can contain up to four teaspoons of sugar. An average 30 g serving of a sugary breakfast cereal such as coco puffs or fruit loops, made up of 40% sugar, equals around three teaspoons of sugar sprinkled on your children's breakfast. Results from a recent nutritional survey found that between 20-30% of Australian children eat confectionery at least four times a week and around 10% of kids eat confectionery daily.[1]

Foods high in refined sugars are energy-dense foods that are usually lacking in vital nutrients. It's a concern that these energy-dense sugary foods are replacing more nutritious foods in your child's diet, which can lead to nutritional deficiencies. These sugary foods are also often notoriously high in saturated and trans-fats and lacking in dietary fibre. Foods rich in refined sugars and low in fibre also fail to create a feeling of satiety (fullness), resulting in children overeating these foods.

When children consume sugar-rich foods they get an artificial high, rapidly raising the levels of sugar in their bloodstream. This can contribute to hyperactivity, anxiety and difficulties concentrating. This rapid rise in blood sugar levels stimulates the release of too much insulin, which causes children's blood sugar levels to plummet, resulting in irritability and tiredness. High consumption of sugar has been associated with exacerbating children's behavioural problems and ADHD symptoms, and can effect a child's learning ability.[2,3] The regular consumption of these foods can lead to children becoming overweight or obese, which is a risk factor for developing type-2 diabetes.

Children consuming diets rich in sugary foods are at an increased risk of developing cardiovascular disease and atherosclerosis later in life. [4,5] Excessive sugar can raise blood triglyceride levels (blood fats), reduce HDL 'good' cholesterol and raise LDL 'bad' cholesterol.[6-8]

Excessive sugar consumption has a suppressive effect on the immune system, suppressing the ability of white blood cells to function. Sugar competes with vitamin C uptake into immune cells, leaving children vulnerable to infections and viruses.[9,10] Large amounts of sugar in the diet can also interfere with the absorption of calcium, increasing the risk of osteoporosis.[11,12] High consumption of sugar and refined foods can increase the excretion of zinc out of the body, which could lead to a deficiency. Frequent consumption of sugary foods and beverages is one of the leading causes of tooth decay in children.

Understanding ingredient and nutrition panels

To reduce sugars in your child's diet it is important to know how to interpret ingredient and nutrition panels, and be able to distinguish between total sugars and added sugars on processed or packaged foods. If a food contains more than 10 g of added sugars per 100 g, this is a lot and should be limited in the diet. To give you an idea of how much sugar is added to a food, keep in mind that there is 4 g of sugar in 1 teaspoon. So next time your child is tucking into a brownie (which contains 20 g of added sugar), they are consuming a whopping 5 teaspoons of sugar.

In Australia food labeling laws require manufacturers to list all ingredients from greatest to smallest proportion. However, there might not be a nutrition panel included on packaging as it's not mandatory. Nutrition panels give a breakdown of nutrients present in the product: carbohydrates, protein, fats, total sugar, as well as some vitamins and minerals.

Most nutrition panels found on Australian products, list only the total amount of sugar in the product, listed as 'total sugars' or 'sugars'. This total sugars value includes added refined sugars and natural occurring sugars from fruit and milk components that might be present in that product. It is important to be able to distinguish between total and added sugars.

For example, plain yoghurt has a total sugar value of 7.04g/100g due to the presence of lactose (milk sugar), but no added sugars. Sweetened fruit yoghurt has a total sugar value of 19g/100g and an added sugar value of 11.4g/100g due to sugar being added. Freshly squeezed orange juice has a total sugar value of 8.4g/100g due to its fructose content but has no added sugars. Low-fat milk has a total sugar value of 5.06g/100g due to its lactose content but it contains no added sugars.

Most processed or packaged foods have sugars present, in some form, from fruit, milk or honey. However, it's the added refined sugars that we must look out for and limit in children's diets. If a product has a high total sugar value and does not contain fruit or milk in the ingredients, it is likely to be high in added refined sugars.

Added sugar is not always listed as sugar on the ingredient panel. You must also look out for sucrose, glucose, sorbitol, mannitol, corn syrup, malt, malt extract, maltose, rice extract, molasses, honey and golden syrup.

If there is no nutrition panel on the packet and sugar is listed in the top three ingredients on the ingredient panel, this food is more than likely high in added sugars. Be careful of so-called healthy muesli bars that appear to be a wise snack choice, as some can actually contain up to four different types of sugar.

Look out for trick marketing that tries to make products sound more appealing, with words such as healthy, nutritious, good, natural, pure, fresh, low GI, light or low-fat. This doesn't mean the product is healthy. It could possibly be very high in added sugars. For example, it is common to see packets of lollies with '99% fat-free' splashed across the packet. Manufacturers will promote the benefits of the product, such as added vitamins and minerals, to draw attention away from the fact that the product is full of added sugar, fat and sodium. Don't be fooled - read ingredient labels carefully. Terms such as healthy and nutritious are not defined by law so they can legally be applied to pretty much any product.

Sugar content of commonly eaten foods [13]

Food	Serving size	Total sugar (g)	Added sugar (g)
Cookies, brownies	1 cookie (56 g)	20.5	19.8
Cookies, oatmeal, fat-free	1 cookie (56 g)	23.5	14.9
Doughnuts, chocolate, glazed	1 medium (42 g)	13.4	13
Muffins, blueberry	1 muffin (57 g)	11.2	9.4
Soft drink, cola, caffeine	1 can (355 ml)	33.0	33.1
Chocolate syrup	1 tablespoon (19 g)	9.31	9.2
Cereals, corn flakes	1 cup (30 g)	1.71	1.7
Cereals, chocolate puffed corn	1 cup (30 g)	14.1	14.1
Instant oats, cinnamon flavoured	1 packet (46 g)	15.5	15.2
Chocolate milk, reduced fat	1 cup (250 ml)	23.9	14.3
Yoghurt, fruit variety, nonfat	1 cup (250 g)	46.6	27.9
Salad dressing, Caesar, low cal	1 tablespoon (15 g)	2.5	2.5
French low cal, salad dressing	1 tablespoon (16 g)	4.2	3.6
Beans, baked, canned	1 cup (126 g)	11.4	6.1
Snacks, banana chips	20 g	7.07	5.1
Trail mix (nuts, sweetened coconut)	40 g	17.3	14.2
Granola bars, oats, fruits, nuts	1 bar (40 g)	17.4	16.3
Teriyaki sauce	1 tablespoon (16 g)	2.3	2.13
Milk chocolate	1 bar (40 g)	20.6	17.6
Jellybeans	10 large (30 g)	21.0	21.0
Jams and preserves	1 tablespoon (20g)	9.7	8.6
Tomato sauce	1 tablespoon (15 g)	3.4	2.5

"Excessive consumption of sugary foods has a suppressive effect on the immune system, leaving your child more vulnerable to infections."

Tips for reducing your child's sugar intake

1. Your child doesn't have to give up their favourite treats altogether. This book is full of yummy, healthy versions of all their favourites, like chocolate chip cookies, chocolate brownies, cakes, muffins, jelly, cheesecake and milkshakes.

2. Keep extra sugar out of your child's diet by choosing foods with 'no added sugar', 'reduced sugar' or 'low in sugar' on the label. Remember, no added sugar means no sugars were added during the foods manufacturing. It doesn't mean that there are no sugars present (eg. sugars from fruit, milk or honey).

3. Instead of giving your child sweet snacks that are high in added sugar and low in nutrients, offer them healthier naturally sweet foods, such as fruit, a small amount of sun-dried fruit (eg. dates, figs), and unsweetened carob buds. Try dipping sun-dried dates, figs or apricots in melted carob, place on a sheet of grease proof paper and pop in the fridge until set.

4. Watch out for fruit straps that contain added sugars. 100% all natural fruit straps still contain a lot of fruit sugars and can easily be eaten to excess. Give your children small servings of these or sun-dried fruit pieces instead.

5. Replace sugary sweet biscuits with savoury crackers and rice cakes spread with healthy savoury dips or toppings.

6. Jams and other sweet spreads are notoriously high in sugars and should be limited in your child's diet. Use small amounts of homemade fruit purees, or prune or date spreads as a healthy sweet alternative to spread on toast, pancakes, scones, puffed rice cakes and muffins. Mashed banana with a little tahini or nut butter makes a great topping for toast.

7. Choose whole oats, natural muesli, puffed cereals (rice, millet, buckwheat) and other wholegrains for breakfast instead of sugary breakfast cereals. Watch out for some toasted mueslis that are high in added sugars (make your own toasted muesli with a little honey). Sweeten your cereal naturally with fresh or dried fruit, fruit yoghurt or vanilla rice milk.

8. Limit buying commercially made cakes, muffins and biscuits, which usually contain a lot of added sugar and limited nutritional value. Make your own nutritious baked goods from the recipes in this book. Ideal for lunch box snacks and after school munchies.

9. Ice cream is a favourite of most kids but unfortunately contains large amounts of sugar. Once your children taste homemade ice cream they will never turn back. This book contains lots of wonderful, healthy recipes for ice creams and ice blocks that are guaranteed to please. Homemade, frozen yoghurt makes a healthy dessert or summers treat.

10. Look out for added sugars in yoghurt and yoghurt drinks. Most probiotic drinks also contain a lot of added sugar. Look for yoghurts naturally sweetened with fruit or buy plain yoghurt and add your own fresh fruit (mashed banana, grated pear or apple, mixed berries, passionfruit, mango), fruit puree, frozen raspberries and blueberries, date puree, diced sun-dried fruits or some muesli (with no added sugar).

11. Do not pack lollies, chocolate, soft drink, rolled fruit, sugary commercial muesli bars, sugary biscuits or cakes in your child's lunch box as a snack. Most children will fill up on these foods first and leave the more nutritious foods you packed.

12. Watch out for so called health bars and breakfast bars in your supermarket, marketed as healthy snacks or breakfast on the run. They may contain healthy elements such as oats, nuts, seeds and dried fruit but they also contain a lot of sugar and saturated fats. You are best off making your own muesli bars and biscuits for your kids to take to school and for after school snacks.

13. Avoid using cordials as they are a concentrated form of sugar. Use fruit juice (100% with no added sugar) as cordial, diluted with water. Diluted pineapple, apple, mixed berry and tropical juices make healthier substitutes. Make up a jug of weak fruit tea (with no added sugar) and keep in the fridge.

Artificial sweeteners
should NOT be given to children

Artificial sweeteners such as aspartame could potentially be one of the most damaging substances added to foods on the market today. These chemicals have flooded our food supply and could have a significant impact on children's health. Long-term safety of artificial sweeteners are unknown as there has only been a few human trials published. However, studies conducted before the FDA approval of aspartame revealed a high incidence of brain tumours found in animals that had been fed aspartame.[1] A recently published long-term study of aspartame indicated that aspartame caused dose-related and statistically significant increases in the incidence of several types of tumours, which has unfortunately been ignored by food regulators.[2-4]

Aspartame becomes methanol after exposure to heat or during prolonged storage, which is potentially toxic to the brain, retina and nerves.[5] The regular use of these artificial chemicals in a child's diet could therefore disrupt normal growth and development.

Read labels carefully for any added artificial sweeteners. They're hidden in most 'sugar-free' and 'diet' products, including soft drinks, flavoured milks, yoghurts, chewing gum, breakfast cereals, cakes, biscuits, ice cream and frozen desserts, just to name a few.

Artificial sweeteners are not recommended for anyone, especially children. As we don't really know the long-term effects of consuming these artificial sweeteners, why take the chance with your child's health? Use natural alternatives, such as a little raw honey or dried or fresh fruit, to sweeten drinks, desserts and baked goods.

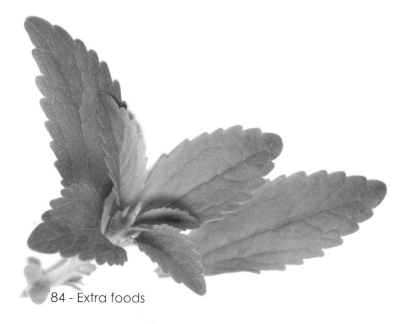

Xylitol and stevia

Xylitol (found in certain fruits and vegetables) and stevia (a South American herb) are two natural sweeteners that are safe for children and suitable for diabetics. These sweeteners do not contain any harmful artificial chemicals and have been shown to help prevent tooth decay in children.[6,7] These sweeteners can be used in cooking or beverages in place of sugar.

Soft drink
should NOT be given to children

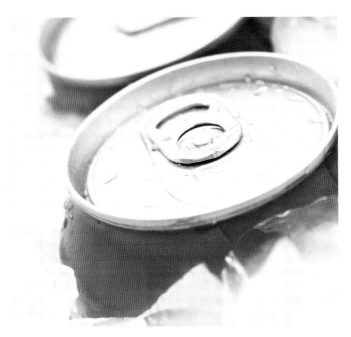

Over the past decade the amount of soft drink consumed by children has greatly increased and is often replacing more nutritious beverages such as milk and possibly fruit juice.[1] The results of a recent survey taken by the 'NSW centre for overweight and obesity' showed that a staggering 60% of boys and more than 40% of girls drink more than 250ml per day of soft drink and a frightening 7-12% of boys and a smaller proportion of girls drink more than 1 litre per day.[2]

These results are of great concern as soft drinks are energy-dense beverages that contain high levels of sugars or artificial sweeteners, caffeine, phosphoric acid and other artificial additives (flavours and colours). Some soft drinks can contain as many as 11 teaspoons of sugar per serving. Soft drink supplies no nutritional benefit to your child's diet and should be severely limited or done without.

Studies have shown that consumption of soft drink is associated with obesity. Obesity rates in children have risen in conjunction with increases in children's soft drink consumption.[3]

Drinking soft drink can be detrimental to the health of children's bones. High doses of sugar present in soft drinks increase urinary excretion of calcium, which can lead to weaker bones, the development of osteoporosis, and kidney stones later in life.

Consumption of cola beverages in particular, has been associated with bone fractures, due to their high phosphoric acid content.[4] Phosphoric acid also robs the body of calcium by increasing the loss of calcium in the urine. The increase in soft drink consumption is a contributing factor in the growing number of people with osteoporosis.

A healthy substitute for soft drink is mixing natural sparkling mineral water with ¼ fruit juice (100% with no added sugar). However, water should always be encouraged as the beverage of choice for children.

How sugary foods and soft drink effect your child's teeth

Teeth are one of your child's most important possessions and how you help your child look after them will make a significant impact on their health and wellbeing. This means not only teaching your child the importance of regular brushing and flossing, but also focusing on cutting down on sugary foods and acidic drinks, which cause permanent damage to teeth.

Dentists have long recognised the link between good oral health and a healthy diet. Good nutrition during childhood is essential, not only for the growth of strong teeth but also to prevent the development of tooth decay and erosion. Children grow their first permanent teeth around the age of six and by the time they're 12 to 13 years of age, most children have 28 permanent teeth. These teeth have to last a lifetime so it is vital that children learn good oral care from an early age. If left untreated tooth decay can cause infection and other dental problems later in life. Dental decay is one of Australia's most expensive diet-related disease.[5]

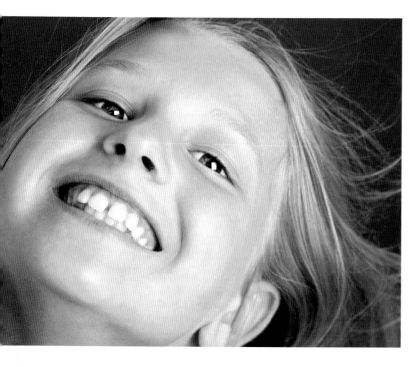

Sugar and tooth decay

Excessive consumption of sugary foods and soft drinks are the leading causes of tooth decay in children.[6] According to a concerning report released by the Australian Dental Association (ADA), tooth decay is on the rise in young Australian children (pre-schoolers).[7] ADA warns that the main culprits are processed sugary snack foods, lower consumption of fruit and vegetables, and an increase in sugary beverages including carbonated and sports drinks.

Tooth decay (also known as dental cavities or caries), is a location on a tooth where so much of the tooth's enamel has been dissolved away that a hole or 'cavity' is formed. Tooth decay occurs when three factors are present: bacteria, sugar and weak enamel. Oral bacteria live in a sticky white film on the surface of teeth, called plaque. Bacteria love sugar, every time your child consumes sugary foods or drinks, bacteria comes in contact with sugar, and produces lactic acid, which attacks the teeth for 20 minutes or more. During this time the hard protective coating on teeth, called 'enamel', becomes softer for a short time and loses some of its mineral content. Saliva will then usually neutralize the acidity and restore it to its natural balance. However, if these acid attacks happen too often, the mouth does not have a chance to repair itself, resulting in tooth decay. Studies have shown the frequency, more so than the quantity, of sugar eaten, is strongly related to tooth decay.[8]

Soft drinks and tooth erosion

Tooth decay and tooth erosion are two different processes that can both permanently damage children's teeth. Unlike tooth decay, tooth erosion occurs across the whole tooth surface and does not involve bacteria or dietary sugars. Tooth erosion is caused by teeth being repeatedly exposed to acids that eventually lead to the enamel being worn away. This results in the sensitive dentine underneath being exposed causing sensitivity and pain. Small pieces of the tooth can also crumble around the biting edge.

It is widely accepted that children consuming acidic foods, in particular beverages, play a major role in the development of tooth erosion. Studies have found that soft drinks, cordials, sports drinks and fruit juices (in particular citrus juices like orange juice) are the worst offenders.[9,10] Most soft drinks, including diet soft drinks, contain phosphoric acid and citric acid which can cause the erosion of tooth enamel.

"Excessive consumption of sugary foods and soft drink are the leading causes of tooth decay in children."

Dietary tips for reducing tooth erosion and decay

1. Reduce your child's intake of soft drinks and sugary foods (especially confectionery). Remember it's the frequency of sugar consumption that causes greatest damage to teeth, so slowly sipping a sugary beverage or picking at sugary snacks throughout the day is going to be worse than consuming them in one sitting.

2. When your child drinks acidic beverages like orange juice, dilute the juice and give them a straw, as this will help reduce the drinks contact with teeth.

3. Give your child a glass of water after having fruit juice.

4. Having acidic drinks only at mealtimes is another way of cutting down enamel erosion. The process of chewing the meal will produce more saliva and neutralize the acid from the drink.

5. Foods that stick to the teeth like chewy confectionery can be even more of a problem because they help bacteria stay on tooth surfaces longer.

6. The sugars naturally found in foods like fruit and vegetables have been shown to have little damaging effect on teeth. It is foods high in added sugars that are most detrimental to teeth.

Caffeine

should NOT be included in a child's diet

Caffeine is a natural stimulant found in foods and beverages such as soft drinks, energy drinks, coffee, tea, cocoa and chocolate. The main source of caffeine in the diets of Australian children is from soft drinks, especially cola types. Soft drinks can contain up to 36 mg of caffeine per 250 ml can.

Caffeine rich energy drinks are not recommended for children, primarily because of their high caffeine content. They can contain up to 80 mg of caffeine per 250 ml can, which is equivalent to a strong cup of coffee.

Tea contains between 10-50 mg of caffeine per 250 ml cup, coffee between 60-120 mg per 250 ml cup, and chocolate around 20 mg of caffeine per 100 g bar.

Caffeine is addictive and considered unhealthy for children. At high doses, caffeine is known to stimulate the central nervous system and can cause irritability, anxiety, increased heart rate and sleeping problems. Regular consumption of caffeine is also linked to hyperactivity, diuresis (excessive urinating), diarrhoea, gastrointestinal disturbances and headaches. Because of their smaller size, children are even more susceptible to caffeine's effects than adults. Excessive and long term consumption of caffeine has the ability to cause a caffeine addiction.

Children's bone health can also be affected by regular caffeine consumption. Caffeine increases calcium excretion from the body and decreases calcium absorption, leading to weak bones and increased risk of osteoporosis in later life.[1,2] The ingestion of caffeine at mealtimes inhibits the absorption of iron and destroys B vitamins.

Chocolate can be included occasionally in your child's diet without any effect on their health. However, carob is a healthier, caffeine-free alternative to chocolate. Carob is high in calcium and contains phosphorus, magnesium, iron and is a good source of B vitamins. Pack some unsweetened carob buds or carob coated rice or buckwheat cakes in your child's lunch box as a treat. Make some carob chip cookies or muffins as after school snacks. Carob powder makes delicious chocolate-like smoothies, cakes and hot drinks.

It is not recommended that children drink coffee. Occasionally however, it is OK for children to have a weak dandelion root or chai tea. Chai tea contains a small amount of caffeine as it contains some black tea, so only make it weak. These healthy alternatives to coffee are delicious made with mostly milk and a little honey to taste.

Herbal teas

Caffeine-free herbal teas are a wonderful alternative to soft drinks and other sugar ladened beverages. Served warm or chilled, herbal teas possess different health benefits such as aiding digestion and helping your child to sleep. Some herbal teas that can be enjoyed by children include calming chamomile (avoid if your child has a ragweed allergy) and lemon balm, peppermint or spearmint, ginger, weak fruit teas, rooibos, rosehip and echinacea (given occasionally as an immune booster). Black tea is not recommended for young children because it contains caffeine and tannins that can be too stimulating and can reduce iron absorption if consumed regularly.

Salt

should be limited in your child's diet

The Australian diet contains an unnecessarily large amount of salt (sodium chloride). Salt, like sugar is difficult to avoid as it's added to most processed foods to make them more flavoursome.

Sodium is naturally found in small quantities in a majority of the foods we eat. We need some sodium in our diet as it helps to balance our body fluids and is necessary to help our muscles and nerves function properly.

Sodium in small quantities is not going to have any detrimental effect on your child's health however, the problem is, a vast majority of children have intakes of sodium exceeding the adult maximum daily recommendations.[1]

The majority of sodium in the diets of Australians comes from processed foods (65-75%), although sodium added to cooking, at the table, and naturally present in food, also contributes to the total dietary intake. Much of the sodium consumed by children comes from foods such as cheese, butter, margarine, spreads and sauces, snack foods like potato chips, convenience foods, processed meats, breakfast cereals and canned foods like baked beans, soups and pasta. A bowl of canned soup can contain more sodium than the daily maximum amount acceptable for a 13 year old. Even processed foods that don't have a salty taste can contain large amounts of added sodium such as desserts and sweet biscuits.

If you take a look at an example of food consumed by an 8 year old, you will see how easy it is to exceed the recommended daily sodium limit.

How much sodium is your child having a day?

Breakfast: Bowl of corn flakes
Lunch: Cheese burger and large fries
Snack: Plain doughnut
Dinner: 1 pork sausage, potato salad, small green salad with French dressing
Dessert: 1 small bowl of vanilla ice cream

The total amount of sodium consumed is approximately 2940 g, which is about 5 times the recommended maximum daily limit of sodium for an 8 year old.

Research has shown that both sodium and chloride can be detrimental to health when consumed in excess.[2] Excessive consumption of salt puts extra pressure on children's kidneys, making them work harder to eliminate the sodium out of the body. High sodium diets have been linked to high blood pressure that can increase the risk of cardiovascular disease later in life.[3] In Australia, hypertension is the most frequently seen problem by general practitioners. Children of hypertensive parents are at particular risk of developing hypertension because of the genetic link and their shared eating environment. High blood pressure is a condition usually only seen in adults. A recent Australian survey has found an alarming one in five secondary school students are already showing signs of health problems such as high blood pressure, putting them at greater risk of developing cardiovascular disease as an adult.[4]

High sodium intake also affects children's bone health as it increases calcium excretion, which could have a detrimental effect on children's bone mass.[5-6] It's during childhood and adolescence that the development of peak bone mass is essential for prevention of osteoporosis later in life.

Children's recommended target intakes of sodium per day [7]
(Aim to keep below these levels)

- Children aged 4–8 years should aim to consume below 300–600 mg/day (13–26 mmol)
- Children aged 9–13 years should aim to consume below 400–800 mg/day (17–34 mmol)

(There is 2325 mg of sodium in 1 teaspoon of common table salt)

Food Standards Australia NZ defines low-salt foods as having a sodium concentration of up to 120 mg/100 g. Most manufactured foods are well over the suggested sodium content limit of 120 mg/100 g, so read labels carefully and choose foods that contain less than 120 mg/100 g.

Most food labels list the sodium content of the food however, if it's shown as 'salt' you can calculate the sodium content by dividing the amount of salt by 2.5.

Iodized salt & iodine deficiency

Iodine, a very important trace mineral, is required by the body for proper thyroid function and for the production of thyroid hormones. Thyroid hormones, produced by the thyroid gland, play a vital role in the regulation of metabolic processes such as growth and energy production, and are essential throughout childhood for normal brain development.

Australian researchers have now discovered almost 50% of Australian children are iodine deficient. The results of the Australian National Iodine Nutrition Study (2003-2004) revealed that almost half of Australian primary school children are mild to moderately iodine deficient.[8]

It is crucial that children have an adequate intake of iodine as iodine deficiency can have a devastating impact on children's growth and development. While goitre (enlarged thyroid gland) is the most visible consequence of iodine deficiency, the most significant and profound consequences are on the developing brain. Even a mild deficiency can lower a child's IQ. Iodine deficiency can cause stunted growth, weight gain, fatigue and depression.

The decline in iodine intake in Australia may appear to be due to changes within the dairy industry (reduced use of iodine-based disinfectants), greater public awareness of the health benefits of reduced salt intake and the change towards a greater consumption of processed foods (few food manufacturers use iodised salt).[9]

To be sure your child is getting enough iodine, include plenty of unprocessed iodine-rich foods in their diet. The richest natural food sources of iodine are seafood (ocean fish) and seaweed (such as kelp and nori). Two or three serves a week of seafood will provide sufficient intake of iodine. Add a sprinkling of seaweed flakes to salads, soups and vegetable dishes or make nori rolls filled with nutritious ingredients.

Sodium (mg) content of commonly eaten processed foods [10]

Food	Serving size	Sodium (mg)
Soup, chicken vegetable, canned	1 cup (250 g)	1068
Macaroni and cheese, canned	1 cup (250 g)	1061
Baked beans, plain	1 cup (254 g)	856
Cheeseburger, with condiments	1 burger (219 g)	1108
Ham, sliced, regular	2 slices (57 g)	739
Bread, white	1 slice (25 g)	170
Cereal, rice bubbles	1 cup (33 g)	314
Cheese, cheddar	28 g	176
Cheese, feta	28 g	316
Cheese, cottage, low fat	28 g	114
Crackers, regular	4 crackers (12 g)	102
French fries	Medium (134 g)	260
Gravy, beef	¼ cup (58 g)	326
Muffins, blueberry	1 muffin (57 g)	255
Pork sausage, cooked	1 sausage (27 g)	202
Salad dressing, Italian	1 tablespoon (15 g)	243
Tomato sauce, canned	¼ cup (63 g)	321
Butter, salted	1 Tbsp (14 g)	82

Reducing your child's sodium intake

1. Prevent children becoming used to the taste of foods with high salt content by giving them low-sodium foods, allowing them to enjoy the fresh natural taste of food.

2. The easiest way to keep salt to a minimum in your child's diet is to look for products labelled 'no-added salt', 'reduced-salt' or 'low-salt'. Choose products with a sodium content of 120 mg/100 g or less. The majority of your child's diet should be made up of fresh food and food processed without added salt.

3. It will be far easier for your child to maintain healthy eating habits if the whole family has the same diet. Children should avoid adding salt to meals and parents should lead by example and not add any extra salt to their food either. Do not leave salt on the table.

4. They may not taste salty, but a lot of commercial breakfast Cereals that kids love, such as cornflakes, nutra-grain, rice bubbles and coco pops contain high levels of sodium and make a hefty contribution to your child's daily sodium intake. Containing 600-800 mg of sodium per 100g cereal, this amounts to more than 30% of the upper level of the daily adequate sodium intake for 4 to 8 year olds. Choose all natural cereal grains such as oats, puffed grains (including brown rice, millet, buckwheat and amaranth), corn or spelt flakes and natural muesli.

5. Instead of using salt to season dishes try using fresh and dried herbs, spices, curry powders, mustards, garlic, onion, lemon, lime, vinegars or fruit juices. They make a wonderful tasty addition to your child's diet with all the added health benefits.

6. Miso paste is also another great way of adding extra flavour and nutrients to meals such as soups, stir-fries, casseroles, sauces and salad dressings. Miso does contain sea salt so you only need to use a small amount.

Make sure you don't over heat miso or it will lose some of its goodness. Add it at the end of cooking.

7. Keep take away foods such as hamburgers, chips, fried chicken and pizzas to a minimum as they contain high levels of salt. Make your own healthy version of these foods from the recipes in this book.

8. Pre-packed microwave popcorn might sound like a healthy snack idea but one single pack contains twice as much fat as a Mars Bar and contains high levels of salt. Make your own air-popped popcorn without butter or salt.

9. Limit your child's intake of salty foods such as crisps, pretzels, salted peanuts and pre-packed biscuit and cheese snacks. Instead give raw, unsalted nuts and seeds and low-salt rice crackers and puffed rice cakes served with a healthy dip (hummus, avocado, baba ghanoush).

10. Replace canned foods, such as baked beans, pasta and soups, that contain added sodium, with healthy homemade versions.

11. Instant noodles contain high levels of saturated fat and sodium and usually contain MSG. Make your own healthy version with thin Asian noodles (eg, ramen, buckwheat), a little miso paste and a handful of diced vegetables.

12. Be careful of some mineral waters. Choose a mineral water that contains 20 mg/litre of sodium.

13. Spreads kids commonly eat on sandwiches and toast, such as peanut butter, yeast spreads (such as Vegemite and Marmite) and mayonnaise are high in sodium. Make your own healthy low-salt mayonnaise. Buy 100% all natural nut butters and tahini. Use hummus, avocado and baba ghanoush as spreads.

Saturated & trans-fats
the 'bad' fats

Children need certain types of fats in their diet for overall good health. However, caution must be taken to ensure your child is getting the right kind of fats.

There are two main types of fats that are considered 'bad' and should be limited in children's diets. These are saturated fats and trans-fats.

Harvard research has shown that it's not so much the amount of fat in the diet that is linked to disease - it's the type of fat in the diet.[1-4] It's becoming clearer that bad fats, meaning saturated and trans-fats, increase the risk of certain diseases while good fats, meaning monounsaturated and polyunsaturated fats, lower the risk.

When reducing fat in a child's diet, careful attention needs to be paid to the importance of a well-balanced diet, taking into account their need for adequate intakes of good fats (unsaturated fats), notably omega-3 essential fatty acids (EFAs). The key is to replace bad fats with good fats in the diet. Young children, two years and under, must not be placed on fat restrictive diets, as it may adversely affect their growth and development.

Saturated fats are unfortunately the most commonly consumed fat in Australian's diets. Nutrition surveys have found that saturated fats account for the highest proportion of fat intake in children of all ages.[5,6] If all parents realised that just one meal from any of the well known fast food chains contains the total recommended daily allowance of saturated fat for an adult, how many parents would still be happy for their children to consume it?

Saturated fats
should be limited in your child's diet

Saturated fats are commonly found in animal based foods such as meat and poultry (especially their fat and skin), sausages, deli meats (pastrami, pepperoni and salami), full-fat dairy products (milk, cheese, yoghurt, cream), butter and most margarines. Saturated fats can also be found in some plant based foods such as tropical plant oils like palm oil, palm kernel oil, coconut oils and cocoa butter.

Most processed and take away foods contain high levels of saturated fats including pastries, creamy foods and sauces, vegetable oil, ghee, lard, pizza, deep fried chicken, hamburgers, hot chips, pies, sausage rolls, potato chips, chocolate and ice cream. These foods should be limited in children's diets. Eaten occasionally these foods will not cause any harm to your child, as long as the majority of their diet is made up of nutritious foods from the five food groups.

Dairy foods such as milk, cheese and yoghurt are valuable sources of calcium and protein in a child's diet. However, excessive consumption of the full-fat varieties can affect your child's health. It is recommended that children (over the age of 2 years old) consume low-fat milk, cheese and yoghurt.

High consumption of saturated fats is strongly associated with childhood obesity. Children consuming diets rich in saturated fat is one of the major contributing factors in the increasing prevalence of childhood obesity. Research shows that a large percentage of Australian children that are overweight or obese also have raised blood cholesterol and triglyceride levels.[7] Some of these children have already started to develop fatty deposits of atherosclerosis, which is usually only seen in adults.[8]

Cholesterol

High levels of blood cholesterol greatly increase the risk of heart disease. One of the most important determinants of blood cholesterol levels is fat in the diet, not total fat, but the specific types of fat consumed. Some types of fat are clearly good for cholesterol levels and others are bad.

Saturated fat and trans-fats are the main dietary factors that raise blood cholesterol levels. It is important to limit the amount of dietary cholesterol your child eats, however dietary cholesterol has much less of an effect on cholesterol levels than the amount of saturated and trans-fats we eat. Animal based foods high in saturated fats usually contain cholesterol, for example meat, poultry, liver, kidney, prawns, egg yolks and whole-milk dairy products. Diets high in saturated fats are associated with increased risk of coronary heart disease, heart attack and certain cancers.

Cholesterol plays an essential role in the formation of cell membranes, some hormones (eg, testosterone) and vitamin D. However, if cholesterol levels in the blood are too high, this can lead to the artery-clogging process known as atherosclerosis that can eventually lead to a heart attack.
There are two main types of blood cholesterol that basically work in opposite directions.
Low-density lipoproteins (LDL) are often referred to as 'bad' cholesterol. When there is too much LDL cholesterol in the blood, it can be deposited on the walls of coronary arteries leading to atherosclerosis.

High-density lipoproteins (HDL), often referred to as 'good' cholesterol has a protective effect against heart disease, making it less likely that excess cholesterol in the blood will be deposited in the coronary arteries.

In general, the higher your LDL and the lower your HDL, the greater your risk for atherosclerosis and heart disease.

Reducing saturated fats in your child's diet will help maintain healthy cholesterol and triglyceride levels which will help reduce their chance of developing cardiovascular disease later in life. Monounsaturated fats and polyunsaturated fats do not raise blood cholesterol levels. Scientific studies suggest that these unsaturated fats actually have a lowering effect on total cholesterol, LDL 'bad' cholesterol levels, and triglyceride level, when eaten as part of a low saturated fat diet.[9]

A recent study has found that the type of fat your child eats may also relate to their cognitive performance.[10] Increasing saturated fat intake was associated with poor short term memory in school aged children and a higher intake of polyunsaturated fats contributed to improved memory recall. These findings reinforce the need to avoid saturated fats in children's diets and the inclusion of foods rich in omega-3 fats. Be aware of some manufacturers trying to get you to buy their products using trick marketing tactics, claiming their products are cholesterol free. Dietary cholesterol is only found in foods of animal origin, not vegetable, so you wouldn't expect to find cholesterol in foods such as vegetable oils (olive, canola), breakfast cereals and rice. That doesn't stop some manufacturers putting 'cholesterol-free' on products that are usually high in saturated fat.

Trans-fats
should be avoided or severely limited in your child's diet

When we look at fats, trans-fats are the worst of them all. Researchers have found that trans-fats are one of the prime culprits in heart disease, having an even more detrimental effect than saturated fats.[11,12] Clinical trials have shown that the consumption of trans-fats actually raises LDL ('bad') cholesterol levels and lowers HDL ('good') cholesterol levels.[13-16] This dangerous combination significantly increases the risk of cardiovascular disease and strokes. A recent study from the Harvard School of Public Health has confirmed this, finding a strong link between high consumption of trans-fats and heart disease.[17] Eating trans fats is also associated with a higher risk of developing type 2 diabetes.[18] High consumption of these fats could have detrimental effects on your child's health.

The majority of trans-fats (or trans fatty acids) are formed in an industrial process called 'hydrogenation', which adds hydrogen to liquid vegetable oils to make them more solid.

Trans-fats are also known as 'partially hydrogenated oils.' Food manufacturers like using trans-fats as they are less likely to spoil, giving food a longer shelf life and a more desirable taste and texture. Many fast-food restaurants use trans-fats to deep-fry foods because oils with trans-fats can be used many times in commercial fryers.

Trans-fats are commonly found in vegetable shortenings, some margarines (hard), commercially baked products (biscuits, cakes, muffins, crackers, doughnuts, pastries, pie crusts, pizza dough), some cereal bars, fried foods (hot chips, hamburgers, fried chicken), cheese spreads, commercial cooking oils used for frying in restaurants and any other foods made or fried in partially hydrogenated oils. A small amount of trans-fat is found naturally, primarily in some meat and dairy products.

The majority of trans-fats consumed in the diet come from commercially baked goods, margarine and fast foods.[19] Trans-fats are detrimental to children's health and should be avoided or severely limited.

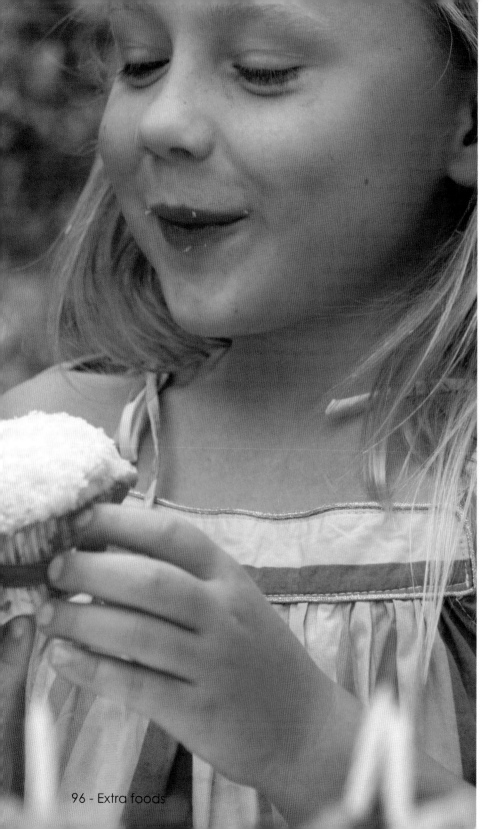

A child eating a doughnut for a mid morning snack and a cheese burger, thick shake and large fries for lunch would ingest a whopping 17 g of trans-fats. The US National Academy of Sciences' Institute of Medicine has suggested that the only safe level of trans-fat is zero and that we should eat as little as possible, consistent with a healthy, balanced diet. Given that a lot of people would eat small amounts of naturally occurring trans-fats every day, there is no place for industrially manufactured trans-fats in the diet.

Unfortunately it is not mandatory for food manufacturers in Australia to list trans-fats on labels unless they make a nutritional or health claim about the food. If they make no claim, they need only give the levels of total and saturated fat on the label and you could be buying a product high in trans-fats. Some processed foods may have 'hydrogenated' or 'partially hydrogenated' vegetable oils on the label. This is an indication that the product contains trans-fats.

Trans-fats are very strictly regulated in many other countries. In the US it is mandatory that trans-fats be listed on all processed foods. Denmark has gone a step further and banned any food products that contain more than 2% trans-fats. We have products in Australia that children consume containing up to 8% trans-fats.

Saturated and trans-fats present in commonly eaten foods [20]

Food	Serving size	Saturated fat (g)	Trans fat (g)
French fries	medium (147g)	7	8
Butter	1 Tbsp	7	0
Hard margarine	1 Tbsp	2	3
Soft margarine	1 Tbsp	1	0.5
Shortening	1 Tbsp	3.5	4
Potato chips	small packet (42.5 g)	2	3
Doughnut	1	4.5	5
Cookie, cream filled	3 (30 g)	1	2
Chocolate bar	40 g	4	3
Cake, pound	1 slice (80 g)	3.5	4.5

How much fat is OK for children to consume?

- For children between the ages of 5-14 years, saturated fats should make up only 10% of their diet, preferably less.[21]
- Trans-fats should be avoided where possible or kept to an absolute minimum.

"Make nutritious treats for your kids, free from harmful fats. All the muffins and cakes in this book use healthy olive oil instead of butter or vegetable oils."

Reducing saturated and trans-fats in your child's diet

1. Replace saturated and trans-fats in your child's diet with healthy monounsaturated and polyunsaturated fats.

2. Encourage your child to reduce their use of high fat sauces, salad dressings and spreads. Make your own healthy sauces, dressings and spreads using beneficial unsaturated oils such as olive oil and flaxseed oil.

3. Limit the use of butter and margarine in their diet. Use flaxseed oil or avocado instead of butter on toast. Only buy soft margarines with no trans-fats, non-hydrogenated and low in saturated fats.

4. Trim any visible fat from meat and remove the skin off chicken.

5. Give your child low-fat dairy products (milk, cheese and yoghurt).

6. Limit the use of processed meats such as hot dogs, luncheon meats and sausages. Choose low-fat sausages made from quality, lean mince. Using left over lamb or roast chicken slices is a healthy alternative to deli meats. Choose good quality deli meats that are low in fat and nitrite-free.

7. Limit deep-fried, take away foods such as hot chips, pies, fried chicken or fried fish. Homemade healthy versions of these foods from this book, not only taste better, but are actually good for your kids.

8. Do not cook with saturated fat vegetable oils. Use olive oil (monounsaturated oils) instead. Don't be fooled by some vegetable oils that declare that they're 'light'. This could refer to its colour and taste, not fat content. Read the small print.

9. Limit commercially made baked goods such as cakes, muffins and biscuits that contain partially hydrogenated oils and trans-fats. Bake your own healthy goodies from this book. All of the muffins, cakes, biscuits and slices are made with olive oil.

10. When eating out ask what type of cooking oil they use.

"Flaxseed oil or avocado make a healthy alternative to butter for toast or sandwiches."

Chapter 5:
Super foods
optimum nutrition for kids

Your child's health depends on the proper functioning of their brain and on the health of their immune and digestive systems. Kids have specific needs with regard to the development and maturation of their digestive and immune systems as well as brain growth and development.

The following group of 'super foods' all have special health promoting qualities and contain specific vitamins, minerals or phytochemicals. Regularly including these 'super foods' in a child's diet will help them reach optimal health.

Antioxidant-rich
Berries

Antioxidants are important disease-fighting compounds that include vitamins A, C and E, the mineral selenium and phytochemicals found in plant foods. Antioxidants help prevent damage from oxidation, a natural process in the body that occurs during normal cell function. A small percentage of cells become damaged during this process and turn into free radicals, which can start a chain reaction, harming other cells in the body. Cell damage from free radicals has been implicated in many chronic diseases such as cancer, heart disease, Alzheimer's, and Parkinson's disease.[1]

Recent studies have demonstrated that environmental pollutants, radiation, chemicals, deep fried foods, as well as physical stress can produce large amounts of free radicals, resulting in cellular damage throughout the body.

Antioxidants help to strengthen the immune system and are particularly important during phases of rapid growth in children. Antioxidants are best taken in combination with each other. Consuming a diet rich in a variety of antioxidant foods will provide your child with protection against a number of diseases.

Luscious, bright coloured berries bursting with flavour can brighten up any kid's meal. Perfect in breakfast cereals, smoothies, muffins or on their own, these tiny fruits not only taste delicious but they contain some of the highest levels of antioxidants of all fruit and vegetables. The red, blue and purple colour in berries signifies the presence of an important group of phytochemicals, the anthocyanins, which act as powerful antioxidants in the body. Anthocyanins, possess a broad spectrum of health benefits relating to their antioxidant activity, having protective effects against cancer and many other diseases.[2-4]

There are a wide variety of berries available most of the year round, such as blueberries, raspberries, strawberries, cranberries and blackberries.

Researchers say that of all the common fruits and vegetables, berries have the highest antioxidant concentration, especially those with dark-coloured skins, one of the highest being blueberries.[5-6] The superior antioxidant content of red and blue berries has been well-studied, however less is known about the so called 'purple berries', such as elderberry, black currant, and chokeberry. These 'purple berries' are 50% higher in antioxidants than some of the more common berry varieties.[7] Goji berries have also become popular over the last couple of years for their abundance in antioxidants and nutrients.

Fish
food for thought

The food your child eats affects the development and performance of their brain. Giving your children the right food containing specific nutrients can boost your child's IQ, allow them to think more quickly, be more coordinated, have better memory, improve concentration and be more emotionally stable.

Children's brains are around 60% fat, so they need to be supplied with the right kind of fats to keep their brains well oiled and functioning properly.

The brain needs omega-3 fatty acids (FAs), in particular docosahexaenoic acid (DHA), found in oily fish, to work properly.[1] The brain and the retina contain the highest content of DHA found in any tissue in the body. Dietary DHA is essential for optimum brain and visual function.

Omega-3 FAs cannot be made by the body, so they need to be supplied through the diet. DHA is not widely found in the diet, but it is present in cold water fish such as salmon, tuna, sardines, trout, herring, halibut and mackerel. DHA can also be made by the body from the omega-3 FA, alpha-linolenic acid, found in high levels in flaxseed oil and in other oils such as canola, soy and walnut. Green leafy vegetables, nuts and seeds, wholegrain cereals and legumes also contain omega-3 FAs.

Omega-3 FAs are essential for optimum brain performance. Children's learning and behavioural problems at school can be due to a lack of omega-3 fats in their diets, according to a study published in the May 2005 edition of Pediatrics.[2] Children lacking in omega-3 fats are susceptible to conditions such as depression, poor memory, low IQ, learning disabilities, dyslexia, and ADD/ADHD.

Studies have shown major improvements in attention, behaviour, IQ, reading and spelling abilities in children who had increased their omega-3 FA intakes.[3-7]

DHA enhances learning and memory by increasing proteins that enhance neural communication. It is believed that in ADHD, deficiencies of DHA may be responsible for abnormal signalling associated with learning disabilities, cognitive deficits and visual dysfunction. These abnormalities can be partially corrected with a diet enriched with DHA.[8]

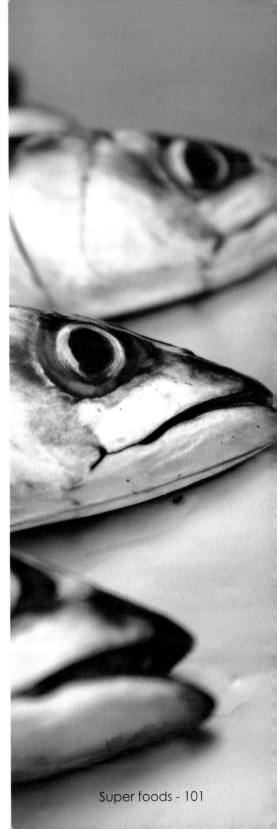

Immune boosting
Garlic

Schools are a favourite place for kids to share infections. Many children repeatedly come down with respiratory, ear and gastro-intestinal infections in these environments. Frequent use of antibiotics and over the counter medications can suppress children's immune systems, making them more vulnerable to these infections. Protect your child and break the vicious cycle of recurring illness by strengthening your child's immunity with immune-boosting foods.

The most commonly known food to help prevent cold and flu and strengthen immune function is garlic. Garlic has a long distinguished history of healing, dating back thousands of years. This pungent herb, which is a member of the onion family, is used widely around the world in cooking and natural medicine.

Garlic contains constituents such as allicin that have powerful immune enhancing actions. Garlic is also a good source of vitamins A, C, E and minerals selenium, sulphur and zinc, which are all needed for healthy immune function.

Garlic protects against infections (bacterial, fungal, parasitic) and viruses. Studies have shown that if garlic is included in the diet you will be less likely to get a cold, recovering faster if infected.[1]

Incorporating garlic into your child's diet not only helps to strengthen their immune system but also enhances the flavour of meals. When cooking add one or two crushed garlic cloves to dishes, add to dips, sauces and salad dressings, or make bruschetta or garlic bread (mix with cold pressed virgin olive oil). Allicin is formed when garlic cloves are crushed, so this is the best way to eat and reap the benefits of garlic.

Other important immune boosting foods & nutrients

Other foods that possess special immune-boosting properties include shiitake mushrooms (considered one of the most powerful immune enhancing foods), yoghurt, miso and sea vegetables. Green tea is another commonly consumed immune-enhancing herb however, due to it containing caffeine it is not recommended for younger children. Adding small quantities of miso, shiitake mushroom and sea vegetables to soups and stir-fries is a nice way to further boost your child's protection from colds and flu during the winter months.

Several important nutrients are also needed to enhance immune health. Without these your child's immune system can become suppressed and deficiency symptoms can occur. For your child to have super resistance, you need to feed them food packed with immune-boosting nutrients. Here are the top five nutrients to help build immunity and protect your child against disease, infections and allergies.

Nutrients to help build immunity

1. Vitamin C: Citrus fruits (oranges, guava) and coloured berries (strawberries, blueberries and boysenberries) are excellent sources of vitamin C. Fruit juices are also good sources of vitamin C if they are vitamin C fortified. Freshly squeezed orange juice is a good source of vitamin C (make sure you drink it soon after squeezing). Vegetables such as red capsicums, parsley, broccoli and cabbage are also rich sources.

2. Zinc: Zinc is found in a wide variety of foods. The best food sources of zinc includes lean meat, chicken, fish, milk and other dairy foods (cheese), brewers yeast, egg yolks, legumes (soy beans, lima beans, lentils, peas), wholegrains (bread), sunflower seeds, pumpkin seeds, pecans and a moderate amount of zinc found in vegetables.

3. Vitamin A and beta-carotene: Milk, egg yolk and cod liver oil contain vitamin A. Beta-carotene is found in high levels in yellow and orange fruits and vegetables such as carrots, sweet potato, pumpkin, butternut squash, apricots, mangoes, and also in green leafy vegetables.

4. Vitamin E: Foods rich in vitamin E include wheatgerm, whole oats, cold pressed olive oil, fruits, dark green leafy vegetables, avocado, fish, poultry, meat, eggs and raw nuts and seeds.

5. Omega-3 FAs: Omega-3 FAs found in oily fish (mackerel, herring, sardines, tuna, trout, salmon), flaxseed oil, canola, soy, and walnut oils, dark green vegetables, parsley, seaweeds, nuts, seeds (pumpkin and sesame seeds, tahini), legumes (hummus), and wholegrain cereals.

"Incorporating garlic into your child's diet will help to strengthen their immune system and help prevent colds and flu."

Yoghurt
probiotic food

Healthy intestinal function is critically important for your child's overall health. The gastrointestinal tract represents a complex ecosystem in which a delicate balance exists between 'friendly' and 'pathogenic' (disease-causing) bacteria. A healthy intestinal tract should contain a large percentage of these 'friendly' bacteria to prevent over-growth of disease-causing bacteria-like salmonella and e-coli.

'Friendly' intestinal bacteria play a major role in children's nutritional status by improving digestion and absorption of nutrients from foods. These 'friendly' bacteria are also involved in the production of certain B vitamins and vitamin K (needed for blood clotting).

Probiotics are live micro-organisms including the commonly known lactobacillus, acidophilus and bifidus, found in fermented foods such as yoghurt. These micro-organisms help promote good health by promoting a healthy balance of 'friendly' bacteria in the large intestine.

Fermented foods have important nutritional and therapeutic benefits. Most cultures around the world use some form of these foods to maintain good health. Other fermented foods include buttermilk, miso and tempeh.

When the balance of intestinal bacteria is disrupted and harmful bacteria start to outnumber beneficial bacteria, a condition known as dysbiosis can occur. Symptoms of dysbiosis include gastrointestinal symptoms such as flatulence, bloating, diarrhoea or constipation, and reflux. Dysbiosis may predispose children to infections, allergies, inflammatory conditions, and behavioural and learning disorders. The gastrointestinal tract plays a major role in the development and functioning of your child's immune system.

There is strong scientific evidence demonstrating yoghurt's ability to enhance and promote healthy immune function.[1,2] Researchers attribute yoghurt's health-promoting effects to the live bacteria present in yoghurt. Caution must be taken however when purchasing yoghurt, as not all yoghurt contains live bacteria. In heat-treated yoghurts, the live and active bacteria have been killed off during the heating process. Other products that don't contain live and active bacteria include yoghurt-covered confectionery, muesli bars and yoghurt salad dressings. Make sure you are getting the most out of yoghurt. Look for the 'live & active cultures' or 'live & active bacteria' seal on the yoghurt you buy.

The best way to include immune-boosting yoghurt in your child's diet is served on breakfast cereal, mixed into porridge or Bircher-style muesli, as a topping on pancakes and muffins, and in home made salad dressings, dips and smoothies. Include other fermented foods by adding a small amount of miso paste to stir-fries and soups (make sure you add it at the end of cooking). Add tempeh to salads and stir-fries and for a lovely tangy flavour add low-fat buttermilk to mashed potato.

Chapter 6:
Building healthy bones
for a lifetime

Unfortunately, bone health is rarely thought of until later in life, when it can be too late. During our growing years, while we are young, we accumulate bone mass. Skeletal growth increases dramatically during childhood and adolescence with about 90% of bone laid down by 17.[1,2] Bone mass development usually reaches its peak around age 20. Another 10% can be added up to the age of 30 [3,4], with a slow and steady decline each year thereafter. This is why it's imperative that bone health is addressed in childhood. Increasing your child's bone mass to peak capacity at an early age provides them with a lifetime of skeletal health and reduces their risk of developing bone diseases such as osteoporosis and fractures later in life.

Bone is made of calcium and other minerals such as magnesium and phosphorus. The structural framework of bone is made up of collagen protein. Bone is a living tissue that is constantly being broken down and built up again. It's part of the normal aging process to gradually lose bone mineral content as we get older. Osteoblasts are bone cells that lay down new bone and osteoclasts are bone cells that break down bone. During childhood and adolescence, osteoblastic activity is greater and therefore more bone is built. During adulthood however, osteoclastic activity increases, resulting in more bone being lost.

Osteoporosis

It's vital that a strong bone foundation is laid in childhood and adolescence to prevent osteoporosis and fractures later in life. Early dietary and lifestyle habits have a huge effect on bone health in later years, to the point where osteoporosis is considered a pediatric disease with geriatric consequences.

Osteoporosis, a disease that affects about 10% of the Australian population, is a condition where bones become fragile and brittle, making bones more susceptible to fracture.[5] Osteoporosis occurs when there is a loss of mineral content from bone,

mainly in the form of calcium as well as architectural loss of normal bone structure. Among children and teens we are already seeing an increase in bone fractures and a rise in rickets (a bone disease related to vitamin D deficiency).[6]

Calcium for strong bones

Calcium is the most abundant mineral in the body and one of the most important minerals for bone health. With 99% of calcium being stored in bones, calcium's primary function in the body is the building up and maintaining of bone. Through childhood and into our teens, skeletal growth is dramatic and there is a need for a continuous supply of calcium in the diet to obtain peak bone density.

It has been estimated that children need two to four times (per body weight) as much calcium as adults.[7] Recent research shows that including a supplement with calcium during times of rapid growth in girls age 8 to 13 for seven years increased their bone mass. This might help prevent osteoporosis later in life. Because 37% of bone mass accumulates during the pre-adolescence growth spurt, this might represent the highest need for calcium during a person's life.[8,9]

An Australian survey found that about 20% of children in year 1, 50% in year 5, and more than half in year 10 have inadequate calcium in their diets.[10] Diets inadequate in calcium were more common in girls than boys. Calcium deficiency in children can lead to rickets, which results in bone deformities and growth retardation.

The primary food source of calcium is dairy products such as milk, cheese and yoghurt. Other food sources rich in calcium include almonds, sesame and sunflower seeds, canned salmon (with bones), legumes, green leafy vegetables (kale, spinach, bok choy, turnip greens, mustard greens, dandelion greens), parsley, broccoli, kelp and carob. Children's growing dependence on junk foods and soft drinks has contributed to the increase in bone related diseases such as osteoporosis. Excessive sugars in the diet can interfere with the absorption of calcium, leading to a greater risk of bone loss and increased risk of osteoporosis.[11-13] Children's bone health can also be affected by regular caffeine consumption. Caffeine is readily found in soft drinks, energy drinks, coffee, tea and chocolate. Caffeine increases calcium excretion from the body and decreases calcium absorption, leading to weakened bones and increased risk of osteoporosis.[14,15]

Other vital nutrients for bone health

The body needs not only calcium, but many other vitamins and minerals to lay down quality bone.

Providing your children with all the key elements for good bone health during childhood and adolescence is extremely important for preventing bone disease later in life. Other essential nutrients required for strong healthy bones include vitamin D, C and A, magnesium and phosphorus.

VITAMIN D also known as the 'sunshine vitamin', is produced when the skin is exposed to sunlight. Vitamin D is needed for the proper absorption of calcium and phosphorus. This vitamin is crucial for building strong, healthy bones in childhood.

Recently, there has been some concern that children are not getting enough vitamin D through sun exposure, because of our extensive use of sunscreens. Sunscreens with a sun protection factor (SPF) of 15 reduces the capacity of the skin to produce vitamin D by about 98%. Wearing sunscreen is extremely important to help prevent skin cancer and other problems associated with excessive sun exposure. However, minimal sun exposure (without sunscreen), only about 10-15 minutes a day, on the face, arms, hands or feet before and after the hottest part of the day, is important for sufficient vitamin D production. Studies have found that the prevalence of vitamin D deficiency in Australian children appears much higher than previously thought.[16] Vitamin D deficiency is associated with high bone turnover, reduced bone density and is an important risk factor in the development of osteoporosis and fractures in adulthood.[17]

Vitamin D deficiency in childhood is associated with a type of bone disease called rickets. Until recently the incidence of rickets in Australia was not common.[18] Due to reduced sun exposure and children's diets lacking in vitamin D we are now seeing an emergence of this type of bone disease. Rickets is characterised by an inability to calcify bone, resulting in softening of the skull bones, bowing of legs, spinal curvature and increased joint size.

Good food sources of vitamin D (which should be included in children's diets) are dairy products (fortified with vitamin D), cod liver oil, cold-water fish (salmon, tuna, herring, sardines, mackerel), egg yolks and vitamin D fortified almond and rice milks.

PHOSPHORUS AND CALCIUM are two nutrients that work together to build healthy, strong bones. Both calcium and phosphorus are needed to support an increased bone mass. Phosphorus makes up more than half the mass of bone mineral. Therefore, the diet needs to have sufficient phosphorus in order to have healthy bones. Bone diseases, such as osteoporosis, can develop when calcium and phosphorus are not balanced in the body and in adequate supply.

High and low levels of phosphorus can cause problems with regard to bone health. Too much phosphorus in the body can leech calcium from the bones, which can result in bones becoming brittle. High consumption of phosphoric acid in the diet, through the consumption of cola beverages in particular, has been associated with bone fractures.[19,20] The increase in soft drink consumption has been thought to be a contributing factor in the growing number of people developing osteoporosis.

Good sources of phosphorus include milk and dairy products such as cheese and yoghurt, which are also excellent sources of calcium and vitamin D. Other sources of phosphorus include corn, dried beans, nuts, oatmeal, spinach, sardines and sweet potato.

MAGNESIUM is one of the most important nutrients linked to bone strength. It assists in the delivery and laying down of calcium in the bones. Latest studies reveal that balanced amounts of dietary calcium and magnesium in the diet result in a better accumulation and maintenance of bone density, when compared to a diet emphasising calcium alone.[21,22] Osteoporosis is not always a problem of insufficient calcium intake but incorrect calcium utilisation. Magnesium is needed for the correct utilisation of calcium in the body.[23]

If you are deficient in magnesium, calcium will not be correctly deposited into bone and instead will deposit in soft tissue, causing kidney stones and gallstones, joint discomfort and other calcification problems, as well as increased atherosclerotic plaque.[24] When magnesium is deficient, abnormally shaped bones are formed that appear dense but are weak and break easily.

The best food sources of magnesium include vegetables (especially green leafy vegetables), wholegrains, legumes, nuts and seeds, and fruits. Always choose wholegrain since 80% of magnesium is lost when wholegrains are refined into white flour.

VITAMIN A is needed for the healthy growth and development of bones. Vitamin A assists in protein synthesis and the maturation of bone cells.

The best food sources of vitamin A are whole milk and fortified low-fat and skim milk, while the best sources of beta-carotene (pro-vitamin A) are dark green leafy vegetables (collards and spinach), yellow and orange vegetables (carrots, sweet potatoes and squash) and orange coloured fruits (mangoes and apricots).

VITAMIN C plays an important role in bone health as it is needed for the forming of collagen in bones.

The best food sources of vitamin C are citrus fruits (orange, lemon, lime, grapefruit and tangerine) and vegetables such as broccoli, capsicums, potatoes and brussel sprouts.

Exercise for bone health

Exercise is not only vital for children to stay a healthy weight and for overall health, but also for growing strong healthy bones. Physical inactivity during growth in childhood and adolescence has been identified as a risk factor for osteoporosis.

Regular exercise and weight bearing activities can slow bone mineral loss and maintain a healthy bone mass.[25] Children who exercise regularly significantly increase their bone density and bone strength and therefore reduce the risk of developing osteoporosis. The more weight-bearing exercise children do, the stronger their bones will get. The best types of bone building exercises include walking, running, dancing, tennis, gymnastics, soccer, frisbee, skipping rope and basketball.

It is possible to have a healthy diet without consuming foods derived from animal sources. However, children have special nutritional requirements so care is needed when planning a nutritionally balanced, vegetarian diet. If well planned, a vegetarian diet can provide your child with all the nutrients they need to grow up healthy. When certain foods are excluded, ensure that you're adding lots of equally nutritious foods back in to your child's diet. Childhood is such a critical period of body building, so much so that if your child's diet is lacking in certain nutrients, it can affect their health for the rest of their lives. Parents must be aware of the nutritional value of different foods to ensure that their child is not missing out on vital nutrients needed for healthy growth and development.

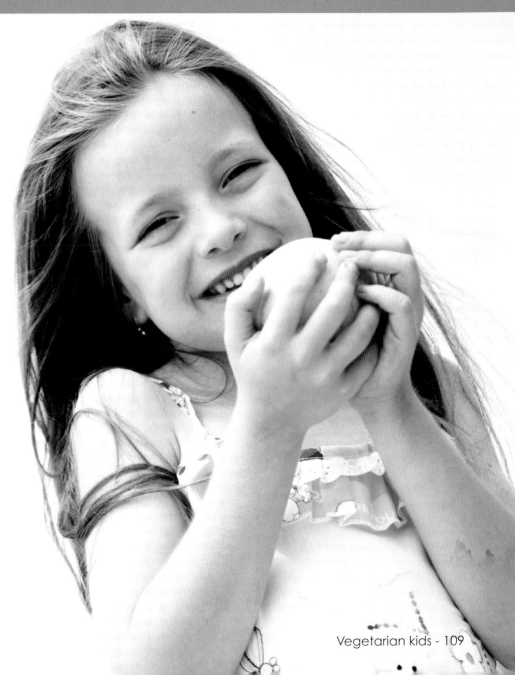

A vegetarian diet that is adequate for adults is not necessarily suitable for children. It might be helpful to see a nutritionist that specialises in vegetarian diets for children, especially if your child is on a very restrictive vegetarian diet. A children's multi-vitamin is also recommended for vegetarian children (especially vegans), along with a well balanced diet, to ensure they are getting adequate levels of all the macro and micro nutrients they need to flourish.

Different types of vegetarians

Vegetarians are people who consume mainly plant foods, including vegetables, fruit, legumes, grains, seeds and nuts. However, there are actually many different types of vegetarians, whose diets can differ greatly. Vegetarian diets can be classified into two major groups - lacto-ovo vegetarians and vegans. The nutritional differences between these two diets are of great importance when it comes to vegetarian children.

Lacto-ovo vegetarians avoid all animal flesh, including meat, poultry and fish. They still include dairy (lacto) and egg (ovo) products as part of their diet. Many vegetarians avoid cheese made from animal-based rennet, but can eat vegetarian cheeses which are made using rennet produced by the fermentation of a fungus. This type of vegetarian diet, if planned properly, provides adequate nutrition and will satisfy children's nutrient requirements.

Vegans avoid all foods of animal origin, including meat, poultry, fish, eggs, dairy, gelatin and honey. Vegans can eat a vegetable-based substitute cheese which is usually soy based. This diet is not advisable for children as great care must be taken to ensure an adequate intake of protein, energy, and vitamins and minerals, such as vitamin B_{12} and iron.

The optimum vegetarian diet for kids should include a variety of foods such as eggs, dairy products (milk, cheese and yoghurt), legumes (hummus, beans, peas and lentils), nuts and seeds (including nut spreads and tahini), fruits and vegetables, and wholegrain cereals (bread, pasta, noodles and breakfast cereals). Vegetarian kids will particularly benefit from an organic diet, as organic produce generally has a higher nutrient content.

Problems with vegetarian diets

If not planned carefully, vegetarian diets can lead to nutritional deficiencies and health problems in children. The main problems associated with extreme vegetarian diets, such as vegan diets, is children not getting enough energy and protein from foods such as fruits, vegetables, and cereals. Children become full very easily on these high fibre foods before their nutrient needs can be met. These children will risk stunted growth, low weight for height, muscle wastage, anaemia and fatigue. You must make sure your child is gaining weight, developing normally and is active with lots of energy.

Health benefits of a vegetarian diet

Vegetarian diets can provide several health benefits, including a lower incidence of several chronic diseases. Some vegetarian communities have been shown to have health advantages over the general population, notably the cardiovascular area, with reductions in risk factors such as high cholesterol and high blood pressure.[1-6]

Vegetarian diets tend to be lower in total and saturated fat, dietary cholesterol, and higher in fibre and polyunsaturated fats, which promotes good bowel health and helps lower LDL 'bad' cholesterol levels. Studies have found that vegetarians have lower rates of certain types of cancers, possibly due to vegetarians consuming more antioxidants, lower fat consumption, and increased fibre.[7] Vegetarians are also less likely to suffer from obesity and type-2 diabetes.

Planning a vegetarian diet

Important nutritional aspects must be addressed when planning a vegetarian diet for your child. There are several micronutrients for which meat, fish, and poultry are the most bioavailable source. Care needs to be taken if these foods are excluded from your child's diet. These micronutrients are vitamins B_{12} and D, and minerals iron, zinc and calcium. Protein quality and essential amino acid profile of vegetarian protein sources is also a concern with regards to vegetarian diets.

Vegetarians and protein

Proteins are made from amino acids, which are important body builders necessary for sustaining growth. When protein foods are consumed, the body breaks them down into amino acids, which are then used to make proteins in the body for muscles, bones, skin, hair, nails, and antibodies, to name a few.

There are 23 amino acids, 15 of them non-essential, which means they can be made by the body. There are eight essential amino acids that cannot be made by the body, so they must be obtained from the diet. Whenever a protein is made in the body, for example when a muscle needs to be repaired, the body needs a variety of amino acids (essential and non-essential) for the protein making process. If there is a shortage of an essential amino acid, which is common in low protein diets, the building of proteins in the body stops and the body suffers.

For non-vegetarians this is not a concern, since meat, fish, poultry, cheese, eggs and milk are 'complete' proteins, which contain all eight essential amino acids. On the other hand, plant proteins are called 'incomplete' proteins, because they are missing one or more essential amino acids. These plant proteins are found in a variety of foods, including wholegrain cereals, legumes (peas, lentils and beans), hummus, oven baked falafels, nuts and seeds (tahini and nut butters), and to a lesser extent green leafy vegetables.

All soybean products (tofu, tempeh, milk and yoghurt) are protein sources, however there has been some questions raised recently in regards to the safety of children consuming soy foods. Soybeans and soy products contain chemicals called isoflavones that exert a weak oestrogenic effect on the body. There are concerns that these isoflavones could potentially have a negative effect on children's growth and development if eaten to excess. Organic soy products can still be enjoyed by children, in moderation, as part of a well-balanced diet. Soy foods can often dominate the diet of vegetarians so be mindful not to over do them in your child's diet.

Lactose-free milk and protein enriched rice milks are also now available for people who are unable to drink cow's milk.

Protein complementation

Many vegetarian diet issues relating to insufficient amino acid intake can be overcome by protein complementation. Protein complementation refers to the combining of plant protein sources to achieve a better amino acid balance. Because of differences in amino acid levels in foods, when plant sources are combined, an essential amino acid that is low in one food can be made up by consuming another food that contains an excess of that amino acid. For example, many grains are notoriously low in lysine, but legumes are high in lysine. On the other hand, legumes are low in the sulphur-containing amino acids, while grains like wheat contain good levels. Therefore, by eating legumes and grains together, the strengths of one make up for the deficiencies of the other, making a source of complete protein that is a high-quality substitute for meat, fish or chicken. Complementary vegetarian protein foods do not have to be eaten in the same meal to get a complementary effect, as long as they're consumed within a few hours or even within the same day.

The following table shows foods that complement each other

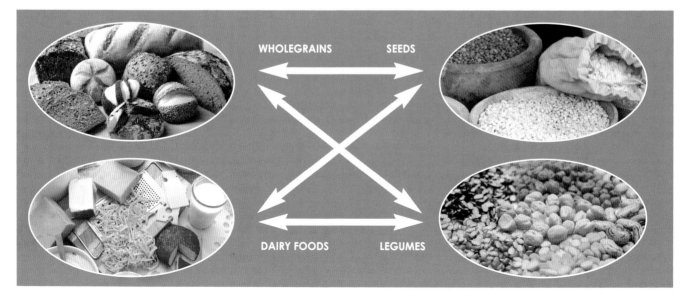

WHOLEGRAINS   SEEDS

DAIRY FOODS   LEGUMES

Lacto-ovo vegetarians who consume dairy foods and eggs regularly, along with plant protein sources should receive adequate amounts of essential amino acids in their diets. Protein combining is important for vegans.

Using almond butters and tahini is a good way of adding extra protein and essential fatty acids (EFAs) to your child's diet. Spread it on sandwiches, toast, muffins, pancakes and biscuits. Sprinkle LSA (ground linseed, sunflower and almond) or raw and unsalted nuts and seeds on their cereal, yoghurt, fruit salad, stir-fries, vegetables, rice dishes or salads.

Legumes are extremely versatile - add them to stir-fries, rice dishes, or salads (with nuts and seeds); make hummus (with tahini); add them to soup served with a wholegrain bread roll.

Vegetarians and vitamin B$_{12}$

Vitamin B$_{12}$ is essential for red blood cell production and for cell growth and metabolism. It also plays an important role in maintaining the nervous system. Vitamin B$_{12}$ helps in nerve conduction by maintaining the protective myelin sheath that surrounds nerve fibres.

Since B$_{12}$ can only be found in animal products, vegans must be particularly concerned with this vitamin. Lacto-ovo vegetarians should receive adequate vitamin B$_{12}$ from milk and eggs. Vegans however, will need to consume reliable food sources of vitamin B$_{12}$, such as fortified commercial cereal products or nutritional yeasts. It is recommended that vegetarians also regularly consume B$_{12}$-fortified food products.[8] Alternatively, children's multivitamins generally contain enough vitamin B$_{12}$ to avoid deficiency.

Vegetarians and calcium

Getting enough dietary calcium is especially important for children to maximize bone mass during growth and to minimize the bone loss that occurs later on in life. Dairy products such as milk, yoghurt and cheese contain the best levels of readily absorbable calcium. Calcium deficiency is generally not a concern for lacto-vegetarians who consume adequate amounts of these foods. However, children who follow a vegan diet can have problems getting adequate calcium.

Although it can be more of a challenge to get the recommended amounts of calcium from a vegan diet, good sources of calcium include dark green leafy vegetables, broccoli, sweet potato, chickpeas, navy beans, and calcium-fortified products, including orange juice, organic soy milk and almond or rice drinks. While these plant foods contain good levels of calcium they often have low absorption rates.

Vegetarians and zinc

Zinc is a particularly important mineral for children as it is involved in the healthy functioning of every cell. Zinc plays a vital role in growth and development and immune function.

Zinc is found in a wide variety of foods. The best vegetarian sources of zinc are milk and other dairy foods (cheese) and eggs. Lacto-ovo vegetarians should get enough zinc through these foods. Zinc is also found in moderate amounts in brewers yeast, legumes (beans, lentils and peas), wholegrains (including bread), sunflower seeds, pumpkin seeds, pecans and a lesser amount found in vegetables. Some foods are also fortified with zinc such as breakfast cereals and breads, which can make an important contribution to your vegetarian child's zinc intake.

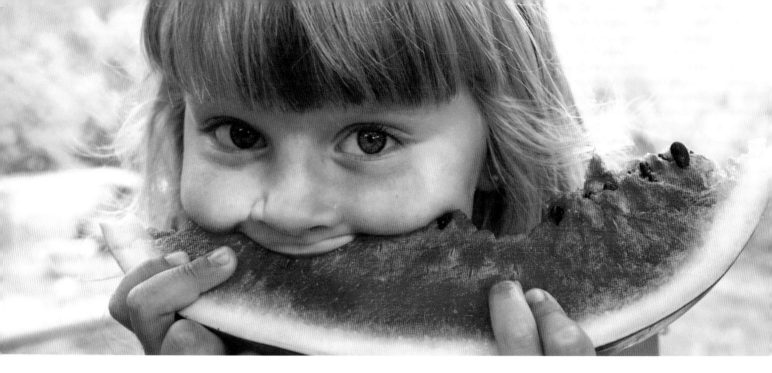

Vegetarians and vitamin D

Vitamin D helps keep children's bones and teeth strong and healthy, as it is responsible for laying down calcium in bones. Vitamin D is also involved in the healthy functioning of a range of body systems including the brain and nervous system, muscles, reproductive organs and some immune system cells.

Vitamin D is present in fortified milk, egg yolks, and fish. If your child is following a vegan diet they might not be getting adequate amounts of vitamin D, so make sure you include vitamin D fortified almond and rice milks in their diet. The body also makes vitamin D when exposed to sunlight, so make sure your child gets their daily dose of sunshine each day.

Vegetarians and iron

Iron is an important mineral for your child's growth and development, for strong muscles and healthy immune function. Iron, essential for red blood cell production, is found in haemoglobin, the component of red blood cells that carries oxygen to different parts of the body.

The absorption of iron from animal based iron sources such as meat, chicken, fish and eggs, is much higher than that of plant based iron sources such as wholegrain breads and cereals, wheatgerm, legumes, nuts and seeds (nut butters, tahini), green leafy vegetables and dried fruits. A wide range of iron-fortified food products, including breakfast cereals and breads are now available and should be used to increase your child's iron intake.

Vegetarian children must regularly consume a wide range of plant based iron sources to receive adequate iron intake. The addition of foods rich in vitamin C to a meal can greatly increase iron absorption from that meal. Ways of including vitamin C rich foods with your meal include having a small orange juice with a meal; adding tomatoes or tomato sauce to wholegrain cereals (pasta or rice) and green leafy vegetables; add fruit to breakfast cereals (oats); baked beans on wholegrain bread; or adding vitamin C rich vegetables to dishes.

Chapter 8:
Kids with food
Allergies & intolerances

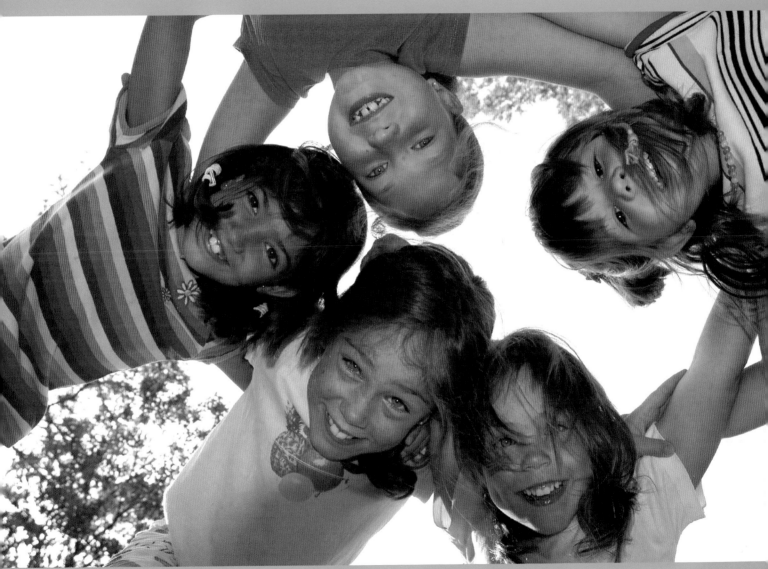

One of the most worrying aspects for parents in regards to feeding their children is when their child is allergic or intolerant to certain foods. Food allergies differ from food intolerances, as food allergies involve an immune response.

Food allergies

There has been a dramatic increase in the incidence of food allergies in children. The number of Australian children with food allergies has doubled in a single generation, with 10% of children currently having some kind of food allergy.

There have been relatively few studies into food allergies in Australia, despite the increasing prevalence and increasing burden this serious condition presents for parents and teachers. Many food allergies are potentially life threatening, in particular peanut allergy. Even a small trace of peanut is enough to trigger symptoms and require medical treatment in peanut-sensitive children.

There are many types of food allergies prevalent in children; the most common are allergies to milk, eggs and peanuts.

Children under the age of three are most likely to develop food sensitivities, probably because their immune systems are not yet able to tolerate a wide range of new substances. Children with a family history of food allergies should not be given these foods or products containing them, until the age of three.

When you're allergic to certain foods, your body thinks they're harmful. The body's immune system is supposed to help fight off intrusion from infectious substances that enter the body, such as a virus or bacteria. But sometimes, as in the case of food allergies, your body's immune system identifies certain food proteins as harmful invaders.

For example, when a child with a milk allergy consumes milk or products containing milk, the immune system responds by creating specific antibodies to that food, which are designed to fight off the 'invader'. These antibodies, called immunoglobulin E (IgE), trigger the release of an army of chemicals, one of which is histamine, to protect the body. The release of these chemicals can cause reactions in the body, affecting the respiratory system, gastrointestinal tract, skin and cardiovascular system. Common symptoms include skin rashes, hives, eczema, nausea, vomiting, stomach cramps, diarrhoea, runny nose, nasal congestion, difficulty breathing and wheezing.

Most children with food allergies will experience some of these reactions, but a few might have a very strong reaction called anaphylaxis. This severe allergic reaction causes swelling of the mouth, throat and airways, resulting in difficulty breathing and a dangerous drop in blood pressure, which can make a child dizzy and pass out, and can quickly lead to shock. Peanut allergies are commonly associated with anaphylaxis, although it can happen with other food allergies.

If you suspect your child might have a food allergy it is recommended having tests done to detect any offending foods, which should be taken out of their diet. When removing several important nutritious foods from your child's diet such as milk, wheat, or eggs, care must be taken to replace these foods with equally nutritious substitutes. A naturopath, nutritionist or dietician will be able to help you plan a suitable diet for your child, to make sure they are not missing out on essential nutrients needed for their growth and development.

Managing children's food allergies
(avoidance, awareness, preparedness & education)

AVOIDANCE: Children should completely avoid foods that they are allergic to. This means not eating or coming in contact with anything that has even minute traces of the food. Allergenic foods can leave residue on utensils and containers, so caution also must be taken to carefully clean cooking and serving utensils to ensure they don't have traces of foods your child could react to.

For someone with a food allergy, even a pinch can be too much, so read food labels carefully. For example, even if a peanut-free product is run on the same line as a peanut containing product, you may get trace amounts of peanut in the peanut-free product due to cross-contamination. So, when in doubt, don't use the product or phone up the company and ask. In cases of severe allergies, avoiding those products altogether is the safest option.

In Australia it is mandatory for foods or food ingredients that can cause severe adverse reactions in some individuals, to be declared on the label, however small the amount.

AWARENESS & PREPAREDNESS: It is important to inform school teachers, your child's friends and their parents, and other caregivers of your child's food allergy. Inform them of the potential dangers involved and what to do in case of an allergic attack. If your child is going to a birthday party or sleep over, always inform the parents of your child's allergy, and make up a plate of food for your child to take and share with the other kids. You don't want your child feeling left out or different because of their allergy, so always be prepared and have something on hand for them to take. When eating out, inform café or restaurant staff of your child's allergy.

EDUCATION: Parents should educate their children about foods they should avoid. Parents should teach their allergic child to ask about foods they are offered and, if possible, have an adult read the ingredients label.

Kids with milk allergies

Cow's milk is the most common cause of food allergy (and food intolerance) in children. Unlike milk intolerance, which is usually a reaction to the sugar lactose, milk allergies are usually reactions to the proteins found in milk.

Cow's milk is a common cause of food allergy in infants. In Australia 1 in 50 babies are allergic to cow's milk and dairy products. Although a lot of children out-grow cow's milk allergy by the age of 4, it can persist into later childhood. If your child hasn't grown out of it by then, they will probably be sensitive to cow's milk for life. True cow's milk allergy affects 2-5% of children.

Milk has several components, these include lactose (milk sugar), fats and up to four varieties of casein and other milk proteins. Casein should not be confused with lactose. Most people who have difficulty digesting milk are lactose intolerant, which is not life threatening. However, a casein allergy can manifest as breathing difficulty, hives,

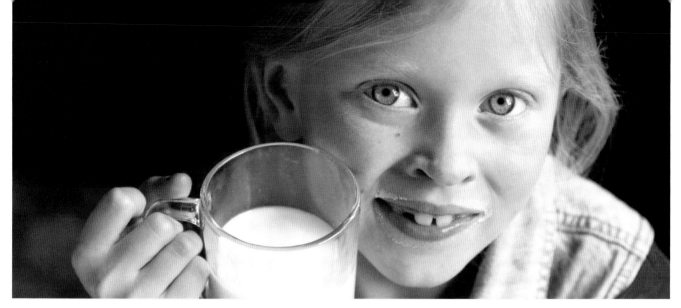

rashes, serious stomach pain and reduced ability to breakdown and absorb nutrients properly from foods, which can result in dangerous weight loss. Some children might even experience anaphylaxis.

It is very important to make sure your child avoids milk and all foods containing milk proteins. You should carefully read ingredient panels of all processed foods. You will be amazed at the number of foods that contain milk products. Obvious forms of milk to avoid are cheese, cream, butter, ice cream and yoghurts. Milk proteins can also be hidden in foods, listed as something other than milk, such as whey, curds, casein, caseinates, hydrolysates, lactose, lactalbumin, lactoglobulin or milk solids.

The words 'non-dairy' on a product label indicates it does not contain butter, cream or milk. However, this does not necessarily indicate it does not have other milk-containing ingredients, so care must still be taken with these products. The Kosher food labelled 'pareve' or 'parve' almost always indicates that the food is free of milk and milk products. A 'D' on a product label next to the circled K or U indicates the presence of milk protein and should be avoided.

Milk and dairy products are important sources of protein, calcium and vitamin D for children.

Therefore, if these foods are removed from your child's diet you will have to replace them with foods equally rich in these nutrients so your child doesn't develop nutritional deficiencies.

When choosing an alternative to cow's milk you must consider the health benefits and nutritional balance of the milk. Soy, rice and almond milks do not contain the calcium content of cow's milk so calcium fortified varieties are recommended. Rice milk is not normally a good source of protein, however protein enriched varieties are now available. Vitamin D fortified soy, rice and almond milks are also available.

There is a wide selection of non-dairy frozen desserts (ice cream, sorbets, ice blocks) and puddings available from supermarkets (these products can contain a lot of sugar so should be eaten only occasionally).

All the recipes in this book can be made without milk or milk products. Make your child delicious homemade cakes, muffins and cookies using olive oil and almond or rice milk. Make your own milk-free sauces, dressings, quiches, ice cream and desserts all using almond, soy milk, rice milk and vegan cheeses. Buy dairy-free breads or make your own. Bread machines are a great investment.

Foods that contain milk and milk products that should be avoided

• All milks (buttermilk, evaporated, condensed, powdered, lactose-free), yoghurt, cream, all cheeses, custard, ice cream, butter and margarine.

• Commercially baked goods such as breads, cakes, muffins, pancakes, doughnuts, biscuits, crackers, quiches and pastries (brushed with milk).

• Puddings, junket, milk-based desserts and custard powder.

• Some soy cheeses.

• Confectionery made with milk such as chocolate, fudge, caramels, nougat, sherbet and yoghurt topped muesli bars.

• Processed meats, including hot dogs, sausages and luncheon meats, frequently contain milk or are processed on milk containing lines.

• Malts and all beverages made with milk or milk products.

• High protein cereals (often 'high protein' or 'protein enriched' products have added milk protein).

• Some chewing gums. Recaldent is an ingredient found in some chewing gums which is milk-derived.

• Very sensitive people may react to hydrolyzed vegetable protein (HVP) since the processing phase may utilize casein.

• Salad dressing or mayonnaise containing milk, milk solids or milk products.

• Breaded meats, meatloaf, croquettes and hamburgers (unless made without milk).

• Frozen fries sprayed with lactose.

• Bisques, chowders, creamed soups, some chicken broth or bouillon can contain milk solids.

• Some canned tuna contain 'hydrolized caseinate'. However, the low sodium ones in spring water are generally milk free.

• Chocolates and carob. Even dark chocolate is often run on the same production line as milk chocolate, so the risk of cross-contamination is high if your chocolate bar comes from the beginning of the run. You might want to check out soy based or kosher pareve chocolates.

• Vinegar flavored potato crisps. The vinegar may actually be a milk-derived ingredient.

• Cheese flavoured snacks.

Kids with egg allergies

There are many different types of proteins in eggs, primarily in the whites, to which children may be allergic. Cooking can break down some of the proteins, although not all the proteins are broken down and can still cause an allergic reaction. Egg allergy usually first appears when kids are very young and most outgrow it by the time they're five years-old.

Eggs are a great source of many nutrients including protein, fat, and vitamin B2 and B12. When you take eggs out of your child's diet you have to replace them with foods equally as rich in these nutrients.

Children with egg allergies must avoid eating eggs and products made with eggs.

Products that contain egg and should be avoided

• Commercially baked goods (cakes, muffins, biscuits, pastries, pancakes, waffles, doughnuts and desserts).

• Commercial breads and bread products made with egg or brushed with egg (glazing), bread crumbs and foods containing them (meat balls, stuffed chickens, sausage rolls, meat and vegetable patties) and some sausages.

• Sauces and salad dressings such as mayonnaise.

• Pretzels.

• Quiches, soufflés.

• Egg noodles.

• Sherbet, creamy centre of chocolates, marshmallows and icing.

• Puddings, custard and ice cream.

• Baking powder containing egg white or egg albumin.

Most of these products can be made at home without eggs. Health food stores and supermarkets sell 'egg replacer' products. These products contain no egg protein and can be eaten by people with egg allergies and used in recipes in place of eggs. Make sure you buy egg-free baking powder to bake with.

Check ingredient labels carefully for any presence of egg. Sometimes they can be hard to detect. Avoid any products that list any of the following: egg, egg white, egg yolk, dried egg, egg powder, egg solids, egg substitutes, albumin, baking powder, globulin, mayonnaise, ovalbumin, ovomucin, ovovitellin, livetin, ovoglobulin, vitellin, meringue or ovomucoid.

Kids with peanut allergies

Of all the food allergies, peanut allergy is one of the most dangerous and the leading cause of anaphylactic reactions. Unlike milk and egg allergies, children tend not to grow out of peanut allergies.

Peanuts are a cheap source of dietary protein, predominantly ingested as peanut butter, but one of the world's most allergenic foods. Peanuts are, unfortunately, progressively finding their way into more and more food products, either directly, or by indirect contamination of food products during the manufacturing process. You might have noticed some foods that have a label indicating 'may include peanuts' or 'processed in a plant containing peanuts'.

Children with peanut allergies are not necessarily allergic to all nuts and might be able to eat other nuts such as walnuts, almonds and cashews. However, it is safer to avoid nuts altogether as they may have been contaminated by traces of peanuts.

It is important to realise that for the sensitive person, this is a lifelong allergy, and that even trace amounts can be detrimental. An accidental casual contact with peanuts, or even inhaling small amounts of peanut particles, can cause a severe allergic reaction and even death for those who suffer from this condition. Read product labels of all foods and avoid obvious sources of peanut protein, such as peanut butter and peanut flour. Foods that contain peanuts or peanut products might be labelled using words like peanut extracts, ground nuts, mixed nuts, hydrolyzed vegetable protein (HVP), or natural flavouring. Be especially aware of packaged and processed foods because they might contain hidden peanuts. Most schools have a 'no nut policy' due to the fear of triggering an anaphylactic reaction in pupils with nut allergies.

Foods that contain peanuts that must be avoided

• Avoid any product that says NUTS (ground or crushed nuts, peanut butter and nut flour).

• Peanut oils should also be avoided, even though they are theoretically free from peanut protein, they still might contain traces. Thai and Chinese cooking often uses peanut oils, so it would be wise to avoid these restaurants.

• Some individuals also must avoid other foods in the legume family to which nuts belong eg. soya bean, pea, and garbanzo (chickpea), if an allergy to these has been previously demonstrated.

• Chocolate bars and commercially baked products (muffins, cakes and pastries) and ice creams can easily be contaminated.

• Peanut butter can sometimes be used in chilli, or for thickening frosting for cakes or cupcakes.

• Hydrolyzed plant or vegetable protein will probably be marked if it is made from peanuts.

• Peanuts can also be found in some commercially made cereals, ice cream, dips, curry pastes and pasta sauces.

Food intolerances

Food intolerances differ from food allergies as they do not involve an immune response. Food intolerances are more common than food allergies. Two common food intolerances among children are lactose intolerance and gluten intolerance.

Rather than thinking about all the foods your child can't have, focus on all the nutritious foods they can have. This will make you experiment with different foods such as gluten-free grains like quinoa and millet. These days, due to the increasing number of food intolerances, food companies have developed increasing ranges of gluten-free and lactose-free products. Following these types of diets has become a lot easier.

If you suspect your child has an intolerance to a certain food, try keeping a food diary. Record everything your child consumes for a couple of weeks. Include any symptoms your child experiences, such as digestive complaints (bloating, flatulence, constipation and diarrhoea), stomach cramps, headaches or skin rashes. After a couple of weeks remove the food you think might be causing problems, making sure you replace it with an equally nutritious alternative. If your child's symptoms improve after removing the suspected food, your child probably has an intolerance to that food.

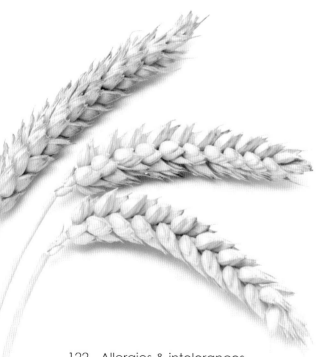

Kids with gluten intolerance (Coeliac disease)

Coeliac disease is characterized by a hypersensitive reaction to gluten, which results in damage to the small intestine. This damage interferes with the body's ability to absorb nutrients. Gluten is a protein found in wheat, rye, barleyand oats. Gluten causes leavening and gives elasticity to baked goods such as breads, cakes and muffins.

The small intestine is lined with tiny fingerlike protrusions called villi. Nutrients from food are absorbed into the bloodstream through these villi. Without them a child will become malnourished resulting in weight loss and deficiencies in vitamins and minerals. When a child with this disease eats food containing gluten, the villi lining their small intestine become damaged and flattened and less able to absorb nutrients. This causes the child to become susceptible to a variety of other conditions related to malabsorption. Malnutrition is a serious problem for anyone, particularly for children, because they need adequate nutrition to grow and develop properly.

The symptoms can vary with each individual, ranging from no symptoms at all to quite severe. The classical symptoms of children with gluten intolerance is poor weight gain and delayed growth, chronic diarrhoea, behavioural changes, irritability, flatulence, abdominal distention, buttocks thin and wasted, tiredness, pallor and large offensive smelling stools. Other symptoms include: abdominal pain, anaemia, bone or joint pain, muscle cramps and mouth ulcers.

A gluten-free diet is essential for children with gluten intolerance. If left untreated they could become malnourished and develop complications associated with nutrient malabsorption. Due to decreased iron, folate and vitamin B_{12} absorption, children with untreated coeliac disease can develop anaemia (low red blood cell count). A damaged small intestine might not absorb fat and fat soluble vitamins (A, D, E and K), zinc or protein properly, resulting in weight loss and impaired growth in children. Due to decreased calcium absorption, children with this disease have an increased risk of osteoporosis (weak, brittle bones due to poor calcium absorption) and certain cancers that can develop in the intestine. Short stature results when childhood coeliac disease prevents nutrient absorption during the years when nutrition is critical to a child's normal growth and development.

The only treatment for children with coeliac disease is a strict adherence to a gluten-free diet, avoiding all foods containing gluten. The gluten-free diet is a lifetime requirement. Eating any gluten, no matter how small an amount, can damage the intestine. An adherence to a gluten-free diet however, can prevent almost all complications caused by the disease, heal existing intestinal damage and prevent any further damage.

The villi of a child recovers quite rapidly, with improvements seen within days or weeks of starting the diet, whereas adults can take a couple of years to fully recover. By establishing good dietary habits and strictly adhering to a gluten-free diet early on in childhood, a pattern will be set and should continue with ease into adulthood.

Coeliac disease is genetic but might not manifest itself in all generations. If a parent has coeliac disease there is a 1 in 10 chance that their child will also develop gluten intolerance. As a parent it is good to be aware that some children born with a tendency to develop coeliac disease might not develop symptoms until later in life, although damage to the small intestine might already be taking place.

Be aware that lactose intolerance is also common in people with undiagnosed or newly diagnosed coeliac disease. This is because their damaged gut lining is unable to break down lactose (sugar in cow's milk), which leads to symptoms such as abdominal bloating and pain after dairy products are consumed. Initially your child may also have to follow a lactose-free diet too, making sure they include plenty of calcium and protein rich foods in place of dairy foods.

There is a difference between being gluten intolerant and intolerant to wheat. People with wheat intolerance only have to avoid wheat and any product containing wheat. This is less restrictive than a gluten-free diet where you have to avoid wheat and any other grains containing gluten.

"Rather than thinking about all the foods your child can't have, focus on all the nutritious foods they can have."

GLUTEN-FREE DIET

AVOID
all foods that contain
WHEAT, RYE, BARLEY & OATS

• Reading food labels is important. Remember, products labelled wheat-free are not necessarily gluten-free.

• Avoid wheat, including grains related to the wheat family such as spelt, kamut or durum (triticale), farina, semolina, couscous, wheat germ and bulgur.

• Avoid barley. Barley is present in many commercial products as malt, and is used as a flavour enhancer. Some soy milks contain malt.

• Gluten is found in all products made from these gluten containing grains, including breakfast cereals, breads, tortillas, pasta, biscuits, cakes, pancakes, muffins and flour.

• Avoid durum wheat pasta and wheat flour noodles (instant, udon and hokkien).

• Hydrolyzed vegetable protein (HVP) may contain gluten.

• Steer clear of fast food and a lot of foods from the freezer department (chips, chicken nuggets and fish fingers), these foods generally contain gluten.

• A lot of processed foods are thickened with flour. Be careful of products such as baked beans, soups, sauces (oyster, Worcestershire, soy sauce), yeast extract spreads (vegemite, marmite or promite), salad dressings, mustard and desserts.

• Avoid bread crumbs and products containing them such as patties, sausage rolls, sausages, meatballs, stuffed chickens and meats.

• Other products to watch are processed meats, confectionery, potato chips and some medications use gluten as a binder.

• Other products that might contain gluten include: some baking powders, corn flakes, corn tortillas, gravy mixes, instant dried mashed potato, tinned baked beans, custard and custard powder, and some yoghurts.

GLUTEN-FREE DIET

INCLUDE
foods made from gluten-free grains
RICE, MILLET, BUCKWHEAT, QUINOA & AMARANTH

• Include breads (including flat breads), flour and baked goods made from these gluten-free grains. Corn, potato, arrowroot, legumes (chickpeas - besan), and nuts can also be used to make flour, breads, muffins and other baked goods. You can buy gluten-free all-purpose flours made from a combination of gluten-free grains, ideal for cooking cakes and muffins.

• Use gluten-free corn tortillas and taco shells to make healthy nachos and tacos.

• Use arrowroot and corn flour (cornstarch – without added wheat starch) to thicken soups, casseroles and sauces.

• Use gluten-free grains for breakfast cereal including gluten-free muesli, puffed grains (brown rice, amaranth, buckwheat, corn and millet), rolled rice and corn flakes. Instead of oats, make creamy porridges with quinoa, buckwheat, rice flakes or millet.

• Serve rice crackers with healthy dips or puffed corn and rice cakes spread with your kid's favourite toppings (avocado, nut butters or hummus).

• Buy gluten-free pasta (spaghetti, macaroni and lasagna sheets) made with rice.

• Make desserts with tapioca (cassava), sago and rice.

• Add buckwheat, millet, quinoa, and brown rice to salads such as tabouli (instead of couscous).

• Add quinoa to soups instead of barley.

• Make creamy polenta (cornmeal) or millet mash (great mash potato alternative) or make a polenta slice.

• Gluten-free noodles include rice, buckwheat (soba), mung bean vermicelli and rice paper.

• Use wheat-free tamari instead of soy sauce. Balsamic and wine vinegars can be added to salad dressings.

• Psyllium and rice bran can be added to breakfast cereals and baked goods for extra fibre.

Helpful tips for parents with coeliac kids

• Prepare gluten-free meals for the whole family, so your child doesn't feel different.

• Make sure you have lots of healthy gluten-free snacks on hand for your kids to grab.

• Bake your own healthy gluten-free cakes, muffins, breads and biscuits.

• Make gluten-free bread crumbs by placing gluten-free bread in the oven on low to dry, until they turn golden. Place in a processor or place in a bag and crush with a rolling pin.

• When your child is attending birthday parties, provide a plate of gluten-free foods for them to share with everyone.

• Teach your child which foods contain gluten and which foods they are allowed.

• Encourage your child to make simple gluten-free food choices so they can learn to take responsibility for their own diet. That way they will feel confident to make the right food choices away from home, when at school and at friends' places.

• Inform your child's teacher. Your child's friends and their parents should also be informed. If your child is going to stay at a friend's place, pack some gluten-free goodies for them to take and share.

• If your child is going somewhere for lunch, packing some gluten-free bread is a good idea. Cafes and take away sandwich bars usually don't mind you supplying your own gluten-free bread.

• When making gluten-free baked goods, using a combination of different gluten-free flours will improve the texture. You can buy gluten-free flour mixtures from the supermarket and health food store. It is helpful to add ½ - 1 teaspoon of xanthan gum to baked goods as it acts like gluten, helping to prevent crumbling.

• To learn more about the disease and your child's new dietary requirements, get in contact with your local coeliac disease support organization. They will also be able to tell you which local restaurants and cafes in your area cater for gluten-free diets.

A gluten-free diet can be complicated at first as it requires a completely new approach to eating. With practise however, following a gluten-free diet will become second nature for your child. Children with coeliac disease have to be extremely careful about what foods they buy at school and when eating away from home. These children need to learn to read ingredient panels and get into the habit of asking people if the food contains gluten.

As long as your child's diet is nutritionally well balanced, following a gluten-free diet will not affect their growth or development. In today's multicultural society with such a variety of foods, going gluten-free is not so different. Look out for gluten-free products in your local supermarket or health food store. Be aware that 'wheat-free' does not mean 'gluten-free', as wheat-free products can be made from grains that contain gluten. These days there is a wide selection of gluten-free products available. Gluten-free meals and snacks are easy to prepare and delicious to eat - your child won't be able to taste the difference. All the recipes in this book are designed to be easily changed to gluten-free. These meals can be enjoyed by the whole family so you won't need to prepare separate meals for your gluten intolerant child.

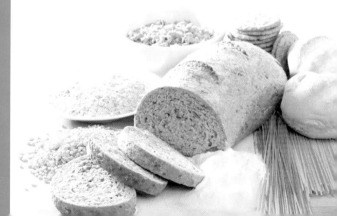

Kids with lactose intolerance

People sometimes confuse lactose intolerance with cow's milk allergy because the symptoms are often the same. However, lactose intolerance and cow's milk allergy are not related. An allergy to cow's milk is an allergic reaction triggered by the immune system. Whereas lactose intolerance is a problem caused by the digestive system, and does not involve an immune response like milk allergy.

Lactose intolerance is the inability to digest significant amounts of lactose, the predominant sugar of milk. This inability is caused by a shortage of the enzyme lactase, which is normally produced by the cells that line the small intestine. Lactase breaks down milk sugars into simpler forms that can be absorbed into the bloodstream. When there is not enough lactase to digest the amount of lactose consumed, it results in uncomfortable gastrointestinal symptoms that are not dangerous and will not cause anaphylaxis. Because the body cannot digest the lactose properly, the bacteria in the intestine ferments the sugar into gasses that can cause abdominal discomfort, flatulence, pain, cramps, diarrhoea and other distressing symptoms, which can begin about 30 minutes to 2 hours after eating or drinking foods containing lactose. The severity of symptoms varies depending on the amount of lactose each individual can tolerate.

With a well balanced diet and equally nutritious substitutes for milk and dairy foods, lactose intolerance need not pose a serious threat to your child's good health. Younger children with lactose intolerance should avoid food containing lactose. Older lactose intolerant children need not avoid lactose foods completely. They can learn which dairy products and other foods they can eat without discomfort and which ones they should avoid. Individuals differ in the amounts of lactose they can handle, so dietary control of lactose intolerant children depends on learning through trial and error how much lactose they can handle.

Many children will still be able to enjoy small amounts of cow's milk, yoghurt and hard cheeses. Yoghurts and hard cheeses are usually tolerated better than milk, as they contain less or easier to digest lactose than cow's milk. Goat and sheep's milk (cheese and yoghurts) can sometimes be well tolerated by lactose intolerant people, even though they still contain lactose.

Lactose-free alternatives

Lactose-free dairy products (milk, cheese and yoghurt) are widely available in supermarkets and health food stores. They contain the same amount of nutrients as the lactose-containing variety, so your children will be able to enjoy dairy products and reap the health benefits they offer.

Milk and dairy products are important sources of protein, calcium and vitamin D for children. Therefore, if these foods are removed from your child's diet you will have to replace them with foods equally rich in nutrients so they don't develop deficiencies.

Soy products are an alternative to dairy food, however, there has been some questions raised recently in regards to the safety of children consuming soy products. Soybeans and soy products contain chemicals called isoflavones that exert a weak oestrogenic effect on the body. There are concerns that these isoflavones could potentially have a negative effect on children's growth and development if eaten to excess. Organic soy milk and soy products can still be consumed by children in moderation. Introduce your child to a variety of different milks that are lactose-free so their diet is not dominated by soy. Some soy cheeses contain milk, so read the labels carefully. Vegan cheeses are lactose-free.

When choosing an alternative to cow's milk you must consider the health benefits and nutritional balance of the milk. Soy, rice and almond milk contain little calcium so calcium fortified varieties

Lactose-containing foods

• Lactose is found in dairy products, milk (buttermilk, evaporated, condensed and powdered), cheese (especially softer cheeses), cream, butter, margarine, ice cream and yoghurts.

• Yoghurts that contain active cultures are easier to digest and much less likely to cause lactose problems, due to the bacteria present having partially broken down the lactose already. Several studies have demonstrated improved lactose digestion and absorption when consuming yoghurt with live cultures, along with the reduction of digestive symptoms associated with lactose intolerance.[1,2]

• Cheese can still play an important role in lactose intolerant children's diets. New research has found that most people who are lactose intolerant can digest some dairy foods, such as hard cheeses, daily. Hard, aged cheeses are lower in lactose than softer cheeses. Most of the lactose found in cheese is removed with the whey during the manufacturing process. Most aged cheeses such as cheddar and Swiss contain about 95% less lactose than whole milk. Other cheeses with small amounts of lactose that can usually be tolerated in small amounts are brie, colby, edam, fetta, gouda, havarti, mozzarella and parmesan. Avoid softer cheeses like cream cheese, processed cheese, cheese spread, cottage and ricotta cheese, as these contain higher levels of lactose.

• Lactose can also be hidden in foods listed as something other than milk such as whey, curds, casein, caseinates, hydrolysates, lactose, lactalbumin, lactoglobulin or milk solids.

• Commercially baked goods made with milk include breads, cakes, muffins, pancakes, doughnuts, biscuits, crackers, quiches and pastries (brushed with milk).

• Dairy based puddings, junket and desserts.

• Confectionery made with milk such as chocolate, fudge, caramels, nougat and sherbet.

• Malted beverages made with milk or milk products.

• Some breakfast cereals and yoghurt topped muesli bars.

• Creamed soups, mayonnaise, and other sauces and dressings.

• Flavoured chips and cheese flavoured snacks.

are recommended. Rice milk is not a good source of protein, however protein enriched varieties are now available. Vitamin D fortified soy, rice and almond milks are also available.

There is a wide selection of non-dairy frozen desserts (ice cream, sorbets, ice blocks) and puddings available from supermarkets (these products can contain a lot of sugar so should be eaten only occasionally).

All recipes in this book can be made without milk or milk products. Make your child delicious homemade cakes, muffins, and cookies using olive oil and lactose-free milk. Make your own lactose-free sauces, dressings, quiches, ice cream and desserts. Buy lactose-free breads or make your own. Bread machines are a great investment.

Lactase drops and tablets are also available from health food stores. Taking a product like this before a lactose-containing meal, or adding a few drops into milk, helps digest the lactase and improves any digestive symptoms associated with lactose intolerance. Children with lactose intolerance can then still enjoy dairy products and benefit from the calcium and protein they contain.

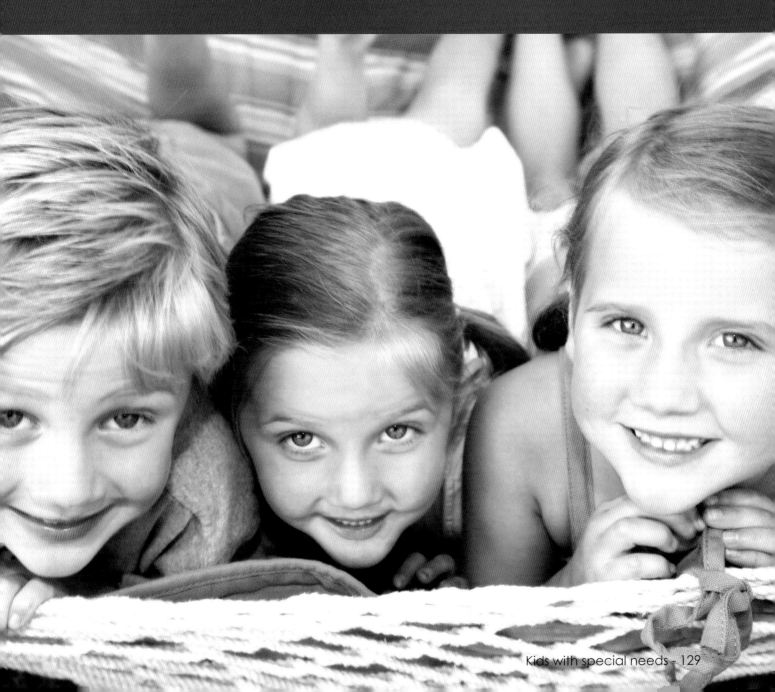

Chapter 9:
Kids with special needs

Childhood obesity

One in four Australian children are either overweight or obese. These recent statistics are of a great concern, indicating that the future health of our children is in jeopardy. The number of Australian children obese or overweight is now comparable to that in the UK or the United States.

Over the last 20 years, rates of childhood obesity have risen at an alarming rate in many countries around the world, including Australia. There is evidence that childhood obesity in Australia has increased dramatically over the past two decades and is still increasing.[1-3]

Obesity is the most common medical problem in Australia and a major, global public health concern. Being overweight or obese substantially increases the risk of both acute health problems and the chronic diseases that account for a high proportion of illness, disability and premature death. Cardiovascular disease and type-2 diabetes are strongly associated with obesity and are two of Australia's major health priorities.[4]

A recent Australian study by the NSW Centre for Overweight and Obesity has shown some disconcerting findings on the eating habits of Australian children. Researchers found that almost a quarter of children aged 5 to 16 were overweight or obese. These figures were much greater than figures from similar surveys in 1985 and 1997. The prevalence of children overweight and obese had risen from 11% in 1985, to 20% in 1997, to 25% in 2004 (similar alarming statistics have been found in the United States and the UK).[5]

Where genetic susceptibility can play a part, the underlying reasons for this global obesity epidemic in children is attributed to a changing lifestyle of reduced physical activity, and increasing consumption of energy-dense, processed foods, containing high amounts of sugars and saturated fats.[6,7] People in westernised countries also tend to eat out of the home more often and these foods are likely to be energy-dense fast foods that are processed and packaged for convenience. The media, social and economic influences also contribute to this rising incidence of our children becoming overweight and obese.

High consumption of unhealthy foods and soft drink results in excess energy (calorie) intake, resulting in weight gain. These energy-dense foods also displace more nutritious foods in a child's diet, like fruits, vegetables and wholegrain cereals. A diet rich in these energy-dense foods will also contribute towards the early development of adult-onset diseases such as heart disease, cancer, fatty liver and type-2 diabetes.[8-11]

The current trend towards 'super sized meals' has lead to an increase in the amount of food we consume. Portion size has been identified as an important environmental factor that influences calorie intake and could lead to weight gain and obesity.[12]

"One in four Australian children are overweight or obese"

Prevention remains the key, as treatment and management of obesity can still be difficult, given all the associated physical and psychological problems associated with it. There's good evidence that children who are overweight beyond age seven, are at greater risk of being obese adults. Overweight children with obese parents have a 70% greater risk.[13-15] As obesity in adulthood is related to coronary artery disease and hypertension, the prevention of childhood obesity therefore has the potential of preventing cardiovascular disease in adults.[16]

Treatment of childhood obesity relies heavily on parents. The whole family needs to change their lifestyle towards healthy eating, increased daily physical activity and decreased time doing sedentary activities like watching television and playing computer games. Weight problems can be avoided by helping your child develop healthy eating habits, and teaching them the importance of healthy living and exercise from an early age. Parents need to help their children establish a positive outlook towards food and exercise, and encourage them to have a positive body image without becoming obsessed about weight and dieting (like so many teenagers and adults).

Health risk

What is of great concern is that diseases once seen only in adults, such as type-2 diabetes, are now being seen in increasing numbers in children. One in five secondary students are already showing signs of health problems from being overweight such as high insulin levels, low HDL 'good' cholesterol and high LDL 'bad' cholesterol, high blood pressure and fatty liver, putting them at greater risk of developing heart disease, liver disease and type-2 diabetes.[17]

Evidence is emerging that distribution of body fat is also an important factor. Children with excessive abdominal fat can be at increased risk of developing hypertension, and increased insulin and blood fat levels.[18,19] These symptoms are collectively known as metabolic syndrome.

Childhood obesity can also contribute to orthopaedic complications, sleep apnoea, certain cancers and psychosocial illnesses.

Overweight and obese children are at great risk of developing a range of immediate problems as well as long-term health problems. The main ill-effects of obesity during childhood are social and emotional. Obese children can be teased and socially ostracised, putting them at risk of developing depression and similar psychiatric conditions.

Glycaemic-insulin link

Changes in food processing over the past 30 years, with the addition of sugar to a wide variety of foods and the removal of fibre, have created an environment in which our foods are essentially addictive, encouraging children to be overweight. These processed foods appear to be a major contributor to the increasing obesity epidemic through their effects on the hormone, insulin.[20]

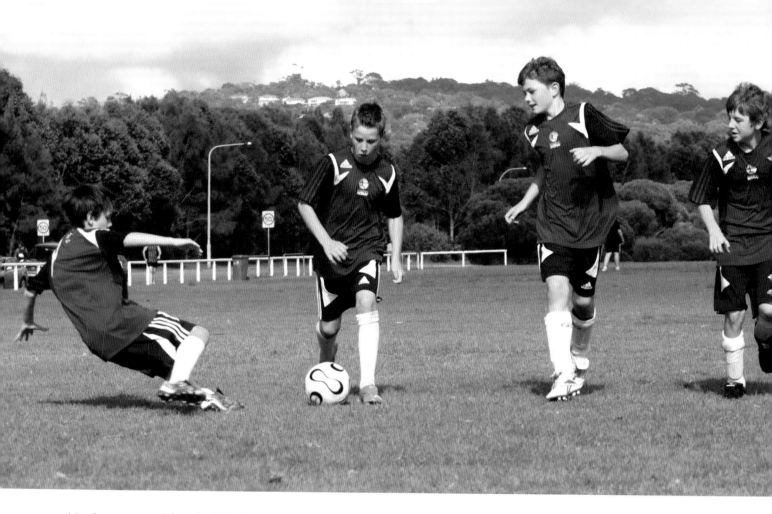

Most processed foods, high in sugar and low in fibre, have a high Glycaemic Index (GI). High GI foods cause blood sugar levels to surge quickly, causing high levels of insulin to be released into the blood stream. Studies have found that a diet rich in high GI foods is associated with weight gain and obesity.[21] Consumption of high GI foods promotes a more rapid return of hunger and therefore increases food and energy intake, leading to overeating and subsequent weight gain.

The hormone insulin plays a primary role in encouraging over-eating. A high level of insulin in the blood suppresses the hormone leptin. Calorie intake and expenditure are normally regulated by leptin. When leptin is functioning properly it increases physical activity, decreases appetite, and increases feelings of wellbeing. However, when leptin is suppressed, feelings of wellbeing diminish, activity decreases and appetite increases, a state called 'leptin resistance'.

A surge of insulin after eating a high GI food encourages over-eating by signalling the release of the chemical dopamine, which gives you a pleasurable dopamine rush.

Importance of exercise

Children should be encouraged to take part in some form of daily exercise, such as a walk with the dog, kicking a football with friends, cycling or walking to school. After school, children should become actively involved in sports such as a swimming club, little athletics or soccer.

Activity patterns developed during childhood carry over to later life and affect health and wellbeing as adults. It is important to ensure children are aware of the important role regular physical activity plays. Not only in terms of fitness and weight control in childhood but also in terms of later susceptibility to chronic disease.

Physical activity provides a mechanism for balancing energy intake and energy output, helping children to maintain a healthy weight. Evidence shows that inactivity is associated with an increased prevalence of obesity.[22,23]

Regular physical activity promotes healthy blood pressure, cholesterol and insulin levels. Physical activity is associated with reduced risk of coronary heart disease and type-2 diabetes.[24]

The Australian Physical Activity Guidelines for Children recommends that children spend at least an hour in moderate-to-vigorous physical activity each day. It also recommends that children should not spend more than two hours per day playing computer games, watching television, or surfing the internet for entertainment. A very high proportion of Australian children spend more than the recommended two hours a day in front of a small screen. Research shows that excessive TV watching and playing computer games is associated with increased risk of becoming overweight and obese.[25]

Should overweight or obese children be put on strict diets?

Overweight or obese children should never be put on strict diets that restrict food intake to promote weight loss. Strict diets like these can compromise a child's growth and health. Some well meaning parents restrict their child's food intake in an effort to control their weight, but research shows that such restrictions can actually have the opposite effect, leading to children overeating and gaining more weight.

When children are forbidden certain foods, these foods become more desirable and can lead to children becoming obsessed by and even binging on these foods. Occasionally allowing your child to have junk food on special occasions, such as birthday parties, is fine, as long as the majority of the time they eat a healthy, balanced diet full of wholesome foods from the five food groups, low in saturated fat, sugar and sodium.

"Children should spend at least an hour a day in moderate-to-vigorous physical activity"

Healthy weight loss tips for overweight and obese children

1. LIMIT SUGARY, PROCESSED & HIGH GI FOODS: High consumption of sugary, processed foods is one of the major reasons for weight gain in children. Limit or avoid processed, high GI snack foods such as cakes, biscuits, chocolates, lollies, commercial muesli bars and chips. Choose wholesome unprocessed low GI snack foods, which are high in fibre and low in saturated fats, sodium and sugars. Have a snack box in the fridge full of healthy snacks: fruit pieces, yoghurt tubs, vegie sticks, hummus and wholemeal muffins.

2. BEVERAGES: Avoid giving your child sweetened beverages such as soft drinks, cordials and flavoured milk drinks. Always offer them water as a first choice, then low-fat milk or small amounts of 100% natural fruit juice diluted with water. Fruit smoothies make a good alternative to flavoured milk. Try a ¼ glass of fruit juice with natural mineral water instead of soft drink.

3. HIGH FIBRE: Include plenty of fibre rich foods in your child's diet. High fibre foods include wholegrain cereals, fresh fruit, vegetables and legumes. Fibrous foods are often bulky and filling and also tend to be low in fat. Soluble fibre forms a gel that slows down the emptying of the stomach and the transit time of food through the digestive system. This will promote a sense of satiety (fullness) after a meal, which will stop children from overeating. This also delays the absorption of sugars from the intestines. This helps to maintain lower blood sugar levels and prevent a rapid rise in blood insulin levels, which has been linked with obesity.

4. SATURATED FATS: In children, strict diets or rigid fat restriction diets are not desirable, but choosing lower fat foods is encouraged. Choose low-fat dairy products (milk, yoghurt and cheese). Children over the age of two can have low-fat milk and dairy foods. Limit foods high in saturated fats such as take away foods (hamburgers, fried chicken, chips, pies, sausage rolls and pizza), chocolate, cakes, muffins, pastries and ice cream. Avoid deep frying food and cooking with butter or vegetable oils. Use olive oil for cooking and baking.

5. GOOD FATS: Nutritious foods should not be eliminated or severely restricted in a child's diet simply because of its fat content. Beneficial unsaturated fats are an essential part of a child's diet, needed for their growth and development. Moderate consumption of monounsaturated and polyunsaturated fats as part of a well balanced, low saturated fat diet, will help your child maintain a healthy weight or assist in weight loss for obese or overweight children.[26]

6. LUNCH BOX: Pack your child healthy nutritious lunches and snacks for school. Don't give them money to buy lunch as they may buy lollies and junk food on the way to school, or pies and sausage rolls from the school canteen. Do not pack lollies, chocolates, soft drinks, flavoured drinks, chips, rolled fruit, sugary biscuits, commercially produced cakes, muffins, or muesli bars in your child's lunch box. They will usually fill up on these foods and leave the other nutritious foods you packed uneaten.

7. PROTEIN: Protein foods have a low GI and help create a feeling of satiety (fullness), preventing children from overeating. This is important for kids trying to lose weight. Add some form of protein in your child's lunch. Example: tuna, chicken, low-fat cheese or egg on sandwiches; individual quiches or timbales; hummus with crisp breads; or a tub of low-fat yoghurt (with no added sugars).

8. HEALTHY COOKING: Use healthy low-fat cooking methods such as steaming, light stir-frying with a little olive oil, grilling or baking. Use an olive oil spray instead of coating a pan with oil. You can pour it into a pump bottle, that way you will use far less oil than if you were pouring it out of the bottle (8 sprites equals about ½ teaspoon oil). Use olive oil spray for sautéing, stir-frying, roasting vegies, pita chips, or for greasing pans.

9. SMALLER SERVING SIZES: Don't over fill your child's plate with food. Offer smaller servings and have more available if they want it. Children must learn to listen to their bodies, to stop eating when they have had sufficient food to eat and to eat when they are hungry.

10. REGULAR MEALS AND SNACKS: Overweight or obese children must eat regularly - three main meals and two smaller snacks. Regularly skipping meals could be detrimental to your child's growth and development. If your child reaches a point of excessive hunger it will trigger them to overeat, usually foods containing high amounts of sugar and fat. Having smaller, regular meals will also help your child lose weight by speeding up their metabolism and giving them plenty of energy to take part in physical activities. Make sure your child starts the day with a good nutritious breakfast.

11. BE WARY OF PACKAGED FOODS LABELLED AS 'LOW-FAT': Some products are labelled as 'low-fat' but contain large amounts of added sugars. This type of misleading labeling is contributing to the obesity problems by giving people permission to overindulge. Read labels carefully to detect any hidden sugars.

Children with diabetes

Diabetes mellitus is a disease in which the body does not produce or properly use insulin, a hormone released by the pancreas. After food is eaten it is digested and broken down into glucose, the simple sugar that is the main source of energy for all the cells in the body. Insulin is needed to move glucose from the blood into the cells, where it can be used as energy for working muscles and for the functioning of the rest of the body. However, when the pancreas does not make enough insulin or the body is unable to use the insulin that is present, the glucose cannot get inside the cells and therefore cannot use it for energy. Excess glucose will then build up in the bloodstream, setting the stage for the development of diabetes.

There are two main types of diabetes, which both have different causes. Type-1 diabetes is an autoimmune disease that affects the pancreas and stops the body from producing insulin. It can develop at any age (although it usually develops in children) and is referred to as juvenile-onset diabetes. Until recently, most children with diabetes had type-1, which is one of the most common and increasingly prevalent chronic diseases in children. Type-1 diabetes is also known as insulin-dependent diabetes, because the affected person needs to take an insulin injection every day.

Type-2 diabetes, on the other hand, is a metabolic disease that develops when either the body doesn't produce enough insulin or the cells won't respond to insulin, which prevents glucose from being delivered into the cells. Type-2 diabetes is strongly linked to lifestyle and more closely associated with genetic inheritance than type-1 diabetes. Type-2 diabetes usually occurs later in life and is known as late-onset diabetes or non-insulin-dependent diabetes, as insulin treatment is not always needed. Increasingly however, type-2 diabetes is being reported in children from Australia and other countries including the United States.[1] It is of great concern that this disease, which was once seen only in adults, is now being diagnosed in growing numbers of children.

Among children, the average age of diagnosis of type-2 diabetes is between 12 and 14 years, affecting girls more than boys, and is associated with obesity, poor diet, physical inactivity, a family history of type-2 diabetes and signs of insulin resistance. Family history is an important predictor of type-2 diabetes. A parent having type-2 diabetes must be aware that their children are at increased risk of developing the disease and lifestyle and dietary changes should be made accordingly.

Insulin resistance & obesity

If you have insulin resistance, your cells do not respond to insulin properly. Insulin produced by your pancreas cannot get glucose inside the cells to produce energy. The pancreas tries to keep up with the demand for insulin by producing more. Eventually, the pancreas cannot keep up with the body's need for insulin and abnormally high levels of glucose build up in the bloodstream (hyperglycaemia). Many people with insulin resistance have high levels of blood glucose and high levels of insulin circulating in their blood at the same time.

Being obese or overweight affects the way insulin works in the body. The increasing prevalence of childhood obesity is a major worry as children who are overweight or obese have a higher risk of insulin resistance, because fat interferes with the body's ability to use insulin. Without appropriate intervention, obesity and insulin resistance can progress to type-2 diabetes. A recent increase in childhood type-2 diabetes has been documented in several countries, paralleling the increase in the prevalence and degree of obesity.[2-4] Children having a sedentary lifestyle also aggravates insulin resistance. Regular exercise is important to help insulin work efficiently.

Being insulin resistant can also affect other aspects of your child's health. People who are insulin resistant typically have increased triglyceride levels (blood fat) and a decreased level of HDL 'good' cholesterol. Imbalances in triglycerides and HDL cholesterol increase the risk of heart disease.

Complications associated with uncontrolled type-2 diabetes

Often children with type-2 diabetes have no symptoms. However, if left untreated they may experience symptoms such as increased thirst, increased urination, increased appetite, fatigue, blurred vision, and frequent or slow-healing infections. Even though these symptoms may not be immediately severe, over time, uncontrolled high blood glucose levels can damage smaller blood vessels in the body, leading to complications including irreversible damage to the eyes, kidneys, nerves and other internal organs. Uncontrolled diabetes increases the risk of cardiovascular diseases such as heart attack and strokes.

Importance of a well-balanced diet

A well-balanced healthy diet is especially important for children with type-2 diabetes. Maintaining a healthy weight and physical activity are also essential to help reduce insulin resistance and help stabilise blood glucose levels. Planning meals with the right nutrients, in the right amounts and eating them at the right times is extremely important. A naturopath, nutritionist or dietitian can help you with your child's specific dietary needs.

It's important that diabetic children are educated about their condition and know what foods they should and shouldn't eat. Diabetic children should be shown how to make wise food choices. You should also tell teachers, parents of your child's friends, and organisers of sport and club activities about your child's condition.

For children with diabetes, special occasions like birthday parties require additional planning because of the temptation of extra sweets. Be organised and make a plate of equally delicious, sugar-free, low GI treats for them to take and share with everyone. Use the natural sweetener xylitol instead of sugar or honey and make any of the scrumptious muffins, cakes, cookies or slices from this book. The other kid's won't know the difference.

RESTRICT SUGAR: Diabetic children should reduce their intake of food that will cause a sharp rise in blood sugar levels. Food containing high levels of sugars such as commercially made cakes, muffins, cookies, pastries, desserts, breakfast cereals, muesli bars, soft drinks, ice cream, chocolates and lollies should be reduced or not eaten at all. Diabetic children should eat whole fruit and drink water instead of drinking juice. All the recipes in this book can be altered to be diabetic friendly, using the natural sweetener xylitol. Do not use artificial sweeteners. You can buy xylitol or products such as biscuits made from xylitol from supermarkets and health food stores.

EAT A LOW GI DIET: Diabetic children should follow a low GI diet, limiting their intake of high GI foods. Following a low GI diet will help stabilise blood sugar levels and help your child maintain a healthy weight.

IMPORTANCE OF FIBRE: Dietary fibre has a stabilising effect on blood sugar levels that makes it beneficial in the prevention and management of diabetes.[5] Diabetic children should eat plenty of dietary fibre, especially soluble fibre and resistant starch. A large study in the US found that a lower risk of type-2 diabetes was associated with higher intakes of all wholegrain cereals, and the protective effect was even greater when combined with a low total glycaemic load.[6-8] These types of fibre slow the absorption of glucose, reducing the sharp rise in blood glucose levels, reducing the GI of a meal. Fibre is present in wholegrain cereals, breads, fruit, vegetables and legumes. Use wholemeal flour when baking instead of refined flour.

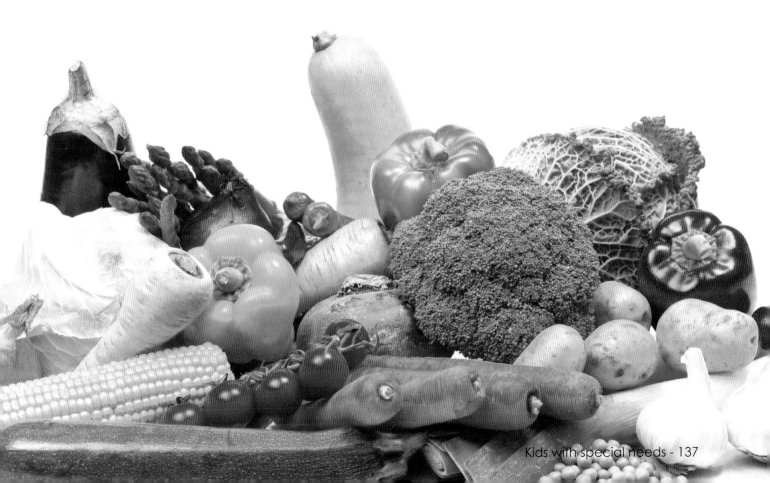

EAT REGULARLY: It is important for your child to eat small meals often (every few hours), so blood sugar levels don't drop too low. By eating 4-5 small meals a day, blood sugar levels will remain stable. It's important that your child has breakfast each morning, otherwise it is too long for the body to go without food (from last night's dinner to the next day's lunch) and their blood sugar levels will drop too low. They will wake up feeling tired, light headed and dizzy. Snacks are also important but can pose a problem if the wrong type of foods are eaten. Snacks should be low in saturated fats and sugar.

INCLUDE PROTEIN-RICH FOODS: Try to include healthy low-fat protein-rich foods with most meals. This will help stabilise blood sugar levels, as protein foods usually have a low GI. Combining these foods with higher GI carbohydrate foods, such as pasta, bread and rice, to help reduce the GI of the meal. Include protein rich foods, such as low-fat dairy products, eggs, nuts, seeds, legumes, lean meats, fish and poultry.

REDUCE SATURATED AND TRANS-FATS: Cut down on saturated fats and eliminate trans-fats from your child's diet. These fats raise blood cholesterol that is a risk factor for heart disease. People with diabetes are at an increased risk of heart disease.

INCLUDE UNSATURATED FATS: Include monounsaturated fats and polyunsaturated fats in your child's diet. Scientific studies have shown monounsaturated fats, such as those found in olive oil and avocado, have a lowering effect on total cholesterol and LDL 'bad' cholesterol levels, as well as reducing triglyceride levels (blood fats).[9] Diets containing monounsaturated fats are associated with a reduced risk of heart disease. Monounsaturated fats have also been found to have beneficial effects on blood glucose levels, making them helpful in the prevention and management of diabetes.[10,11] Moderate consumption of monounsaturated fats as part of a well balanced, low saturated fat diet will help your child maintain a healthy weight, or help with weight loss for obese or overweight children. Polyunsaturated omega-3 fats, found in oily fish (salmon, tuna, sardines, herring, mackerel and trout), flaxseed oil, and nuts and seeds, play an important role in the prevention of type-2 diabetes and cardiovascular disease.[12-15]

"A well-balanced diet as well as maintaining a healthy weight and physical activity are essential for children with diabetes."

Kids with ADHD

Is food affecting your child's behaviour?

Attention deficit hyperactivity disorder (ADHD) is one of the most common behavioural problems seen in children, affecting about 5% of school children. The main symptoms associated with ADHD in children include reduced attentiveness and concentration, and excessive level of activity, distractibility and impulsiveness.

Onset of ADHD usually occurs before the age of four and affects boys 10 times more than girls. Many children outgrow or learn how to control their symptoms, however sometimes ADHD symptoms will persist into adulthood.

ADHD has genetic roots. Children of parents with a history of ADHD have an increased potential to develop the condition.

An increasing number of children being diagnosed with ADHD have been reported in Australia, where it's estimated that at least 50,000 children are now on drugs prescribed for ADHD. The use of Ritalin in Australia has risen from 1.5 million tablets prescribed in 1984 to19.3 million tablets in 2001.[1]

If you suspect that your child is hyperactive it might be related to their diet. Children are unfortunately often misdiagnosed as having ADHD when they're really reacting to certain foods in their diet.

Food additives and ADHD

There is ample evidence to prove a connection between children's behaviour and what they eat, with particular concern regarding food additives and their possible involvement in behavioural disorders such as ADHD.[2,3] Thousands of different chemical additives are used in the manufacturing of processed foods to enhance flavour or colour and to preserve and extend shelf life. An increasing number of children are showing signs of being adversely affected by these chemical additives, with the most common offenders being preservatives and food colourings. Children are particularly susceptible to the adverse effects of these chemicals, partly due to their smaller size, and because their detoxification systems and brains are still immature and developing.

Many parents have witnessed a dramatic change in their children when they consume specific foods containing artificial additives.[4] Research has found that when hyperactive children consume artificial additives they suffer decreased attention spans, irritability, restlessness and disturbance in sleep.[5-7]

Of the identified dietary causes of ADHD, artificial additives in foods, which include preservatives, colourings and flavourings, are most common.

Children's diets today are becoming increasingly reliant on processed foods laden with artificial additives. There are currently about 400 approved artificial food additives in Australia.[8] Many of these have been found to contribute to hyperactivity in children. The worst offenders are the E series, which are banned in baby foods. Several studies have shown that the red food colouring tartrazine, found in cola and other processed foods, has distinct aggravating effects in hyperactive children.[9]

Read ingredient panels carefully and avoid any foods containing the following E series food additives: tartrazine (E102), sunset yellow (E110), carmoisine (E122), ponceau 4R (E124), benzoates

(E210-219), sulphides (E249-252), monosodium glutamate and other glutamates (E621-623), and antioxidants (E310-312, E220, E321).

There is a lot of supportive data suggesting that children with allergies or sensitivity to certain foods may be predisposed to behavioural disorders like ADHD. By omitting the common allergens, milk, wheat, egg, cocoa, corn, sugar and food colourings, researchers have found that about half the ADHD children in the study noticed improvements after seven days.[10] If you suspect your child might have a food allergy it is worthwhile having tests done to detect any offending foods, which should be taken out of their diet. When removing several important nutritious foods from your child's diet, such as milk, wheat or eggs, care must be taken to replace these foods with equally nutritious substitutes. A naturopath, nutritionist or dietician will be able to help you plan a suitable diet for your child, to make sure they are not missing out on essential nutrients needed for their growth and development.

The role diet plays in ADHD

The majority of parents of hyperactive children will agree that sugar plays a big part in aggravating their children's symptoms. When children consume sugar rich foods they get an artificial high, their blood sugar levels rise quickly and so does adrenaline levels, contributing to hyperactivity, anxiety and difficulties in concentrating. This rapid rise in blood sugar levels stimulates the release of too much insulin, which causes their blood sugar levels to plummet, resulting in irritability and crankiness. High consumption of sugar can exacerbate children's behavioural problems and ADHD symptoms.[11] Reduce your child's consumption of processed foods which contain high levels of sugar and artificial additives and replace them with fresh, natural foods from the five food groups. Buying organic food is recommended for children with ADHD as it's free from artificial additives (preservatives, colourings and flavours) and harmful pesticides.

Nutritional deficiencies are commonly seen in children with ADHD, having significantly lower levels of omega-3 essential fatty acids (EFAs).[12] The health of your child's nervous system and brain function can greatly affect their behaviour. The health and function of cell membranes, especially those of the nervous system, are dependent upon adequate EFA intake. EFAs are also required for prostaglandin production, namely PGE1, which is needed for controlling biochemical processes in the brain. If your child's diet is deficient in EFAs an apparent deficiency may lead to ADHD symptoms.[13] Children with ADHD with lower compositions of total omega-3 EFAs have significantly more behavioural problems, temper tantrums, and learning, health and sleep problems than those with high proportions of omega-3 FA.[14]

Reduce your child's saturated and trans-fat intake, replacing them with foods rich in omega-3 EFAs such as oily fish (mackerel, herring, sardines, tuna, trout and salmon), flaxseed oil, dark green vegetables, parsley, seaweeds, nuts, seeds (pumpkin, sesame seeds and tahini), legumes (hummus)and wholegrain cereals.

Behavioural disorders, including hyperactivity, are known to be associated with low zinc status. Research on ADHD children has shown them to be zinc deficient and this to be a contributing factor in their condition.[15] The best food sources of zinc include lean meat, chicken, fish, milk and other dairy foods (cheese), brewers yeast, egg yolks, legumes (beans, lentils and peas), wholegrain bread, sunflower seeds, pumpkin seeds, pecans and a moderate amount of zinc found in vegetables.

Chapter 10:
Packing a safe lunch box
avoid food contamination by preparing and storing your child's food safely

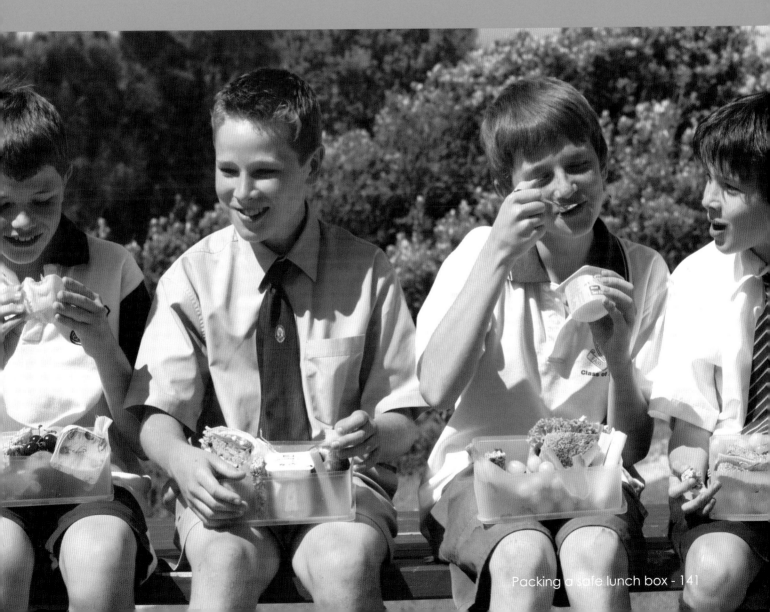

Once food is removed from the fridge, freezer or pantry for long periods of time, it can become contaminated with bacteria. Children's lunches sit in their bags, usually at room temperature for several hours until lunch, which poses a real risk of food poisoning. Care needs to be taken when packing your child's lunch box, especially in warm weather, to minimise the risk of bacterial contamination.

Bacteria that cause food poisoning grow more easily on some foods than others. These high risk foods include meat, poultry, seafood, dairy products, eggs, deli type meats, and prepared salads like coleslaw, pasta and rice salads.

There are many different varieties of bacteria that cause food poisoning. The worst offenders are staphylococcus (found in meat, fish, poultry, dairy products and salads), E. coli (found in raw meats and poultry, but can be eliminated through cooking), salmonella (found in raw or partially cooked eggs and chicken) and listeria (found in cooked meats or seafood, prepared salads, soft cheeses, unpasteurised milk and milk products).

Food poisoning symptoms can range from being so mild that they are hardly noticeable to being so severe that hospitalisation is needed. Common symptoms of food poisoning include abdominal pain, nausea, vomiting, diarrhoea, fever and dehydration, or can be as serious as having trouble swallowing, breathing and paralysis.

Packing a safe lunch box

1. Ensure that food preparation surfaces, hands and utensils are clean when preparing and packing your child's lunch. Lunch boxes, drink bottles and other containers should be washed thoroughly.

2. If possible, lunches should be carried in an insulated lunch box.

3. Something cold, such as a frozen water bottle or freezer gel, should be packed with school lunches. You should always pack a bottle of water with your child's lunch. Freeze it overnight so it keeps the rest of their lunch cool and safe from bacteria.

4. Pack perishable foods such as cold meats or egg sandwiches between cold items.

5. Pack salads such as pasta, rice and coleslaw in a separate container next to a frozen drink or gel pack. You could also use a cold thermos for these types of salads.

6. When hot foods like soups and casseroles are taken to school, they should be kept in an insulated bottle or flask. To ensure that the food is kept hot and safe, the flask should be pre-heated by adding hot water, letting it stand for a few minutes then emptying it and filling it with hot food.

7. Freeze tubs of yoghurt. Not only will the yoghurt be nice and chilled in time for lunch, it will keep the rest of their lunch cool and bacteria free.

8. School lunches can safely be made the previous night, provided they are then kept in the fridge or freezer.

Cooking with your kids

It's difficult these days for busy parents to find the time to cook with their children. Letting kids help cook meals does require time, patience, support and some extra clean up however, it's well worth the effort.

Allowing your kids to participate in food preparation helps them become familiar with different foods, which can improve their acceptance of a wider range of ingredients. Having kids involved in choosing recipes for family meals and shopping for food will also help them broaden their knowledge of new foods, which will increase their willingness to try them.

With a little training and supervision, the kitchen can become a place to enjoy special one on one time with your child. Take advantage of this opportunity to teach your children about the importance of healthy eating and the nutritional value of different foods in a fun atmosphere.

Keep reminding your children of the many health benefits they will receive from eating healthy foods, in ways they can understand. You can discuss different ingredients and why they are good for their health. Reinforce that eating healthy foods will help them stay fit, stop them from getting sick, allow them to concentrate better at school and get better grades. Healthy foods will give them more energy to play sport, will help improve their physical health and fitness, and will give them lots of energy to run faster or swim further. Children should know that eating healthy food leads to a healthy weight, clear skin, shiny hair, strong muscles and healthy teeth.

Involving your children in the kitchen will also help them appreciate family meals together. Many families struggle to spend one daily meal together. Acceptance of foods is improved when children see family members enjoying the healthy meals they have prepared. Children are more likely to sit down to a family meal when they have helped prepare it. This will also give them a sense of accomplishment and feeling that they are contributing to the family. Helping in the kitchen will also get them up away from the TV or computer games to do something more constructive and educational.

Remember that time in the kitchen cooking with your kids should always be fun. Eating should be an enjoyable and sociable part of life for everyone in the family. Preparing and sharing meals with family and friends is an important part of your child's social development. If they have fond memories and positive experiences with healthy foods as a child, they will be more likely to continue to choose them as they get older.

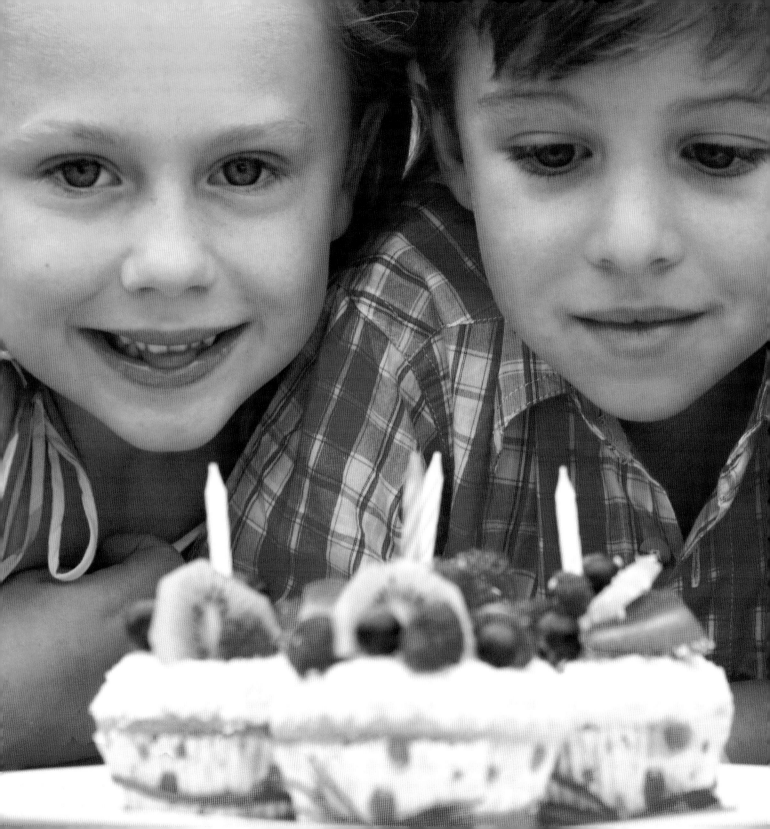

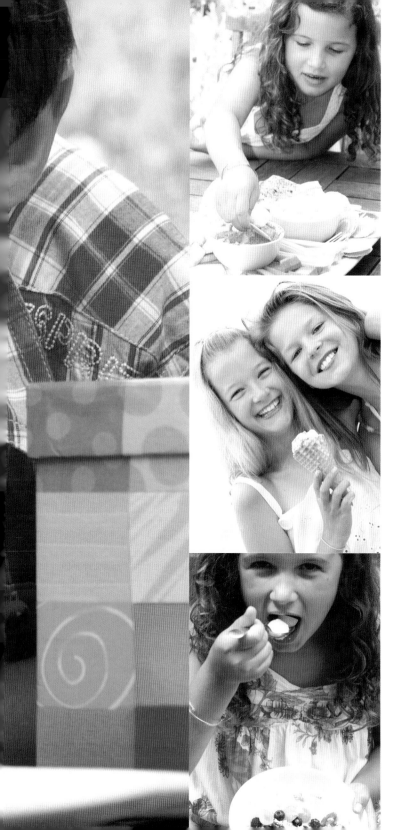

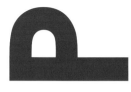

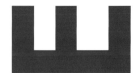
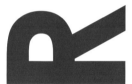

RECIPES

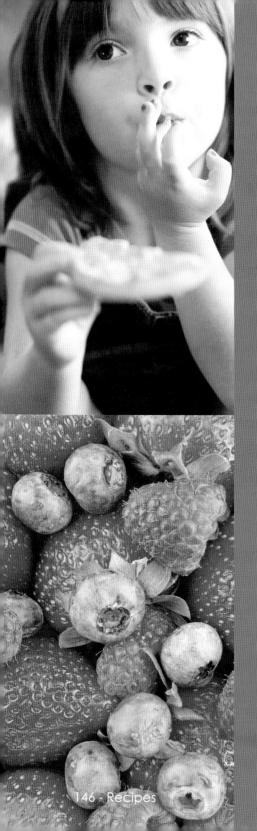

"Children need a nutritious breakfast to fuel their body and brain for the busy day ahead."

Breakfast

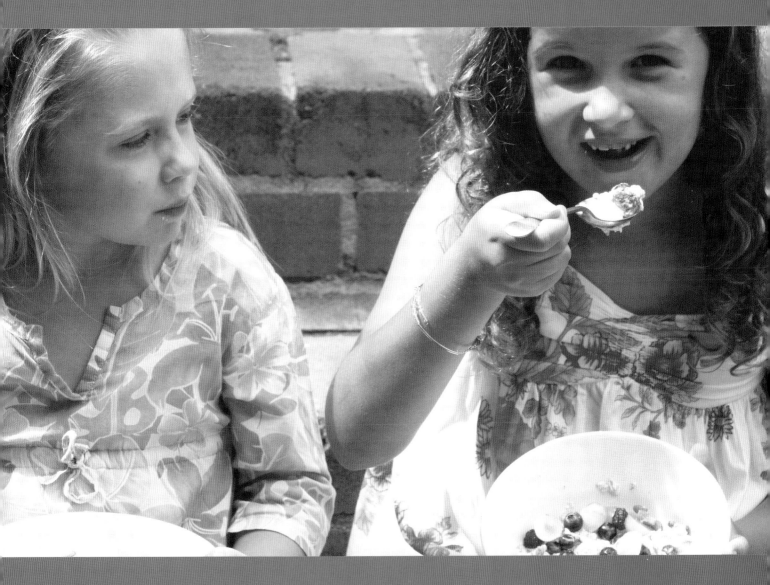

The most important meal of the day

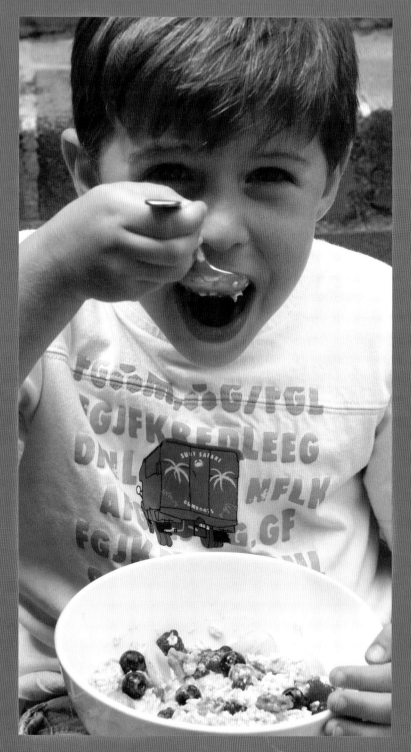

Breakfast is one of your child's most important meals of the day. Breakfast is their first meal after their long fast while sleeping. Children need to replenish their bodies with energy and nutrients for their mentally and physically active day ahead.

Skipping breakfast will lead to your child having a mid-morning energy slump, along with lack of concentration, irritability and those mid-morning cravings for sugary snacks. Children that skip breakfast are more likely to binge later on in the day. Children need a steady supply of nutrients and energy for healthy growth and development. If meals are skipped this will impact on their health. Studies have proven that breakfast consumption is associated with better academic performance, including improved concentration and IQ.[1,2]

Breakfast contributes to around a third of your child's daily nutrient intake of iron, fibre and calcium. These nutrients are found in breakfast foods such as wholegrain bread, oats, muesli, milk, yoghurt, eggs, baked beans and fruit.

If your child will not eat food first thing in the morning, try making them a nutritious smoothie with some skim milk, a teaspoon of LSA (ground linseed, sunflower and almonds), some yoghurt, banana, strawberry (or any other fruit favourites). You could also give your child a healthy snack to have on the way to school. Something like a healthy wholemeal muffin, mini egg frittata, or yoghurt and a piece of fruit; or pack a small tub of Bircher muesli in their lunch box to have when they get to school.

Wholesome muesli

These wholesome mueslis are one of the most nutritious ways your child can start the day. Made with wholegrains these mueslis are packed with energy giving complex carbohydrates, dietary fibre, B vitamins, vitamin E, iron and zinc. Teamed with a combination of fresh seasonal fruits, yoghurt, nuts and seeds, these mueslis are also a good source of vitamin C, calcium, protein and beneficial omega 3 fats.

Berry Bircher-style muesli

This version of a healthy Swiss style muesli makes for a perfect, well-balanced breakfast. Yoghurt is a fabulous addition to a child's diet, full of friendly bacteria that help to promote healthy digestion and immune function. Use any combination of seasonal fruits you like. This muesli also makes a delicious lunch box snack.

2 cups (200 g/7 oz) rolled oats (GF: rice, millet, quinoa or buckwheat flakes)

2 tablespoons almond flakes

2 tablespoons sunflower seeds

2 cups (500 ml/ 17½ fl oz) low-fat milk (LF: rice, soy, almond or lactose-free milk)

¼ cup (63 ml/2¼ fl oz) 100% apple juice

1 grated apple or pear (leave skin on if using organic fruit)

½ cup (125 g/4½ oz) natural yoghurt (LF: lactose-free yoghurt)

1 cup (150 g/5¼ oz) mixed berries (strawberries, blueberries and raspberries)

Soak oats, nuts and seeds overnight in milk and apple juice.

When ready to serve mix through yoghurt and fresh fruit.

Serves 4.

Variations: Use other nuts and seeds such as brazil nuts, pecans, hazelnuts or flaxseeds. Replace berries with other fruits such as diced banana, mango or peach.

Mixed grain natural muesli

This nutritious, earthy muesli is delicious served with milk or used as a topping for yoghurt or fruit salads. Sun-dried fruit gives this muesli a natural sweetness as well as added dietary fibre. Add 1-2 tablespoons of muesli to smoothies to give them a fibre boost.

2 cups (200 g/7 oz) rolled oats (GF: flaked quinoa, millet or buckwheat)

2 cups (125 g/ 4 ½ oz) natural corn flakes

1 cup (30 g/1 oz) puffed rice

½ cup (65 g/2½ oz) oat bran (GF: rice bran or psyllium husks)

½ cup (85 g/3 oz) pepitas (pumpkin seeds)

½ cup (85 g/3 oz) almonds, chopped

3 tablespoons linseeds

¼ cup (40 g/ 1½ oz) sunflower seeds

1 cup (140 g/5 oz) mixed sun-dried fruit (apricot, sultana, dates, banana or apple), chopped - optional

Add all ingredients together and store in airtight container.

This natural muesli will last up to 4 weeks.

When ready to serve, place a cup of muesli in a bowl and add milk.

Makes 16 servings.

Variations: Replace dried fruit with fresh, seasonal fruit (add fruit just before ready to serve). Use other sun-dried fruits such as mango, banana, pear, peach or goji berries.

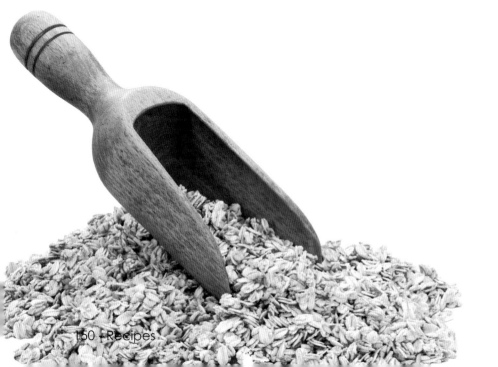

Crunchy toasted muesli

This crunchy, toasted muesli has all the goodness of wholegrains, nuts and seeds, offset with lighter puffed grains. Commercially made toasted mueslis are high in saturated fats and added sugars. This healthier version is lightly toasted in olive oil, which is a good source of beneficial monounsaturated fats, and naturally sweetened with honey and sun-dried fruit. Serve with milk or sprinkle some over yoghurt or fruit salad.

4 cups (400 g/14 oz) rolled oats (GF: flaked quinoa, millet or buckwheat)

¼ cup (40 g/1½ oz) shredded coconut

¼ cup (40 g/1½ oz) sunflower seeds

½ cup (85 g/3 oz) pepitas (pumpkin seeds)

½ cup (85 g/3 oz) almonds

2 tablespoons cold pressed virgin olive oil

¼ cup (63 ml/2¼ fl oz) raw organic honey

1 teaspoon vanilla essence

2 cups (60 g/2 oz) puffed millet

2 cups (60 g/2 oz) puffed rice

1 cup (140 g/5 oz) sun-dried fruit (apricot, banana, apple, pineapple, date, fig or mango), diced - optional

Preheat oven to 180°C (350°F/Gas 4). Line a baking tray with baking paper.

In a large bowl mix rolled oats, coconut, nuts and seeds together.

In a small saucepan over a medium heat, combine honey, vanilla and olive oil, and stir well. Pour honey mixture over oats and gently toss, making sure muesli is well coated. Pour mixture onto baking tray and cook for 15 minutes or until muesli is golden brown and has formed clusters.

Allow muesli to cool then add puffed grains. Add dried fruit pieces if desired. Store in an airtight container in the fridge for up to 4 weeks.

Makes 16 servings.

Banana & berry breakfast smoothie

No more excuses for children missing a healthy breakfast. This quick and easy low-fat smoothie is ideal for kids that don't like to eat first thing in the morning. This delicious smoothie is a meal in itself, rich in protein, complex carbohydrates, dietary fibre, vitamin C and antioxidants. Sweetened naturally with berries and banana, this smoothie provides the perfect opportunity to increase your child's fruit intake. You can use any combination of fruits you like.

1½ cups (375 ml/13 fl oz) low-fat milk (LF: rice, almond, soy or lactose-free milk)

2 tablespoons natural or vanilla yoghurt (LF: lactose-free or soy yoghurt)

1 ripe banana

¼ cup (38 g/1½ oz) berries, (strawberries, raspberries and blueberries) chopped

1-2 tablespoons muesli (GF: gluten-free muesli)

½ cup (125 ml/4½ fl oz) iced water

1 teaspoon raw organic honey - optional

Place all ingredients in a blender and mix until smooth and well combined.

Serve immediately in a tall glass.

Makes 2 glasses.

Variations: Add a couple of ice cubes for a chilled smoothie. Use leftovers to make ice blocks, pour into ice block moulds and freeze.

Perfect porridge

Traditional oatmeal porridge remains a favourite with children during the winter months. Porridge is an excellent source of dietary fibre and energy giving, complex carbohydrates to keep active children going throughout the day. Porridge is not only a delicious winter breakfast, you can also serve it cold during the summer months. Soaking oats overnight is an easy, no fuss way to make porridge.

1 cup (100 g/3½ oz) rolled oats (GF: flaked rice, millet or quinoa)

1 ½ cups (375 ml/13 fl oz) low-fat milk (LF: rice, almond, soy or lactose-free milk) - or use half water

1 tablespoon LSA (ground linseed, sunflower seeds and almonds)

Desired fruit (banana, mango, pear, apple or berries), diced

1-2 teaspoons raw organic honey

In a small saucepan add oats and milk. Cook over a medium heat for 3 minutes, stirring well.

Add diced fruit and LSA and cook for another 3 minutes until porridge has a creamy texture and fruit is cooked through.

Take saucepan off the heat and stir through honey.

Serves 2-3.

Cooking gluten-free grains: Cook flaked millet and quinoa the same as oats. If using rice flakes, add an extra cup of water. Bring to boil, then cover and simmer over medium heat for 20 minutes or until soft and creamy.

Variations: Try adding different combinations like banana, honey and cinnamon; diced mango and almond flakes; pear, dates and sunflower seeds; grated apple, cinnamon and sultanas; or mixed stewed fruit with a dollop of yoghurt.

Baked beans

These homemade baked beans are a healthy alternative to most commercially prepared varieties that contain high levels of sodium. Beans are a major source of dietary fibre, protein, iron and B vitamins. Tomatoes are an excellent source of vitamin A and C, and the antioxidant lycopene.

1 small onion, diced

1 clove garlic, crushed

440 g (15½ oz/2 cups) kidney beans or black eyed peas, rinsed well

400 g (14 oz/2 cups) can tomatoes

1 tablespoon raw organic honey

1 tablespoon lemon juice

1 teaspoon tamari (wheat-free)

2 tablespoons chopped fresh parsley

¼ teaspoon dried thyme

Preheat oven to 180°C (350°F/Gas 4). Lightly spray a casserole dish with olive oil.

Cook beans in a large saucepan of boiling water, according to legume cooking chart.

Lightly spray a frying pan with olive oil and place over a medium heat. Add onion and garlic and cook until tender.

Blend tomatoes, honey, lemon juice and tamari together. Transfer to a casserole dish then add beans, onion, garlic, parsley and thyme, stir until combined.

Bake with the lid on for 40 minutes, stirring occasionally. Add more tomato if beans are too dry, or cook for a further 15 minutes (with the lid off) if beans are too moist.

Serve on wholegrain toast, topped with some grated cheese.

Serves 4.

Serving suggestions: Use as a topping for baked potatoes.

Breakfast cups

Your kids will love these scrumptious breakfast cups packed with protein, fibre and B vitamins. Ideal for breakfast or a quick snack on the run.

12 slices wholegrain bread (GF: gluten-free bread)

300g tin low-sodium baked beans (drain off excess liquid)

¼ cup grated low-fat cheese (LF: vegan cheese)

2 eggs

½ cup low-fat milk (LF: rice, almond, soy or lactose-free milk)

Preheat oven to 200°C (400°F/Gas 6). Lightly grease a 12-hole muffin tray with olive oil.

Cut crusts off bread and place one slice in each hole, pressing down into hole.

Spoon baked beans into each cup.

Whisk eggs and milk together in a small bowl. Pour mixture over each cup.

Sprinkle each cup with cheese and cook for 25 minutes, or until bread is crisp and filling is set and golden brown.

Makes 12.

Breakfast eggs

Eggs make a quick, nutritious meal anytime of the day. Eggs can be enjoyed in a variety of different ways, boiled with toast soldiers, as an omelet or frittata, and scrambled or poached. Eggs are a wonderful source of protein, iron, zinc and B vitamins. Choose free-range organic eggs as they are generally higher in omega-3 fats and are free from antibiotics and other chemicals fed to or injected in chickens.

Perfect poached eggs: Bring to boil 1½ litres (52½ fl oz) of water in a deep frying pan and add 2 tablespoons of vinegar (this will prevent the eggs from spreading too much in the water). Reduce to a simmer then gently stir the water. Break each egg into a cup and slide egg from cup into the middle of the water. Poach for 4 minutes, until eggs are set then remove with a slotted spoon. Use fresh eggs that have plump whites that cling to the yolk, they will hold together better. Serve poached eggs with piece of wholegrain toast or a small bowl of baked beans, roast tomato or avocado slices.

Boiled eggs with toast soldiers: Place whole eggs in a saucepan of boiling water. Simmer for 10 minutes and drain. Serve with wholegrain toast soldiers with a drizzling of flaxseed oil. Boil a couple of extra eggs for school lunches (use for egg sandwiches, egg salad or pack an egg in its shell for a protein snack).

Egg in the hole: With an egg ring press a hole out of the middle of a slice of wholegrain bread. Lightly spray a frying pan with olive oil and place it over medium heat. Place bread in frying pan and crack an egg into the hole. Cook until egg starts to set then flip and cook for another couple of minutes.

Scrambled eggs: Break 2 eggs into a small bowl. Add 2 tablespoons of milk and whisk until well combined. Lightly spray a frying pan with olive oil and place over low-medium heat. Pour egg mixture into frying pan and gently stir with a wooden spoon until eggs are cooked and fluffy. Serve on wholegrain toast with a drizzling of flaxseed oil. Serves 1-2. **Variation**: Add a small handful of baby spinach, diced tomato or finely chopped fresh parsley to mixture.

Fluffy omelet: Whisk 1 egg yolk and 2 tablespoons of milk together in a small bowl. In another bowl, beat 2 egg whites until soft peaks form. Fold yolk mixture and 1 teaspoon fresh parsley into egg whites. Lightly spray a frying pan with olive oil and place over a medium heat. Pour egg mixture into frying pan and cook for a couple of minutes on one side, then flip and cook until omelet is cooked through and tender. Makes 1 fluffy omelet. **Variation:** Add nutritious fillings such as spinach, onion, tomato, mushroom, corn kernels, grated low-fat cheese, tinned salmon or tuna, grated zucchini or fresh basil to the centre of omelet then fold in half.

Breakfast frittata

This tasty frittata is so easy to make and very versatile. Get creative and use any combination of toppings you like. Leftovers make great school lunches or a filling for wraps.

½ cup (100 g/3½ oz) corn kernels (fresh or frozen)

¼ cup (40 g/1½ oz) peas (fresh or frozen)

4 eggs

¼ cup (63 ml/2¼ fl oz) low-fat milk (LF: rice, almond, soy or lactose-free milk)

1 small onion, finely diced

Handful baby spinach

3 cherry tomatoes, halved

¼ cup (30 g/1 oz) grated low-fat cheddar cheese (LF: vegan cheese)

In a small saucepan of water, cook corn kernels and peas for 3-4 minutes until tender.

Place eggs and milk in a small bowl and whisk until well combined. Stir through spinach.

Lightly spray a frying pan with olive oil and place over medium heat. Add onion and cook until tender.

Pour egg mixture into frying pan and cook for 3-4 minutes.

Spread corn, tomato and cheese over the top of frittata. Place frying pan under a griller for 2 minutes, until frittata is golden brown and cheese melted.

Place frittata on a chopping board and cut into triangles.

Serves 4.

Variation: Add diced cooked potato or sweet potato.

Blueberry buttermilk pancakes

These light and fluffy pancakes make a lovely breakfast or after school snack. Blueberries are an excellent source of antioxidants and vitamin C. Leftovers freeze well for lunch box treats. Pop pancakes in the toaster the next day to warm them up.

1 cup (120 g/4½ oz) wholemeal flour (GF: gluten-free plain flour)

1¼ teaspoon baking powder (GF: gluten-free baking powder)

¼ teaspoon baking soda

1 tablespoon raw organic honey

1 cup (250 ml/9 fl oz) low-fat buttermilk (LF: rice, almond, soy or lactose-free milk)

1 tablespoon lemon juice

1 egg

1 cup (150 g/5¼ oz) blueberries (or diced strawberries, banana, peach or pear)

Combine all dry ingredients together in a small bowl.

In another bowl combine liquid ingredients and whisk until well combined.

Make a well in dry ingredients and slowly pour liquid mixture into dry mix, stirring gently until combined. Don't worry if mixture has a few lumps. Over stirring mixture will result in tough pancakes.

Cut fruit into small dices and gently stir through mixture.

Lightly spray a frying pan with olive oil and place over medium heat. Pour spoonfuls of mixture into pan and cook for 2 minutes or until pancake bubbles. Flip and cook for another couple of minutes, until fluffy and cooked through.

Makes 10 medium sized pancakes.

Sweet topping suggestions: Berry puree (you can use frozen raspberries); date or prune spread; sliced fruit; fruit yoghurt; or stewed fruit.

Savoury variation: Replace blueberries and honey with ½ cup (100 g/3½ oz) corn kernels and 2 tablespoons finely sliced shallots. Add ¼ cup (30 g/1 oz) grated low-fat cheese (LF: vegan cheese). Top with avocado.

Tasty toast

When eaten with nutritious toppings, toast can provide a complete, wholesome meal. Wholegrain bread is an excellent source of dietary fibre and energy giving, complex carbohydrates. Choose from a variety of breads: wholemeal, multigrain, rye, spelt, soy and linseed, sourdough, fruit and nut, wholemeal muffins and crumpets, or brown rice and other gluten-free breads.

Flaxseed oil: Flaxseed oil is a healthy alternative to butter or margarine that should be limited in a child's diet. Butter and margarine are a commonly consumed source of unhealthy saturated fats. Flaxseed oil is a rich source of omega-3 fats that are essential for proper brain development and cardiovascular health. Avocado and hummus can also be used as a nutritious substitute. Drizzle 1-2 teaspoons of flaxseed oil on toast.

Toast toppings

- Avocado.

- Hummus.

- Cottage cheese with slices of avocado or tomato.

- Cottage cheese with crushed walnuts and apple slices.

- Baked beans (homemade or tinned salt-reduced).

- Leftover spaghetti.

- Eggs: poached, boiled, scrambled or lightly fried in olive oil.

- Tuna melt: sprinkle of low-fat cheese, flaked tuna and tomato slices.

- Salmon flakes with low-fat cream cheese.

- Low-fat ricotta, banana slices and raw organic honey.

- Mashed banana, sultanas and chopped nuts.

- Fruit bread with nut butter or tahini and a little raw organic honey.

- Almond spread with sliced banana.

- Small amount of date spread with sliced banana, sprinkled with LSA.

Variation: For lactose-free options replace cheese with vegan cheese.

Dips, sauces, salad dressings & chutneys

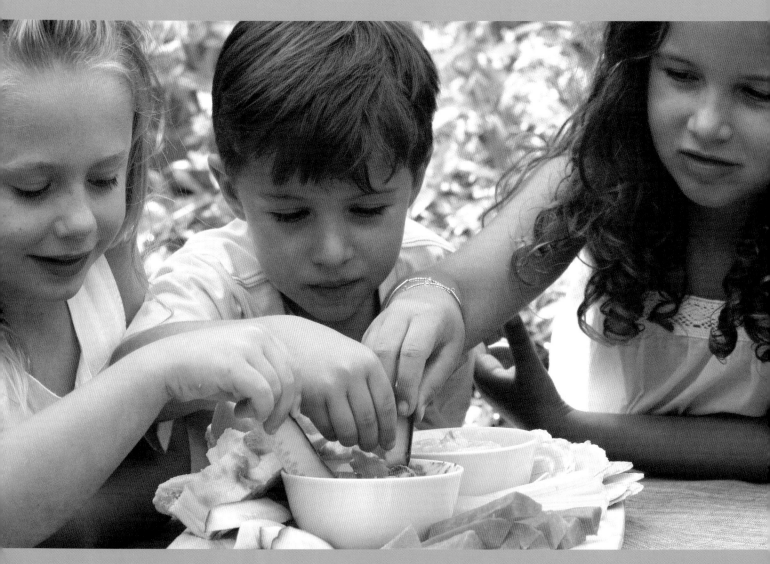

Give meals a flavoursome boost, or turn a boring sandwich into a tasty treat, with these nutritious condiments. These quick and easy recipes will not only add extra flavour to your kid's meals but will also contribute nutritionally to their diet. Most commercially made dips, sauces, salad dressings and chutneys are full of salt, sugar and saturated fats.

Dips & dippers

Your kids will love dipping vegie sticks, crisp breads, crackers and wedges into these nutritious, easy to prepare dips. Packed with healthy ingredients these dips are a great way to include extra legumes and vegetables into your child's diet. These dips can also be used as tasty spreads for toast, burgers, sandwiches, wraps or rice cakes.

Wholesome hummus

This popular Middle Eastern dip made from chickpeas and tahini is rich in protein, dietary fibre and monounsaturated fats. Making your own hummus is so quick and easy and much cheaper than buying it from the supermarket.

2 x 440g (15½ oz) cans chickpeas, drained

2 cloves garlic, crushed

¼ cup (63 ml/2¼ fl oz) lemon juice

¼ cup (63 g/2¼ oz) tahini

2 tablespoons cold pressed extra virgin olive oil or flaxseed oil

Pinch sea salt

1 teaspoon finely chopped fresh parsley or basil

Place all ingredients in a blender and mix until smooth.

If hummus is too firm add a little water.

Store in an airtight container in the fridge for up to 1 week.

Makes 3 cups.

Variation: For a spicy capsicum hummus, add ½ roasted red capsicum and ½ tablespoon cumin. If using dried chickpeas refer to legume cooking chart.

Baba ghanoush

This wonderful Middle Eastern dip contains is a good source of protein and calcium. Immune boosting garlic will help fight off colds and flu during the winter months. This dip makes a lovely spread for wraps and burgers.

1 large eggplant

2 cloves garlic, crushed

¼ cup (63 g/2¼ oz) natural or Greek yoghurt (LF: lactose-free yoghurt)

2 tablespoons tahini

1 tablespoon lemon juice

½ teaspoon ground cumin

¼ teaspoon ground paprika

Pinch sea salt

Preheat oven to 200°C (400*F/Gas 6). Line a baking tray with baking paper.

Cut eggplant into large pieces. Place eggplant and whole cloves of garlic on baking tray and bake for 20 minutes or until eggplant is tender.

When eggplant has cooled remove skin. Place all ingredients in a blender and mix until smooth.

Store in airtight container in the fridge for up 5 days.

Makes 3 cups.

Guacamole

This marvellous Mexican dip made with avocados and tomatoes is packed with healthy monounsaturated fats, vitamins C and antioxidants. Serve guacamole as a dip, filling for baked potato jackets or as a topping for tacos and nachos.

3 ripe avocados, diced

1 clove garlic, crushed

Juice of 1 lime

½ red onion, finely chopped

2 tomatoes, finely diced

2 tablespoons finely chopped fresh coriander

In a medium bowl, combine avocado, garlic and lime with a fork.

Fold in onion, tomato and coriander.

Store in an airtight container in the fridge for up to 1 week.

Makes 4 cups.

Beetroot & cumin dip

Beetroot is such a richly coloured vegetable that brightens up any dish. Beetroots contain powerful antioxidants which help prevent free radical damage in the body. They are also a good source of vitamin C, iron and magnesium. Your kids are going to love this brightly coloured, tasty dip. Ideal spread on sandwiches, wraps and burgers.

4 medium beetroots

2 clove garlic, crushed

3 tablespoons lemon juice

1 tablespoon cold pressed flaxseed or extra virgin olive oil

1 cup (250 ml/9 fl oz) natural or Greek yoghurt (LF: lactose-free yoghurt)

½ teaspoon ground coriander

½ teaspoon ground cumin

½ teaspoon paprika

Boil or bake beetroots until tender.

Boil: Scrub beetroots and cut stems off (leaving a little stem attached). Place in boiling water and cook for around 45 minutes, until tender.

Bake: Preheat oven to 200°C (400*F/Gas 6). Scrub beetroots and wrap individually in foil. Roast for around 1 hour, until tender.

When beetroots have cooled, peel. Skin should rub off easily. You can use rubber gloves for this part as it can get a little messy.

Place cooled beetroots in a blender and process until finely grated.

Add in the remaining ingredients and blend until well mixed.

Store in an airtight container in the fridge for up to 1 week.

Makes approximately 3 cups.

Variations: Add 2 tablespoons of crushed macadamias or walnuts. For a smoother dip add more yoghurt and blend well.

Tzatziki

Tzatziki is a traditional Greek appetizer made from yoghurt, cucumber and garlic. This lovely, light dip contains immune boosting ingredients along with protein and calcium. This dip goes perfectly with curries, or served as a sauce over steamed cauliflower, carrots or roast potatoes.

2 cups finely chopped cucumber
1 clove garlic, crushed
1 tablespoon lemon juice
¾ cup (189 g/6¾ oz) natural or Greek yoghurt (LF: lactose-free yoghurt)

Finely chop cucumber, drain any excess liquid.

Combine all ingredients together in a bowl. For a smooth dip process all ingredients in a blender.

Store in an airtight container in the fridge for up to 5 days.

Makes 2½ cups.

Raw vegetable dippers

What better way of eating vegetables than fresh, raw and crunchy. This is a great way of getting your kids to eat more vegetables, they will love dipping them in their favourite dip. Keep a snack lunch box in the fridge with a combination of these vegie sticks and dip, or pack some in your child's lunch box.

Choose a combination of the following vegetables:
Celery, carrot, zucchini, cucumber, capsicum, snow peas or small broccoli florets
Apple, firm pear slices

Thoroughly wash vegetables. Peel carrots, trim sugar snap peas and lightly stream broccoli. Cut vegetables into thick sticks. Arrange on a plate and serve with your child's favourite dips.

Cut apples into thick wedges and squeeze a little lemon juice over them, to prevent them from going brown. If using organic apples, wash and leave the skin on, otherwise scrub apple well before cutting.

Toasted flat bread chips

These crispy dippers are ideal to serve with dip, soup, nachos, dahl or curries. These baked, flat breads contain monounsaturated fats, making them a healthy alternative to corn chips that are high in salt and saturated and trans-fats.

2 pita bread, tortillas or Lebanese bread (GF: gluten-free flat bread)

2 tablespoons cold pressed virgin olive oil

1 clove garlic, crushed

2 teaspoons dried herbs (basil, thyme, turmeric, paprika, oregano or chives)

Preheat oven to 180°C (350°C/Gas 4). Line a baking tray with baking paper.

Cut bread into wedges and lay on baking tray.

In a small bowl combine olive oil and garlic and brush each piece lightly, then sprinkle with herbs.

Bake for 5-10 minutes until crisp and golden. Serve or store in an airtight container. Serves 2-4.

Baked sweet potato wedges

Potato wedges are always a favourite with kids. Oven baking them with a little olive oil makes them a healthy alternative to deep fried wedges that are high in saturated and trans-fats. Sweet potatoes are an excellent source of beta-carotene, vitamin C, complex carbohydrates and dietary fibre. Serve them with a healthy dip or dipping sauce. You can use a combination of different root vegetables such as potatoes, carrots and parsnips for a variety of colour and flavour.

2 medium sweet potatoes

1 teaspoon ground paprika

2 tablespoons cold pressed virgin olive oil

Preheat oven to 220°C (425°C/Gas 7). Line a baking tray with baking paper.

Peel sweet potato and cut into half, lengthways. Cut into thick wedges. If you're using organic sweet potatoes you can leave the skins on.

Lightly coat wedges in olive oil and paprika and then bake for 40-45 minutes or until golden brown and cooked through. Shake pan occasionally and turn wedges after 25 minutes. Serves 2-4.

Cheese & sesame crackers

These tasty cheese and sesame crackers are fantastic served with dips or on their own. A healthy alternative to a lot of crackers on the market today that are high in sodium and unhealthy fats.

1 cup (120 g/4¼ oz) wholemeal or spelt flour
(GF: gluten-free plain flour)

½ cup (30 g/1 oz) grated low-fat cheddar cheese
(LF: vegan cheese)

1 egg

¼ cup (63 ml/2 fl oz) cold pressed virgin olive oil

1 tablespoon dried basil or chives

2 tablespoons sesame seeds

Preheat oven to 180°C (350°F/Gas 4). Line a slice tray with baking paper.

Place all ingredients (except seeds) in a blender and mix until smooth.

Press mixture into slice tray and mark out squares with a knife. Sprinkle with seeds. Bake for 25-30 minutes until golden brown.

Allow crackers to cool. Cut into squares and serve.

Store crackers in the fridge in an airtight container.

Avocado spread

Rich in monounsaturated fats, avocado is also a good source of vitamin E and many of the B vitamins. This rich, creamy spread makes a wonderful healthy alternative to butter, spread on toast, sandwiches, burgers or wraps. This spread can also be used as a dip or as a topping for baked potatoes.

1 ripe avocado

¼ cup (63 g/2¼ oz) natural or Greek yoghurt
(LF: lactose-free yoghurt)

½ teaspoon finely chopped fresh mint

1 tablespoon lemon juice

1 tablespoon cold pressed flaxseed oil

Place all ingredients in a blender and mix until smooth.

Keep in the fridge for up to 1 week.

Makes 1 cup.

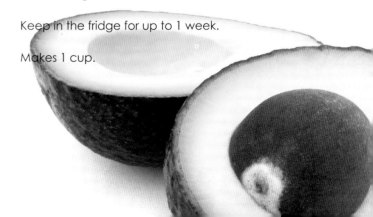

Almond spread

Packed with protein, calcium and beneficial unsaturated fats this nutritious spread is perfect on toast, crackers, puffed rice cakes and muffins. This spread can also be used in dishes such as pad Thai, and used to make salad dressings and sauces. Add a tablespoon of almond spread to muffin, cookie and cake mixtures for added goodness.

300g (10 ½ oz/1 ¾ cup) roasted, unsalted almonds (or walnuts, pecans, cashews or hazelnuts)

½ cup (125 ml/4½ fl oz) cold pressed virgin olive oil or flaxseed oil

Place all ingredients in a blender and mix until smooth.

Keep in an airtight container in the fridge for up to 4 weeks.

Date or prune spread

This delicious, sweet spread is perfect on muffins, pancakes, scones or toast. You can add a tablespoon of this spread to cookie, muffin or muesli bar mixes to give extra sweetness. A little date spread can also be used to sweeten porridge or natural yoghurt. Remember dried fruits are a concentrated source of natural sugar - so don't overdo it.

2 cups (350 g/12¼ oz) sun-dried dates or prunes, pitted

2 cups (500 ml/17¾ fl oz) water

Place dates and water in a small saucepan. Heat gently for 10 min, mash and stir continually until soft and well blended.

This spread can be stored in an airtight container in the fridge for up to 2 weeks.

Fresh tomato sauce

This flavoursome sauce is a healthy alternative to many commercial tomato sauces that are high in salt and added sugar. Tomatoes are an excellent source of lycopene, a powerful antioxidant that helps protect against cancer and heart disease. Tomatoes are also a good source of vitamins A and C. Use this sauce to liven up barbequed meats and burgers or as a base for baked beans or pasta dishes.

3 x 400g (42 oz/6 cups) cans tomatoes
2 tablespoons tomato paste
2 onions, finely diced
1 carrot, finely diced
2 celery sticks, finely diced
1 tablespoon cold pressed virgin olive oil
1 tablespoon lemon juice
4 cloves garlic, crushed
Pinch sea salt and pepper
1 tablespoon finely chopped fresh basil
1 tablespoon finely chopped fresh parsley
¼ teaspoon dried oregano
¼ teaspoon dried thyme
1 tablespoon corn flour (cornstarch) or arrowroot

In a large saucepan over medium heat, sauté onion and garlic in olive oil.

Add diced vegetables and cook for 5 minutes.

Add tomato paste, lemon, herbs, sea salt and pepper then simmer for an hour, stirring occasionally.

For a thicker sauce, mix corn flour with 3 tablespoons of water to make a smooth paste. Add to sauce and keep stirring until thicker consistency reached.

For a smoother texture, place sauce in a blender and mix until sauce is a smooth consistency.

This sauce keeps well in the fridge for up to 10 days or can be frozen for later use.

Makes 8 cups.

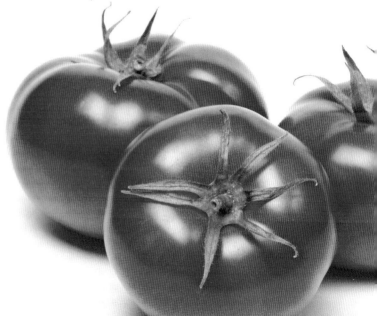

Pesto sauce

This fantastic Italian sauce is rich in healthy unsaturated fats and is a good source of protein, calcium and immune boosting garlic. Pesto can enrich a variety of dishes such as pasta, lasagna, grilled vegetables or bruschetta. For added flavour spread a little pesto on sandwiches, wraps or burgers.

2 cloves garlic, crushed

1 tablespoon finely grated low-fat parmesan cheese (LF: vegan cheese)

2 tablespoons cold pressed flaxseed oil or olive oil

3 tablespoons lemon juice

2 tablespoons pine nuts

150 g (5¼ oz/3 cups) fresh basil leaves

Place ingredients in a blender and mix until well combined.

Keep in an airtight container in the fridge for up to a week.

Creamy mayonnaise

This light and creamy low-fat mayonnaise contains healthy unsaturated fats and immune boosting garlic and yoghurt. Use as a spread for sandwiches, burgers and wraps. This mayonnaise makes a lovely potato or pasta salad, and don't forget the old favourite, egg and mayo sandwiches.

1 teaspoon Dijon mustard

1½ tablespoons lemon juice

1 small garlic clove, crushed

¼ cup (63 g/2¼ oz) natural or Greek yoghurt (LF: lactose-free yoghurt)

Pinch sea salt

2 tablespoons cold pressed flaxseed or extra virgin olive oil

In a small bowl whisk mustard, lemon juice, garlic, yoghurt and sea salt, until well combined.

Slowly pour oil into mixture, whisking until mayonnaise thickens and looks creamy.

Any excess can be stored in an airtight container in the fridge for up to a week.

Makes ½ cup.

Beetroot chutney

This vibrant, red chutney has a wonderful sweet and slightly fruity flavour, making it a perfect accompaniment to salads, sandwiches and burgers. Beetroot is an excellent source of complex carbohydrates, dietary fibre, vitamin C and antioxidants.

4 medium beetroots

1 medium onion, finely sliced

1 medium apple, peeled and finely sliced

2 teaspoons raw organic honey

⅓ cup (83 ml/3 fl oz) apple cider vinegar

2 tablespoons lemon juice

1 teaspoon finely grated fresh ginger

1 clove garlic, crushed

Pinch sea salt

Remove stems from beetroot (leave a little stem so the beetroot doesn't bleed). In a saucepan of boiling water cook whole unpeeled beetroots for 40 minutes.

When beetroots are cooked allow them to cool. Peel and then slice into thin small strips. Use gloves for this part as it can be a little messy.

Place all ingredients in a saucepan over medium heat. Bring to boil and then let simmer for 40 minutes covered, stirring occasionally.

When the chutney is cooked pour carefully into sterilized jars. Immediately seal jars with lids and allow chutney to cool. Chutney keeps well in the fridge for 2 weeks.

Mango chutney

This sweet and spicy chutney is traditionally used in Indian cuisine served with curries and rice. Mangoes are an excellent source of vitamin C and beta-carotene. This chutney can be used as a spread for burgers or sandwiches, or to spice up a stir-fry or homemade pizza.

2 large mangoes

1 medium onion, finely sliced

3 tablespoons finely chopped red capsicum

¼ - ½ teaspoon chilli powder

½ teaspoon finely grated fresh ginger

1 clove of garlic, crushed

¼ cup (63 ml/2¼ fl oz) apple cider vinegar

¼ cup (63 ml/2¼ fl oz) lemon juice

Place ingredients in a saucepan and bring to boil slowly. Cover and simmer for 25 minutes until chutney thickens, stirring occasionally.

Pour carefully into sterilized jars, immediately seal with lids and allow chutney to cool.

Chutney keeps well in the fridge for 2 weeks.

Tahini dressing

This delicious, smooth and creamy dressing made from sesame seed paste contains beneficial unsaturated fats, calcium and protein. Use as a tasty spread for sandwiches, burgers and wraps, or drizzle over salads and vegetables.

¼ cup (63 ml/2¼ fl oz) tahini

¼ cup (63 g/2¼ oz) natural or Greek yoghurt (LF: lactose-free yoghurt)

2 tablespoons lemon juice

2 small garlic cloves, crushed

1 tablespoon cold pressed flaxseed or extra virgin olive oil

1 teaspoon raw organic honey

Pinch sea salt

1 tablespoon finely chopped fresh parsley

1 tablespoon finely chopped fresh basil

In a small bowl whisk all ingredients together until well combined.

Any excess can be stored in an airtight container in the fridge for up to a week.

Makes ½ cup.

Citrus dressing

This tangy salad dressing with a hint of orange is a fantastic way to liven up any salad. This light, healthy dressing works beautifully through bean and beetroot salads.

¼ cup (63 ml/2¼ fl oz) orange juice, freshly squeezed

3 tablespoons apple cider vinegar

1 tablespoon cold pressed flaxseed oil or extra virgin olive oil

2 teaspoons Dijon mustard

Place all ingredients together in a jar and shake until well combined

Any excess dressing can be stored in the fridge for up to a week.

Makes ½ cup.

Vinaigrette herb dressing

This tasty salad dressing can bring any garden salad to life. The apple cider vinegar and lemon juice in this dressing stimulates the production of stomach acids, which helps to improve your digestion.

3 tablespoons cold pressed flaxseed oil or extra virgin olive oil

½ teaspoon tamari (wheat-free)

½ cup (125 m/4½ fl oz) lemon juice

3 tablespoons apple cider vinegar

1 small clove garlic, crushed

1 tablespoon finely chopped fresh herbs (chives, basil or parsley)

Place all ingredients in a jar and shake until well combined.

Any excess dressing can be stored in the fridge for up to a week.

Makes 1 cup.

Wholegrain mustard dressing

This wholegrain mustard dressing is delightful tossed through a garden, roast vegetable or pasta salad.

3 tablespoons cold pressed flaxseed or extra virgin olive oil

2 tablespoons white wine vinegar

3 tablespoons lemon juice

1 heaped teaspoon wholegrain mustard

1 small clove garlic, crushed

2 teaspoons finely chopped fresh parsley

Place all ingredients in a jar and shake until well combined.

Any excess dressing can be stored in the fridge for up to a week.

Makes ½ cup.

Sweet dessert sauces

Here are some healthy alternatives to sugary syrups and dessert sauces. These mouth-watering sauces make delicious toppings for ice cream, pancakes, scones, fruit salads and other desserts. Any excess sauce can be stored for up to a week in the fridge or frozen for later use.

Toasted banana cream: This nutritious topping will add extra protein, calcium and fibre to a meal. Use as a topping for muffins, banana bread, fruit salads or other desserts. It also makes a delicious addition to muesli and porridge. Preheat oven to 200°C (400°C/Gas 6). Line a baking tray with baking paper. Peel 2 large ripe bananas and cook for 20 minutes. Let bananas cool then mash in a small bowl with 2½ cups (625 g/22 oz) natural yoghurt (LF: lactose-free yoghurt), then serve. Makes 3 ½ cups.

Almond cream: This delicious dairy-free cream is thickened with agar-agar, a type of seaweed which acts like a vegetarian gelatin. Heat ½ cup (125 ml/4½ fl oz) almond milk and 1 teaspoon vanilla essence in a small saucepan. In a cup add a little milk to 1 teaspoon of agar-agar powder and stir until dissolved. Add to saucepan and stir until milk starts to thicken. Remove from heat and then stir in 1 teaspoon of raw honey. Keep cream in the fridge until ready to use. Makes ½ cup.

Orange and mango sauce: This sweet and tangy dessert sauce is rich in vitamin C, beta-carotene and antioxidants. Place 1 mango and ½ cup (125 ml/4½ fl oz) freshly squeezed orange juice together in a blender and mix until smooth and well combined. Makes 1cup.

Raspberry sauce: This sweet, richly coloured sauce is abundant in vitamin C and antioxidants, which help protect the body against cardiovascular disease and cancer. Blend 1½ cups (225 g/8¼ oz) raspberries (fresh or frozen) and 1 teaspoon raw organic honey together until well combined. Makes 1½ cups.

Apple and cranberry sauce: Cranberries give this sweet sauce a fresh, slightly tangy taste along with a vitamin C and antioxidant boost. In a saucepan over a medium heat, bring 1 cup (250 ml/9 fl oz) 100% apple juice slowly to boil. Add ½ cup (75 g/2¾ oz) cranberries, 3 grated apples and ½ teaspoon cinnamon. Reduce heat and cook for a further 10 minutes, stirring until fruit is tender and sauce has thickened. Remove from heat and stir through 2 tablespoons raw organic honey and allow to cool. Puree sauce in a blender. Makes 2 cups.

Salads

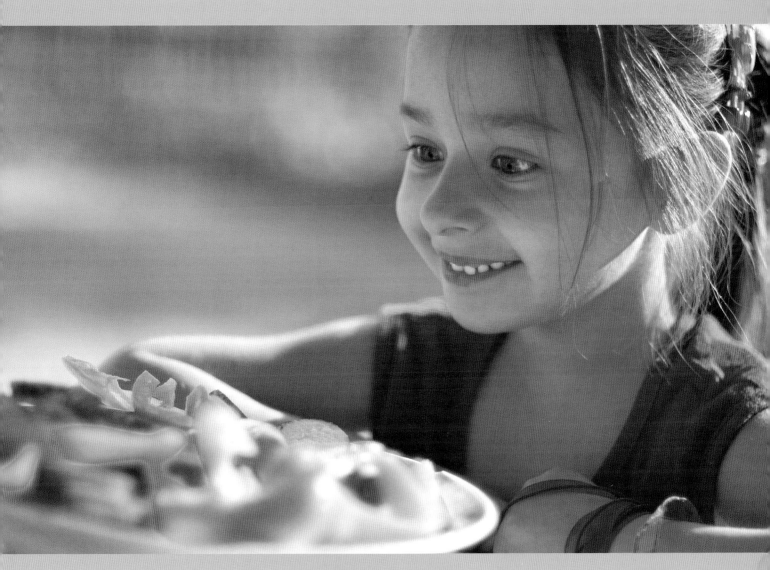

These fresh, healthy salads are jam packed with nutrients and are so versatile and easy to make. A complete
well-balanced meal on their own or perfect served as a delicious side dish. Grilled pieces of fish, meat, chicken or legumes can be tossed through any of these salads to increase their protein content. These salads are ideal for BBQs and picnics. Use leftovers to fill pita pockets and wraps for school lunches. Pack a small container of salad in your child's lunch box for a tasty change from sandwiches.

Lentil rice salad with minted yoghurt

Lentils are an excellent source of protein, dietary fibre and B vitamins. By combining lentils and rice together this salad becomes a 'complete' protein meal. This wonderful, light salad with a hint of lemon goes beautifully with pieces of tuna, salmon or chicken tossed through it. Serve hot or cold with warm wholemeal pita bread.

1 cup (250 g/9 oz) green lentils, rinse well

1 litre (35 fl oz/4 cups) salt-reduced vegetable stock

1 teaspoon ground cumin

1 teaspoon ground coriander

1 bay leaf

1 cup (185 g/6½ oz) brown basmati rice, rinse well

1 tablespoon sunflower seeds

3 tablespoons finely chopped leek or shallots

1 medium zucchini, diced

1 clove garlic, crushed

½ cup (100 g/3½ oz) corn kernels, canned

2 teaspoons organic lemon zest

Juice of ½ lemon

1 tablespoon cold pressed flaxseed or extra virgin olive oil

¼ cup (63 g/2¼ oz) tzatziki (refer to recipe)

Soak rice in water for 30 minutes before cooking (for improved texture and reduced cooking time). Then discard water.

Add vegetable stock to a large saucepan and bring to boil. Add lentils, cumin, coriander and bay leaf.

Reduce heat and simmer covered for 10 minutes.

Add rice to saucepan, cover and simmer for another 20 minutes, stirring occasionally. Add more water if needed.

Let stand covered for 10 minutes.

Lightly spray a frying pan with olive oil and place over medium heat. Add zucchini, corn, garlic, leek and sunflower seeds. Partially cook, then add rice and lentil mixture and gently combine.

Remove from heat and add lemon juice and zest, and flaxseed oil, then toss through salad.

Serve topped with tzatziki.

Serves 4.

Roast vegetable salad with tahini dressing

This colourful, earthy salad is superbly offset by a creamy tahini dressing. Tahini is a wonderful way of adding extra calcium, protein and good fats to your child's diet. This salad can be served warm or cold. Chickpeas can be tossed through to give an added protein boost.

1 large sweet potato

2 medium carrots

3 medium potatoes

1 small bunch broccoli

6 mushrooms

2 medium zucchini

3 tablespoons mixed pepitas (pumpkin seeds)

TAHINI DRESSING:

2 tablespoons tahini

1 tablespoon natural or Greek yoghurt (LF: lactose-free yoghurt)

2 teaspoons lemon juice

Pinch of sea salt

2 teaspoons raw organic honey

Preheat oven to 220°C (425°F/Gas 7). Line a baking tray with baking paper.

Wash and peel vegetables (leave skins on if using organic vegetables), cut into bite size pieces.

Place sweet potato, carrots and potatoes on baking tray.

Lightly spray vegetables with olive oil and bake for 20 minutes.

Add broccoli, mushrooms and zucchini. Bake for a further 15 minutes, until all vegetables cooked through and golden brown. Transfer to a bowl.

Mix dressing ingredients together in a small jar and shake until well combined.

When vegetables have cooled, gently toss through tahini dressing and sprinkle with pepitas.

Serves 4.

Variations: Add chickpeas, or grilled chicken, tuna or salmon pieces.

Cashew & turmeric rice salad

This vibrant, yellow salad is as pleasing to the eye as it is to the palate. Not only is this salad full of flavour, it's also full of nutrients such as energy giving carbohydrates, protein and good fats. Replace the eggs with grilled pieces of chicken or fish for a light summer's lunch or dinner. This salad can be served warm or cold. Pack leftovers in a cool thermos for school lunches.

1½ cups (278 g/9¾ oz) jasmine rice, rinse well

2 cups (500 ml/17¾ fl oz) salt-reduced vegetable stock

½ teaspoon ground turmeric

½ cup (100 g/3½ oz) corn kernels (fresh or frozen)

½ cup (80 g/3 oz) peas (fresh or frozen)

6 cherry tomatoes, halved

2 tablespoons shallots, finely chopped

Handful fresh herbs, roughly chopped

Pinch sea salt

Juice of ½ lemon

½ cup (85 g/3 oz) cashew nuts, raw and unsalted

2 hard boiled eggs, quartered

In a large saucepan add rice, vegetable stock and turmeric. Place over medium heat and bring to boil.

Reduce heat and simmer covered for 15 minutes until rice is tender and water absorbed.

Add corn and peas, and cook for another 3 minutes.

Transfer to a bowl and add lemon juice, herbs, shallots, sea salt, cashews and tomato. Gently combine all ingredients together then toss through egg quarters.

Serves 4.

Variations: Replace egg with 150 g (5¾ oz) grilled chicken breast, tuna, salmon or firm tofu.

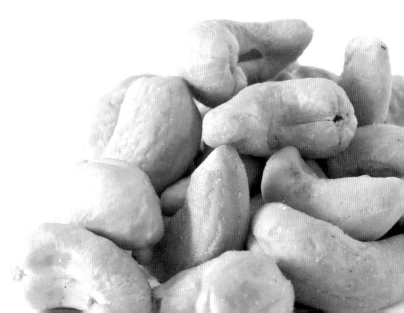

Bean tuna salad

This salad is a nutritious melody of beans, jam-packed with fibre, protein and B vitamins. Beans are also a good source of iron, needed for red blood cell production and healthy immune function.

½ cup (63 g/2¼ oz) green beans

440g (15 ½ oz) can 3 bean mix, drain and rinse

220g (7¾ oz) tin light tuna, drain

½ red capsicum, finely diced

½ cup (25 g/1 oz) chopped fresh herbs (coriander, basil or parsley)

¼ cup (63 ml/2¼ fl oz) citrus vinaigrette (refer to recipe)

Sesame seeds

Trim green beans and cut into small lengths.

Lightly steam green beans.

Combine all ingredients together in a bowl.

Add dressing and gently toss. Sprinkle with sesame seeds.

Serves 4.

Variation: Replace tuna with salmon, grilled chicken or firm tofu pieces.

Beetroot, pumpkin & goats cheese salad
with citrus dressing

This delightful beetroot salad has a lovely citrus flavour, teamed with smooth goat's cheese and crunchy walnuts. This salad will supply your child with complex carbohydrates, dietary fibre, protein, iron and calcium. The rich, red colour of beetroot indicates the presence of antioxidants that help protect the body against disease.

6 baby beetroots

300g (10½ oz) pumpkin, cut into small wedges

4 cups (320 g/11¼ oz) baby spinach

440g (15½ oz/2 cups) can chickpeas, drained

⅓ cup (100g/3½ oz) goat's cheese, crumbled (LF: vegan cheese)

¼ cup (45 g/1½ oz) walnut pieces

¼ cup (63 ml/2¼ fl oz) citrus salad dressing (refer to recipe)

Handful fresh mint, roughly chopped

Preheat oven to 220°C (400°F/Gas 6). Line a baking tray with baking paper.

Cut stems off beetroot, leaving skin on. Wrap each beetroot in foil and bake for 30 minutes.

Place pumpkin on baking tray and return both to oven for another 20 minutes, or until beetroot and pumpkin are cooked through.

Wait until beetroot has cooled, then rub off skin.

Place beetroot, pumpkin, spinach, chickpeas, and mint in a bowl and toss citrus vinaigrette through gently.

Top with crumbled goat's cheese and walnuts, then serve.

Serves 4.

Variation: If using dried chickpeas refer to legume cooking chart. Add cooked quinoa to salad for extra complex carbohydrates.

Potato salad with egg & fresh herbs

What would a BBQ or picnic be without potato salad? This salad is tossed with fresh herbs and a light, tangy mayonnaise rich in healthy omega-3 fats. Potatoes are a good source of complex carbohydrates. Eggs and seeds give this salad an extra protein boost.

4 large potatoes

1 tablespoon finely chopped shallots

1 tablespoon finely chopped fresh mint

1 tablespoon finely chopped fresh parsley

2 tablespoons toasted sunflower and sesame seeds

2 boiled eggs, diced

¼ cup (63 g/2¼ oz) creamy mayonnaise (refer to recipe)

Peel and wash potatoes. Cut into bite size pieces and steam until cooked through. Make sure potatoes are not overcooked and mushy. Transfer to a bowl and place in the fridge to cool.

Add shallots, mint, parsley, egg and seeds.

Gently stir mayonnaise through salad.

Serves 4.

Variation: Add a small tin of salmon or tuna, tin of legumes or shredded chicken.

Buckwheat tabouli

Buckwheat is a highly nutritious grain that is gluten-free and a good source of protein. This salad is made with parsley, which is an excellent source of iron, and garlic to help strengthen your child's immune system. Serve as a side dish with grilled meat, fish and chicken, or as a filler for pita pockets, wraps and burgers.

½ cup (100 g/3½ oz) cracked buckwheat, rinse well

3 tomatoes, chopped

¾ cup (120 g/4¼ oz) finely diced cucumber

3 cups (200 g/7 oz) finely chopped fresh parsley

1 cup (50 g/1¾ oz) finely chopped fresh mint

1 red onion, finely chopped

2 cloves garlic, crushed

⅓ cup (83 ml/3 fl oz) lemon or lime juice

2 tablespoons cold pressed flaxseed or extra virgin olive oil

Pinch sea salt

Bring 1 cup (250 ml/9 fl oz) of water to boil in a saucepan and add buckwheat. Turn down the heat, cover and simmer for 15-20 minutes.

Once buckwheat has cooked, transfer to a bowl and allow to cool.

Lightly mix cucumber, tomatoes, parsley, mint and onion through buckwheat.

Add garlic, lemon, oil and sea salt together in a small jar and shake until well combined, then toss through salad.

Variation: Replace buckwheat with burghul, quinoa, millet, couscous or brown rice (refer to grain cooking chart).

Chickpea, pineapple & tomato couscous salad

Packed with sweet, juicy pineapple and cherry tomatoes, this salad is a taste of the tropics in every mouthful. Couscous, a North African grain made from ground durum wheat, will supply your child with energy giving complex carbohydrates. This salad also boosts an array of nutrients including vitamin C, protein, calcium and B vitamins.

¾ cup (140 g/5 oz) couscous (GF: quinoa or millet)

¾ cup (188 ml/6½ fl oz) salt-reduced vegetable stock

220g (7¾ oz) can chickpeas, drained

Handful small cherry tomatoes, cut in half

3 thick slices fresh pineapple, cut into small pieces

¼ cup (43 g/1½ oz) blanched almonds

Juice of 1 lemon

Handful fresh parsley, finely chopped

Handful mint, finely chopped

In a small saucepan bring vegetable stock to boil and add couscous. Remove from heat, cover and let stand 5 minutes. Fluff with a fork before serving.

Transfer couscous to a bowl and allow to cool. Gently toss through chickpeas, tomatoes, pineapple, almonds, herbs and lemon juice.

Serves 4.

Variations: Add cooked chicken breast, salmon, tuna for added protein. If using dried chickpeas refer to legume cooking chart.

Carrot, apple & capsicum coleslaw

This tangy coleslaw is crunchy and light with a sweet apple twist. Cabbage is an excellent source of vitamin C, folate and antioxidants. Most commercially prepared coleslaw contains mayonnaise high in saturated fats and salt. This coleslaw is tossed with a low-fat mayonnaise rich in beneficial omega-3 fats.

2 cups (125 g/4½ oz) shredded cabbage

2 celery stalks, thinly sliced

¼ cup (40 g/1½ oz) thinly sliced red capsicum

1 cup (150 g/5¼ oz) grated carrot

¼ cup (30 g/1 oz) thinly sliced shallots or leek

2 tablespoons finely chopped fresh parsley

¼ cup (43 g/1½ oz) pecans, chopped

1 large apple, grated (leave skin on organic apples)

2 tablespoons orange juice, freshly squeezed

2 tablespoons lemon juice

½ cup (125 g/4½ oz) natural or Greek yoghurt (LF: lactose-free yoghurt)

In a large bowl combine cabbage, celery, capsicum, carrot, leek, parsley, pecans and apple.

In a jug add orange juice, lemon juice and yoghurt, whisk until well combined.

Lightly toss dressing through salad.

Serves 4.

Salmon & pesto pasta salad

This delicious creamy pasta salad is bursting with flavour and important nutrients such as omega-3 fats, protein and complex carbohydrates. Salmon is a rich source of omega-3 fats, essential for brain development and cardiovascular health. Salmon is also a good source of zinc and iron.

2 cups (180 g/6 oz) small wholemeal pasta shells (GF: gluten-free pasta shells)

½ cup (100 g/3½ oz) frozen corn kernels

220 g (7¾ oz) can salmon, drained with large bones removed

½ cup (80 g/3 oz) diced red capsicum

¼ cup (30 g/1 oz) finely chopped leek

2 tablespoon pine nuts

2 tablespoon natural yoghurt (LF: lactose-free yoghurt)

3 tablespoons pesto (refer to recipe)

Cook pasta in boiling water according to packet directions. Add frozen corn for the last 3 minutes of cooking.

Drain and allow pasta to cool.

Add flaked salmon, red capsicum, leek and pine nuts to pasta and gently toss.

In a jug add yoghurt and pesto, whisk until well combined.

Pour dressing over pasta and gently toss.

Serves 4.

Chicken salad with wholegrain dressing & baked crotons

This delicious chicken salad is topped with oven baked crotons and a wholegrain mustard dressing. This well-balanced salad will supply your kids with protein, healthy monounsaturated fats, calcium and complex carbohydrates.

2 thick slices wholemeal bread (GF: gluten-free bread)

2 teaspoons cold pressed virgin olive oil

1 small clove garlic, crushed

1 cos lettuce, roughly chopped

1 small red onion, finely sliced

2 boiled eggs, quartered

300g (10 ½ oz) chicken breast, strips

Handful fresh mint and parsley, chopped

½ cup (125 g/4½ oz) natural or Greek yoghurt (LF: lactose-free yoghurt)

3 tablespoons wholegrain mustard

2 tablespoons lemon juice

Preheat oven to 180°C (350°F/Gas 4). Line a baking tray with baking paper.

Lightly brush both sides of bread with olive oil.

Cut bread into squares and place on a baking tray, bake for 5 minutes until toasted and golden. Turn after 3 minutes.

Lightly spray a frying pan with olive oil and place over a medium heat. Cook chicken strips and garlic until golden and cooked through.

In a large bowl lightly toss lettuce, onion, chicken, herbs, toast squares and egg.

Whisk yoghurt, mustard and lemon juice together in a small bowl, drizzle over salad and gently toss.

Serves 4.

Char grilled beef & vegetable quinoa salad

This filling salad is a complete nutritious meal on its own. Quinoa has a unique, nutty flavour and provides energy giving complex carbohydrates and dietary fibre. This salad is also an excellent source of protein, iron and zinc.

1 cup (200 g/7 oz) quinoa, rinsed well

2 small zucchini's, sliced length ways

1 red capsicum, thickly sliced

¼ pumpkin, cut into slices

400g (14 oz) lean beef, strips

1 teaspoon tamari (wheat-free)

1 clove garlic, crushed

1 teaspoon finely grated fresh ginger

½ cup (25 g/1 oz) fresh basil and parsley, roughly chopped

½ organic lemon juice and zest

3 teaspoons sesame seeds

¾ cup (188 g/6½ oz) tzatziki (refer to recipe)

Bring 2 cups (500 ml/17¾ fl oz) of water to boil in a saucepan. Reduce heat then add quinoa. Cover and simmer for 15 minutes. Remove from heat and let stand for 5 min, then fluff with a fork.

While quinoa is cooking, lightly spray a frying pan with olive oil and place over medium heat. Cook vegetables in batches, then beef strips in tamari, garlic and ginger.

Transfer quinoa to a bowl and gently stir through mixed herbs, lemon juice and zest.

Gently toss vegetables and meat slices through quinoa.

Serve topped with a spoonful of tzatziki and a sprinkling of sesame seeds.

Variations: Use different grains such as couscous, millet or buckwheat (refer to grain cooking chart). Replace beef strips with lamb, chicken, fish, tofu or tempeh.

Winter soups

Winter wouldn't be the same without warm, wholesome soup. Served with wholegrain toast, these soups can make a meal on their own. Pack leftovers in a warm thermos with a crusty bread roll for school lunches, or freeze for future meals.

Lentil soup

This rich and nourishing lentil soup is perfect served with pita chips. Lentils are an excellent source of protein, fibre and B vitamins.

4 cups (1 Litre/35 fl oz) salt-reduced vegetable stock

2 cups (500 g/17¾ oz) red or green lentils, rinse well

2 onions, finely chopped

½ red capsicum, diced

1 carrot, diced

1 clove garlic, crushed

1 teaspoon finely grated fresh ginger

1 teaspoon ground cumin

2 bay leaves

Pinch marjoram and oregano

2 tablespoons red wine vinegar

Lentils do not need to be soaked before cooking.

In a large saucepan bring vegetable stock to boil.

Add all ingredients (except vinegar) and simmer covered for 45 minutes. Add more water if needed, however this soup should be thick.

Take soup off the heat, remove bay leaf and stir through vinegar.

Serve with either a dollop of natural yoghurt or a sprinkling of parmesan cheese.

Serves 2-4.

Pumpkin & leek soup

This hearty pumpkin soup is rich in beta-carotene, which is needed for good eyesight and healthy immune function. Top with some natural yoghurt to give this soup an added probiotic boost.

1 small leek or onion, finely slice

1 clove garlic, crushed

½ butternut pumpkin

3 cups (750 ml/26¼ fl oz) salt-reduced vegetable stock

2 tablespoons natural yoghurt (LF: lactose-free yoghurt)

Low-fat milk (LF: almond, soy or lactose-free milk) – optional

1 tablespoon chopped fresh parsley

Lightly spray a saucepan with olive oil then place over a medium heat. Add leek and garlic, cook until tender.

Add vegetable stock and bring to boil. Add pumpkin and simmer on low heat until pumpkin is soft and well cooked.

Blend soup until a smooth consistency. If you would like a thinner soup add some milk.

Serve with a spoonful of natural yoghurt stirred through the top and sprinkle with fresh parsley.

Serves 2-4.

Variations: Add 1½ teaspoons of basil, ½ teaspoon of oregano, a bay leaf or ½ teaspoon of curry powder.

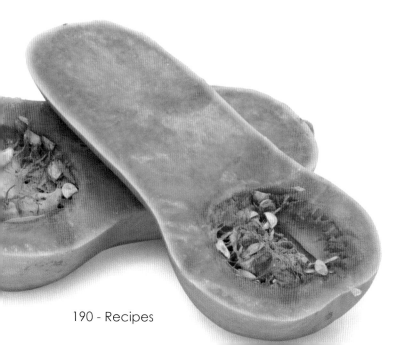

Minestrone soup

This classic soup is a favourite with the whole family. Packed with legumes, vegetables and wholemeal pasta this soup makes a hearty lunch or dinner. Tomatoes are rich in the phytochemical lycopene, which acts as a powerful antioxidant in the body. This soup is an ideal way of giving your child a variety of different vegetables, use any combination you like.

1 onion, finely diced

1 clove garlic, crushed

1 cup (160 g/5½ oz) diced carrots

1 cup (160 g/5½ oz) diced zucchini

1 cup (160 g/5½ oz) diced celery stalks

1 large potato, diced

1 cup (83 g/3 oz) diced green beans, trim and cut into short lengths

10 cups (2½ Litres/875 fl oz) salt-reduced vegetable stock

1 cup (100 g/3½ oz) canned bean mix, drained

400 g (14 oz/2 cups) can tomatoes, chopped

2 tablespoons tomato paste

1 tablespoon chopped fresh parsley

2 teaspoons dried mixed Italian herbs

¼ teaspoon ground thyme

3/4 cup (68 g/2½ oz) wholemeal pasta shapes (GF: gluten-free pasta)

Lightly spray a large saucepan with olive oil and place over a medium heat. Add onion and garlic and cook until tender.

Add vegetables, stock, legumes, tomatoes, tomato paste and herbs. Bring to boil, simmer covered for 40 minutes.

Add pasta and cook for a further 12 minutes.

Add more water if needed. For a thicker soup add 1 teaspoon of arrowroot or corn flour.

Serve with a sprinkling of parmesan cheese and fresh herbs.

Serves 2-4.

Variation: Add lamb or beef cubes for added iron and protein.

Carrot, orange & tomato soup

This brightly coloured orange soup is jam-packed with vitamin C, beta-carotene and antioxidants. This soup is beautifully complemented by the subtle sweetness of fresh orange juice.

1 onion, finely chopped

1 clove garlic, crushed

3 large carrots, chopped

3 medium ripe tomatoes, no skin

1 orange's juice

½ teaspoon ground cumin

½ teaspoon finely grated fresh ginger

1 cup (250 ml/9 fl oz) salt-reduced vegetable stock

Handful fresh parsley to garnish

Lightly spray a saucepan with olive oil and place over medium heat. Add garlic and onion, cook until tender.

Add remaining ingredients and bring to boil. Reduce heat and simmer covered, for 30 minutes.

Blend soup until smooth and well combined.

Serve topped with a spoonful of natural yoghurt and a sprinkling of parsley.

Serves 2-4.

Vegetable stock

This versatile vegetable stock is low in sodium and big on flavour. Commercial stocks are usually very high in salt and can contain MSG and other artificial additives. Use this stock to enrich the flavour of soups and other dishes from this book.

2 cloves garlic, crushed

1 large onion, roughly chopped

2 large carrots, sliced

3 stalk of celery, sliced

2 bay leaves

1 teaspoon black peppercorns

Pinch of sea salt

Large handful of parsley, roughly chopped

3 litres (105 fl oz/12 cups) water

Lightly spray a large saucepan with olive oil and place over a medium heat. Add garlic, onion, carrot and celery. Cook for 2 minutes until tender.

Add water, bay leaves, peppercorns, sea salt and parsley to saucepan and bring to the boil. Reduce heat, cover and simmer for 30 minutes.

Strain through a sieve and use. Leftover stock can be kept in an airtight container in the fridge for 3 days or frozen for later use.

Vegetable miso soup

Miso soup is a traditional Japanese soup made from fermented soy beans. This soup contains immune boosting miso, shiitake mushrooms, seaweed and garlic. Light but extremely nourishing, this soup is perfect for warding off colds and flu during the winter months. Serve a small bowl before a main meal or as a light winter's lunch. Add Asian noodles to this soup for extra complex carbohydrates.

¼ cup dried shiitake mushrooms, thin pieces

2 strips wakame or kombu seaweed

1 clove garlic, crushed

1 teaspoon fresh ginger, finely grated

1½ cups (113 g/4 oz) chopped vegetables (leek, onion, carrot, cabbage, turnips, potatoes or sweet potatoes)

5 cups (1¼ Litres/43¾ fl oz) water

3 tablespoons miso paste (gen mai)

Cut mushrooms and seaweed into small pieces. In a small bowl of boiling water, soak mushrooms and seaweed for 20 minutes.

Lightly spray a saucepan with olive oil and place over a medium heat. Cut seaweed into small pieces. Add garlic, ginger, seaweed, mushrooms and vegetables to pan, and cook for a couple of minutes.

Add water and bring to boil. Reduce heat and simmer covered for 10 minutes.

Cream miso in a little broth and return to soup. Do not overheat miso as it will destroy the active lactobacillus (beneficial bacteria). Remove from heat and garnish with sesame seeds and chives.

Serves 4.

Variation: Add small dices of firm organic tofu.

Green pea & potato soup

This vibrantly coloured soup has a wonderful creamy texture with lots of flavour. For children that love peas this recipe is a good way to sneak some extra green leafy vegetables into their diet. This soup provides dietary fibre, vitamin C, B vitamins and antioxidants. Try adding some grated zucchini, broccoli or a small tin of legumes to this soup.

1 clove garlic, crushed

2 tablespoons finely chopped leek

2 cups (500 ml/17¾ fl oz) salt-reduced vegetable stock

3 cups (465 g/16¼ oz) peas (fresh or frozen)

2 small potatoes

1 cup (63 g/2¼ oz) shredded spinach

½ cup (40 g/1½ oz) shredded white cabbage

1 stalk of celery, finely sliced

1 tablespoon chopped fresh mint

1 tablespoon chopped fresh parsley

⅓ cup (83 ml/3 fl oz) low-fat milk (LF: almond, soy or lactose-free milk)

Lightly spray a large saucepan with olive oil and place over a medium heat. Add leek and garlic, cook for 1-2 minutes until tender.

Add vegetable stock, peas, potato, spinach, cabbage, celery and herbs to pot. Bring to boil and simmer covered for 20 minutes. Add more water if needed.

Add milk and blend until smooth and well combined.

Serve topped with a spoonful of natural yoghurt and a sprinkling of sesame seeds and fresh herbs.

Serves 2-4.

Variation: For a pea and ham soup, add 1 thick slice of leg ham, diced (nitrite-free).

Baked goods & party treats

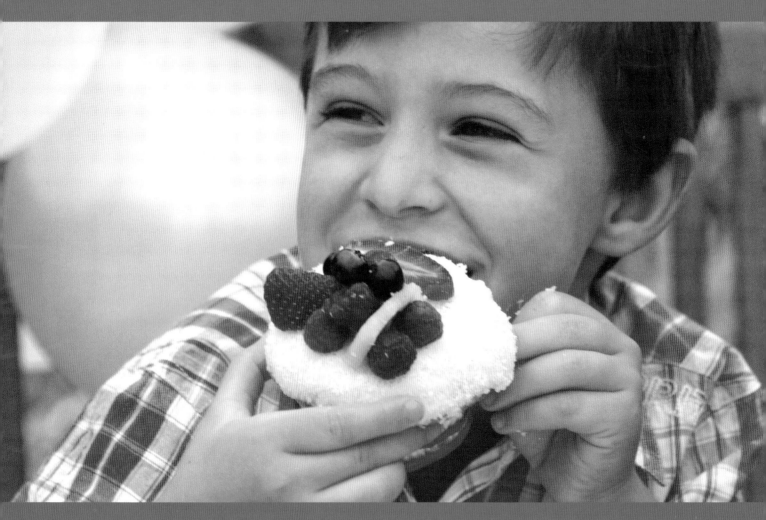

There's nothing better than coming home from school to the smell of freshly baked muffins. Packed with energy giving complex carbohydrates and dietary fibre these goodies are a great way to increase your child's fruit intake. These wholesome recipes are a healthy alternative to commercial baked goods that are generally high in saturated fats, trans-fats and refined sugars. These recipes use olive oil (rich in healthy monounsaturated fats) instead of butter, and are naturally sweetened with raw honey and fruit. So simple and easy to make, these baked goodies make perfect party treats or healthy snacks. Try heating up a muffin with custard for dessert, or freeze leftovers for lunch box treats.

Vanilla coconut icing

This is a healthy alternative to commercially prepared icing that is made basically of sugar. You still get the same delicious icing effect and taste without all the calories. Add some carob powder for a chocolate-like icing or some passionfruit for a fruity flavour.

1½ cups (375 ml/13¼ fl oz) low-fat milk (LF: rice, almond, soy or lactose-free milk)

1 vanilla bean

1 tablespoon tapioca flour or agar-agar

½ cup (80 g/2¾ oz) desiccated coconut

2 teaspoons raw organic honey

Using a sharp knife slice vanilla bean in half, lengthways. Using the tip of the knife scrape out vanilla seeds and place in a small bowl.

Place milk and vanilla seeds in a small saucepan over a medium heat.

Mix tapioca flour with a little cold water until dissolved. Add to saucepan and stir well.

Add coconut to saucepan and leave on the heat for 5 minutes. Stir often until icing starts to thicken.

Take off the heat and stir through honey.

Allow icing to cool a little. It's important to wait until cake or muffins have cooled completely before spreading icing, otherwise icing will not set.

Variations: For carob icing, add 1 teaspoon of carob powder. For passionfruit icing, add 1-2 passionfruits. For lemon icing, add 2 tablespoons of lemon juice. For fruit icing, only use 1¼ cups of milk.

Other icing suggestions: Melt 2 cups of carob buds in a water bath and dip the top of each muffin into the melted carob. Spread evenly with a knife and wait until set. You can sprinkle iced muffins with carob bits, crushed nuts, diced sun-dried fruit, coconut or sesame seeds. Place a whole carob bud in the centre of each muffin or top with small dices of fruit (banana, kiwi fruit, strawberries, blueberries or raspberries).

Pear & carob chip muffins

These deliciously light muffins are a healthy alternative to commercial chocolate chip varieties. Ripe, succulent pear partnered beautifully with carob and vanilla - guaranteed to be a winner with the kids. Pears are a good source of vitamin C and antioxidants, both important for healthy immune function.

1 cup (120 g/4¼ oz) wholemeal flour (GF: gluten-free plain flour)

1 cup (120 g/4¼ oz) spelt or plain flour (GF: gluten-free plain flour)

1 tablespoon baking powder (GF: gluten-free baking powder)

1 teaspoon vanilla essence or seeds

1 egg

⅓ cup (83 ml/3 fl oz) raw organic honey

½ cup (125 ml/4½ fl oz) light olive oil

1 cup (250 ml/9 fl oz) low-fat milk (LF: rice, almond, soy or lactose-free milk)

1 ¼ cups (188 g/6½ oz) diced pear (canned or fresh)

¼ cup small carob chip pieces, unsweetened (LF: soy carob)

Preheat oven to 180°C (350°F/Gas 4). Place muffin cases in a 12-hole muffin tray.

Place all dry ingredients into a large bowl, mix until well combined.

In another bowl add all liquid ingredients, whisk until well combined.

Slowly pour liquid into dry ingredients and gently combine. Be careful not to over mix as this will result in a heavy muffin.

Gently fold in pear and carob chips.

Spoon mixture into muffin holes and bake for 30 minutes, until muffins have risen and are golden brown.

Allow muffins to sit for 5 minutes on a cooling rack.

Makes 12 medium sized muffins.

Tip: If making gluten-free muffins add ½ teaspoon of xanthan gum.

Using vanilla beans: Using a sharp knife slice vanilla bean in half, lengthways. Scrape out the vanilla seeds with the tip of the knife.

Almond, coconut & peach muffins

These delightfully moist muffins just melt in your mouth. Made from sweet, juicy peaches rich in vitamins A and C. Almonds give these muffins an extra protein and calcium boost. If peaches are not in season you can use tinned (in natural juice).

2 cups (240 g/8 ½ oz) wholemeal flour (GF: gluten-free plain flour)

1 tablespoon baking powder (GF: gluten-free baking powder)

¼ cup (40 g/1½ oz) desiccated coconut

1 egg

1 teaspoon vanilla essence or seeds

½ cup (125 ml/4½ fl oz) raw organic honey

⅓ cup (80 ml/2¾ fl oz) light olive oil

1 cup (250 ml/9 fl oz) low-fat milk (LF: rice, almond, soy or lactose-free milk)

¼ cup (43 g/1½ oz) almond flakes

1 ¼ cups (188 g/6½ oz) diced peach (canned or fresh)

Preheat oven to 180°C (350°F/Gas 4). Place muffin cases in a 12-hole muffin tray.

Place all dry ingredients in a large bowl, mix until well combined.

In another bowl add all liquid ingredients, whisk until well combined.

Slowly pour liquid into dry ingredients and gently combine. Be careful not to over mix as this will result in a heavy muffin.

Gently fold in peach pieces and almonds.

Spoon mixture into muffin holes and bake for 30 minutes, until muffins have risen and are golden brown.

Allow muffins to sit for 5 minutes on a cooling rack.

Makes 12 medium sized muffins.

Tip: If making gluten-free muffins add ½ teaspoon of xanthan gum.

Using vanilla beans: Using a sharp knife slice vanilla bean in half, lengthways. Scrape out the vanilla seeds with the tip of the knife.

Blueberry wholemeal muffins

Luscious, fresh blueberries together with a touch of lemon zest make these muffins a treat for the eyes and the taste buds. Blueberries are one of the best sources of anthocyanins, an antioxidant that helps prevent free radical damage in the body. Blueberries are also a very good source of vitamin C.

2 cups (240 g/8 ½ oz) wholemeal flour (GF: gluten-free plain flour)

1 tablespoon baking powder (GF: gluten-free baking powder)

1 egg

½ cup (125 ml/4½ fl oz) raw organic honey

½ tablespoon lemon zest

⅓ cup (83 ml/3 fl oz) light olive oil

1 cup (250 ml/9 fl oz) low-fat milk (LF: rice, almond, soy or lactose-free milk)

1 teaspoon vanilla essence or seeds

¼ cup (43 g/1½ oz) almonds flakes

1 ¼ cups (188 g/6½ oz) fresh or frozen blueberries

Preheat oven to 180°C (350°F/Gas 4). Place muffin cases in a 12-hole muffin tray.

Place all dry ingredients in a large bowl, mix until well combined.

In another bowl add all liquid ingredients and lemon zest, whisk until well combined.

Slowly pour liquid into dry ingredients and gently combine. Be careful not to over mix as this will result in a heavy muffin.

Gently fold in almonds and blueberries so they don't burst.

Spoon mixture into muffin holes and bake for 30 minutes, until muffins have risen and are golden brown.

Allow muffins to sit for 5 minutes on a cooling rack.

Makes 12 medium sized muffins.

Tip: If using frozen blueberries do not thaw, add to mixture frozen. If making gluten-free muffins add ½ teaspoon of xanthan gum.

Using vanilla beans: Using a sharp knife slice vanilla bean in half, lengthways. Scrape out the vanilla seeds with the tip of the knife.

Apple, sultana & cinnamon muffins

The delicate flavour of cinnamon goes perfectly with sultanas and apple in these tasty, fibre-rich muffins. Apples are a rich source of antioxidants and vitamin C, needed for healthy immune function.

2 cups (240 g/8 ½ oz) wholemeal flour (GF: gluten-free plain flour)

1 tablespoon baking powder (GF: gluten-free baking powder)

1 egg

½ cup (125 ml/4½ fl oz) raw organic honey

⅓ cup (83 ml/3 fl oz) light olive oil

1 cup (250 ml/9 fl oz) low-fat milk (LF: rice, almond, soy or lactose-free milk)

1 ¼ cups (188 g/6½ oz) small dices of apple

¼ cup (27 g/1 oz) sun-dried sultanas

2 tablespoons sunflower seeds

Preheat oven to 180°C (350°F/Gas 4). Place muffin cases in a 12-hole muffin tray.

Place all dry ingredients in a large bowl, mix until well combined.

In another bowl add all liquid ingredients, whisk until well combined.

Slowly pour liquid into dry ingredients and gently combine. Be careful not to over mix as this will result in a heavy muffin.

Gently fold in apple and sultanas.

Spoon mixture into muffin holes and sprinkle with sunflower seeds. Bake for 30 minutes, until muffins have risen and are golden brown.

Allow muffins to sit for 5 minutes on a cooling rack.

Makes 12 medium sized muffins.

Tip: If making gluten-free muffins add ½ teaspoon of xanthan gum.

Carob & raspberry muffins

These more-ish carob and raspberry treats are a healthy alternative to chocolate muffins. Carob, not only gives these muffins a chocolate appearance, it's also caffeine-free and a good source of calcium. If raspberries are not in season use frozen berries.

2 cups (240 g/8 ½ oz) wholemeal flour (GF: gluten-free plain flour)

1 tablespoon baking powder (GF: gluten-free baking powder)

1 egg

½ cup (125 ml/4½ fl oz) raw organic honey

½ tablespoon lemon zest

⅓ cup (83 ml/3 fl oz) light olive oil

1 cup (250 ml/9 fl oz) low-fat milk (LF: rice, almond, soy or lactose-free milk)

1 teaspoon vanilla essence or seeds

¼ cup (43 g/1½ oz) almonds flakes

1 ¼ cups (188 g/6½ oz) fresh or frozen blueberries

Preheat oven to 180°C (350°F/Gas 4). Place muffin cases in a 12-hole muffin tray.

Place all dry ingredients in a large bowl, mix until well combined.

In another bowl add all liquid ingredients and lemon zest, whisk until well combined.

Slowly pour liquid into dry ingredients and gently combine. Be careful not to over mix as this will result in a heavy muffin.

Gently fold in almonds and blueberries so they don't burst.

Spoon mixture into muffin holes and bake for 30 minutes, until muffins have risen and are golden brown.

Allow muffins to sit for 5 minutes on a cooling rack.

Makes 12 medium sized muffins.

Tip: If using frozen blueberries do not thaw, add to mixture frozen. If making gluten-free muffins add ½ teaspoon of xanthan gum.

Using vanilla beans: Using a sharp knife slice vanilla bean in half, lengthways. Scrape out the vanilla seeds with the tip of the knife.

Banana & walnut muffins

Creamy, sweet bananas are a favourite with most kids and these scrumptious muffins will definitely bring a smile to their faces. Bananas are one of the best sources of potassium (needed for maintaining normal heart function), B vitamins and energy giving complex carbohydrates. Bananas are considered a prebiotic food as they help nourish friendly bacteria in the colon. Walnuts are a good source of omega-3 fats that are needed for cardiovascular health and proper brain function.

2 cups (240 g/8 ½ oz) wholemeal flour (GF: gluten-free plain flour)

1 tablespoon baking powder (GF: gluten-free baking powder)

1 egg

1 teaspoon vanilla essence or seeds

⅓ cup (83 ml/3 fl oz) light olive oil

½ cup (125 ml/4½ fl oz) raw organic honey

1 cup (250 ml/9 fl oz) low-fat milk (LF: rice, almond, soy or lactose-free milk)

½ cup (85 g/3 oz) walnuts pieces

2 large ripe bananas, diced

2 tablespoons linseeds

Preheat oven to 180°C (350°F/Gas 4). Place muffin cases in a 12-hole muffin tray.

Place all dry ingredients in a large bowl, mix until well combined.

In another bowl add all liquid ingredients, whisk until well combined.

Slowly pour liquid into dry ingredients and gently combine. Be careful not to over mix as this will result in a heavy muffin.

Gently fold in banana pieces and walnuts.

Spoon mixture into muffin holes and sprinkle with linseeds. Bake for 30 minutes, until muffins have risen and are golden brown.

Allow muffins to sit for 5 minutes on a cooling rack.

Makes 12 medium sized muffins.

Tip: Use ripe, slightly browned bananas as they are sweeter and softer. Keep browned bananas in the freezer for baking. If making gluten-free muffins add ½ teaspoon of xanthan gum.

Using vanilla beans: Using a sharp knife slice vanilla bean in half, lengthways. Scrape out the vanilla seeds with the tip of the knife.

Apple & zucchini carrot loaf

This delicious, moist and incredibly tasty loaf is a healthy alternative to commercially made carrot cakes (high in saturated fats and sugar). This wholesome loaf is a great way of getting extra vegetables into your children's diet without them knowing. Carrots are the richest source of beta-carotene, needed for healthy immune function and vision. This loaf is also a good source of dietary fibre and beneficial unsaturated fats.

2½ cups (300 g/10 ½ oz) wholemeal flour (GF: gluten-free plain flour)

1 tablespoon baking powder (GF: gluten-free baking powder)

1 teaspoon cinnamon

3 eggs

½ cup (125 ml/4½ fl oz) light olive oil

½ cup (125 ml/4½ fl oz) raw organic honey

1 cup (150 g/5¼ oz) grated carrot

1 cup (150 g/5¼ oz) grated apple

1 cup (150 g/5¼ oz) grated zucchini

½ cup (83 g/3 oz) chopped pecans

½ cup (54 g/2 oz) sun-dried sultanas

Preheat oven to 180°C (350°F/Gas 4). Line a loaf tin with baking paper.

Place all dry ingredients in a large bowl, mix until well combined.

In another bowl add all liquid ingredients, whisk until well combined.

Slowly pour liquid into dry ingredients and gently combine.

Gently stir in carrot, zucchini, apple, sultanas and pecans.

Pour into loaf tin and bake for 60-70 minutes. When lightly browned cover with foil. When cooked an inserted skewer should come out cleanly.

Tip: If making a gluten-free loaf add ½ teaspoon of xanthan gum.

Apple & beetroot carob brownies

These decadent carob goodies are a healthy alternative to chocolate brownies - your kids won't be able to tell the difference. These brownies are a perfect way of sneaking extra fruit and vegetables into your child's diet. Beetroot is a rich source of complex carbohydrates, dietary fibre, vitamin C and antioxidants.

2½ cups (300 g/10 ½ oz) wholemeal flour (GF: gluten-free plain flour)

1 tablespoon baking powder (GF: gluten-free baking powder)

½ cup (60 g/2¼ oz) carob powder

3 eggs

½ cup (125 ml/4½ fl oz) raw organic honey

1 teaspoon vanilla essence or seeds

½ cup (125 ml/4½ fl oz) light olive oil

1 cup (250 ml/9 fl oz) low-fat milk (LF: rice, almond, soy or lactose–free milk)

1 cup (150 g/5 ¼ oz) grated beetroot

1 cup (150 g/5 ¼ oz) grated apple

⅓ cup (57 g/2 oz) walnut or pecan pieces

Preheat oven to180°C (350°F/Gas 4). Line a lamington tray (13" x 9" x 2" pan) with baking paper.

Place all dry ingredients in a large bowl, mix until well combined.

In another bowl add all liquid ingredients, whisk until well combined.

Slowly pour liquid into dry ingredients and gently combine.

Gently fold in apple, beetroot and walnuts.

Pour into lamington tray and bake for 30-35 minutes. When cooked an inserted skewer should come out cleanly.

Leave brownies to cool and cut into squares.

Tip: If making gluten-free brownies add ½ teaspoon of xanthan gum.

Using vanilla beans: Using a sharp knife slice vanilla bean in half, lengthways. Scrape out the vanilla seeds with the tip of the knife.

Date wholemeal scones

These scrumptious, fibre-rich scones make a delightful morning tea treat or wholesome lunch box snack. Perfect anytime of the day served warm with fresh strawberries and a dollop of natural yoghurt. Delicious drizzled with flaxseed oil and a little raw honey or fruit puree.

2 cups (240 g/8 ½ oz) wholemeal flour (GF: gluten-free plain flour)

1 tablespoon baking powder (GF: gluten-free baking powder)

½ teaspoon all-spice

⅓ cup (83 ml/3 fl oz) light olive oil

2 tablespoons raw organic honey

1 cup (250 ml/9 fl oz) low-fat milk (LF: rice, almond, soy or lactose-free milk)

½ cup (54 g/2 oz) diced sun-dried dates

Preheat oven to 220°C (425°F/Gas 4). Line a baking tray with baking paper.

Place all dry ingredients in a bowl and combine well.

In a smaller bowl whisk liquid ingredients together. Pour liquid into dry ingredients and gently combine. Fold through dates.

Place dough on a well floured board. Roll dough out until 1 ½ inches (4 cm) thick, then cut into 10 equal squares.

Place squares on tray and lightly brush tops with milk. Bake for 12-15 minutes, until lightly browned.

Tip: If making gluten-free scones add ½ teaspoon of xanthan gum.

Variation: Replace dates with ½ cup (88g/3 oz) diced sun-dried apricots, sultanas, figs, apple or pear.

Savoury spicy pumpkin & corn muffins

These wholesome savoury muffins are packed full of fibre and beta-carotene. Serve warm with soup or as a snack spread with avocado or hummus. Pepitas give these muffins an added zinc and protein boost.

1 cup (180 g/6 ½ oz) wholemeal flour (GF: gluten-free plain flour)

1 teaspoon ground cinnamon

½ teaspoon ground coriander

1 tablespoon baking powder (GF: gluten-free baking powder)

1 cup (170 g/6 oz) small dices of pumpkin

2 eggs

⅓ cup (83 ml/3 oz) light olive oil

¼ cup (63 ml/2¼ fl oz) raw organic honey

¾ cup (188 ml/6½ fl oz) low-fat milk (GF: rice, almond, soy or lactose-free milk)

2 tablespoons pepitas (pumpkin seeds)

¼ cup (50 g/1¾ oz) corn kernels, canned

Preheat oven to 180°C (350°F/Gas 4). Place muffin cases in a 12-hole muffin tray.

Place all dry ingredients in a large bowl, mix until well combined.

Place pumpkin and all liquid ingredients together in a blender, mix until well combined.

Slowly pour liquid into dry ingredients and gently combine. Be careful not to over mix as this will result in a heavy muffin.

Gently fold in corn kernels.

Spoon mixture into muffin holes and sprinkle with pepitas. Bake for 30 minutes until muffins have risen and are golden brown.

Allow muffins to sit for 5 minutes on a cooling rack.

Makes 12 medium sized muffins.

Tip: If making gluten-free muffins add ½ teaspoon of xanthan gum.

Crunchy nut muesli bar

These nutritious muesli bars are a healthy alternative to commercially made varieties that are full of sugar and saturated fats. These delicious bars are packed with protein, beneficial fats and complex carbohydrates to keep active kids going throughout the day. Balanced with puffed rice and a mix of nuts, these bars have a lovely light and crunchy texture.

⅓ cup (83 ml/3 fl oz) light olive oil

½ cup (125 ml/4½ fl oz) raw organic honey

½ cup (125 ml/4½ fl oz) almond butter or tahini

1½ cups (45 g/1½ oz) puffed brown rice

2 cups (200 g/7 oz) rolled oats (GF: flaked millet or quinoa)

1 cup (170 g/6 oz) crushed mixed nuts (almonds, cashews, hazelnuts, walnuts or pecans)

2 tablespoons sun-dried sultanas or date – optional

Preheat oven to 160°C (325°F/Gas 2). Line a slice tray with baking paper (or for individual muesli cups place muffin cases in a 12-hole muffin tray).

In a small saucepan add oil, honey and nut butter and place over a medium heat. Stir until melted and well combined.

Place oats, puffed rice, nuts and sultanas in a large bowl and combine well.

Pour honey mixture over oats and stir until oats are well coated.

Pour mixture into slice or muffin tray and press down firmly. Bake for 30 minutes.

Leave to cool then place in the fridge for 30 minutes before cutting into bars, to prevent crumbling.

Store in an airtight container in the fridge.

Makes 12 bars.

Variation: Add ¼ cup of crushed, unsweetened carob buds to mixture or drizzle melted carob over cooled bars.

Apricot seed bar

These delicious energy bars make a nutritious easy snack anytime of the day - your kids won't be able to get enough of them. These well-balanced bars provide energy giving complex carbohydrates, dietary fibre, protein and healthy fats. You can use any combination of sun-dried fruits for this recipe.

½ cup (125 ml/4½ fl oz) almond butter or tahini

½ cup (125 ml/4½ fl oz) raw organic honey

⅓ cup (83 ml/3 fl oz) light olive oil

3 cups (300 g/10½ oz) rolled oats (GF: flaked millet or quinoa)

¼ cup (40 g/1½ oz) sesame seeds

¼ cup (40 g/1½ oz) sunflower seeds

¼ cup (40 g/1½ oz) pepitas (pumpkin seeds), crushed

¼ cup (40 g/1 ½ oz) coconut flakes

½ cup (88 g/3 oz) sun-dried apricot, diced (or date, fig, mango or apple)

Preheat oven to 160°C (325°F/Gas 2). Line a slice tray with baking paper (or for individual cups place paper muffin cups in a 12-hole muffin tray).

In a small saucepan add oil, honey and nut butter, place over a medium heat. Stir until melted and well combined.

Place oats, seeds, coconut and dried fruit in a large bowl and combine well.

Pour honey mixture over oats and stir until oats are well coated.

Pour mixture into slice or muffin tray and press down firmly. Bake for 30 minutes.

Leave to cool then place in the fridge for 30 minutes before cutting into bars, to prevent crumbling.

Store in an airtight container in the fridge.

Makes 12 bars.

Variation: Add ¼ cup of crushed, unsweetened carob buds to mixture, or drizzle melted carob over cooled bars.

Fig & date energy bars

These rich, fruity bars with a crunchy oat base are simply irresistible. Figs and dates are excellent sources of energy and dietary fibre, helping to keep kids regular. These bars also contain protein and healthy fats.

BASE:

1 ¼ cups (150 g/4 oz) oat flour (GF: almond meal)

1 ¼ cups (150 g/4 oz) wholemeal flour (GF: gluten-free plain flour)

100 ml (3 ½ fl oz) light olive oil

2 ½ tablespoons water

TOPPING:

1 cup (160 g/5½ oz) finely chopped sun-dried figs

4 sun-dried dates, finely chopped

¼ cup (63 g/2¼ oz) almond butter or tahini

½ cup (85 g/3 oz) crushed macadamia nuts (raw and unsalted)

1 cup (250 ml/9 fl oz) low-fat milk (LF: rice, almond, soy or lactose-free milk)

Juice and zest of 1 small organic orange

2 tablespoons wholemeal flour (GF: gluten-free plain flour)

¼ cup (40 g/1½ oz) shredded coconut (plus extra for topping)

Preheat oven to 180°C (350°F/Gas 4). Line a slice tray with baking paper.

In a large bowl mix all dry base ingredients together until well combined. You can make your own oat flour by processing rolled oats in a blender.

Add oil and water to flour mixture. With your hands combine mixture until it resembles crumbly dough.

Press mixture into slice tray and prick top with a fork several times. Bake for 10 minutes, remove from oven and allow base to cool.

Place all topping ingredients in a saucepan. Place over medium heat and cook for 5 minutes. Stir frequently until mixture is thick and well combined.

Spoon mixture onto base and sprinkle with extra coconut. Press down lightly with a fork.

Bake for 30 minutes.

Allow to cool then place in the fridge for 30 minutes before cutting into bars.

Makes 24 small bars.

Carob chip oatmeal cookies

These more-ish bite sized cookies just melt in your mouth. Crammed with carob buds, oats and nuts these cookies make a nutritious guilt-free treat for your kids.

½ cup (60 g/2 oz) oat flour (GF: gluten-free plain flour)

½ cup (60 g/2 oz) spelt or wholemeal flour (GF: gluten-free plain flour)

½ cup (50 g/1¾ oz) rolled oats (flaked millet or quinoa)

1 tablespoon tahini or nut butter – optional

¼ cup (63 ml/2¼ fl oz) light olive oil

¼ cup (63 ml/2¼ fl oz) raw organic honey

¼ cup (63 ml/2¼ fl oz) low-fat milk (LF: rice, almond, soy or lactose-free milk)

½ cup carob chips, unsweetened (LF: soy carob)

2 tablespoons almond flakes

Preheat oven to 180°C (350°F/Gas 4). Line a baking tray with baking paper.

In a bowl add all dry ingredients and mix until well combined. You can make your own oat flour by processing rolled oats in a blender.

In another bowl add all liquid ingredients and whisk until well combined.

Pour liquid into dry mixture and combine.

Gently fold in carob chips and almond flakes. You can place larger carob buds in a plastic bag and crush into smaller chips with a rolling pin.

Use 1 tablespoon of mixture for each cookie and place them on baking tray. Press the top of each cookie down with the back of a fork then bake for 15-20 minutes.

Variation: If making gluten-free cookies add ½ teaspoon of xanthan gum. Add a pecan half to the top of each cookie.

Earth cookies

These earthy cookies are an excellent way of increasing your child's fibre intake. These cookies are jam-packed with oats, rich in energy giving complex carbohydrates, B vitamins and vitamin E.

1 cup (120 g/4¼ oz) wholemeal flour (GF: gluten-free plain flour)

2 cups (200 g/7 oz) rolled oats (GF: flaked millet or quinoa)

1 teaspoon cinnamon

½ cup (125 ml/4½ fl oz) raw organic honey

2 tablespoons tahini

½ cup (125 ml/4½ fl oz) light olive oil

1 ripe banana, diced

½ cup (125 ml/4½ fl oz) low-fat milk (LF: rice, almond, soy or lactose-free milk)

½ cup (88 g/3 oz) diced sun-dried apricots

¼ cup (43 g/1½ oz) sunflower seeds

Preheat oven to 180°C (350°F/Gas 4). Line a baking tray with baking paper.

In a bowl add all dry ingredients and mix until well combined.

In another bowl add all liquid ingredients, whisk until well combined.

Pour liquid into dry mixture and combine.

Gently fold in apricots, banana and sunflower seeds.

Use 1 tablespoon of mixture for each cookie and place them on baking tray. Press cookies flat with the back of a fork and pat them around the edges to make perfectly round cookies. Bake for 25 minutes or until lightly browned.

Makes 30 medium sized cookies.

Apricot protein balls

These tasty treats are a great source of protein for healthy growth and development, beta-carotene and dietary fibre. For a nutritious snack, pack some in your child's lunch box.

1 cup (175 g/6 oz) chopped sun-dried apricots

½ cup (108 g/3¾ oz) sun-dried sultanas

½ cup (125 ml/4½ fl oz) boiling water

3 tablespoons sunflower seeds

¼ cup (63 g/2¼ oz) ground almonds

1 cup (60 g/2 oz) skim milk powder (LF: rice based protein powder)

½ cup (80 g/3 oz) desiccated coconut (plus extra for coating)

2 teaspoons lemon juice

Place dried fruit in a bowl of boiling water and leave to soak for 10 minutes.

Place soaked fruit, seeds, lemon juice, milk powder, almonds and coconut in a blender, mix until well combined.

Roll mixture into a 5 cm wide log, then cut into bite size pieces. Roll each piece in a ball and roll in coconut.

Place balls on a plate covered with plastic and place in the fridge to set.

Keep in an airtight container in the fridge for up to a week.

Carob coconut roughs

These irresistible carob treats are a healthy alternative to giving your child chocolate. Pack a couple in your child's lunch box as a special treat or as an after dinner surprise.

375g (13¼ oz) carob buds, unsweetened (LF: soy carob)

4 large puffed rice cakes, crushed into small pieces

½ cup (85 g/3 oz) crushed nuts (almonds, cashew or hazelnut)

½ cup (80 g/3 oz) desiccated coconut

½ cup (88 g/3 oz) small dices of sun-dried fruit (apricots, dates or sultanas) - optional

Line a baking tray with baking paper.

Place a deep frying pan (a third full of water) over a medium heat. Bring to boil and reduce heat to a simmer.

Place carob buds in a small bowl and place in pan, making sure water does not spill into the bowl.

Gently stir carob as it melts. When melted add rice cake pieces, nuts, coconut and dried fruit, and gently combine.

Place bite size spoonfuls on tray and place in the fridge until set. Keep in an airtight container in the fridge.

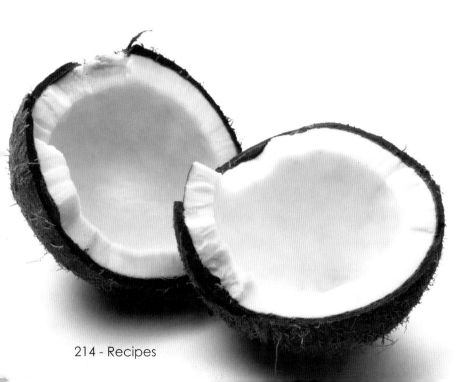

Lunch & dinner

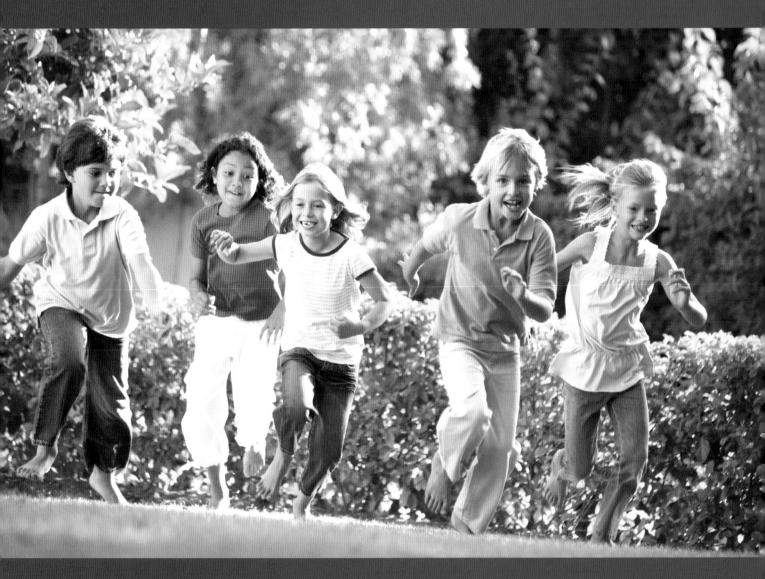

These nutritious lunch and dinner recipes will have your family and friends coming back for seconds. Made from only fresh, wholesome ingredients, these recipes take the guess work out of planning well-balanced meals.

Baked potato jackets

Baked potato jackets are so quick and easy to prepare. By adding nutritious fillings they are ideal for weekend lunches or a light dinner served with a salad. Flaxseed oil gives this dish an extra omega-3 boost. Let your kids create their own potato jackets from the filling suggestions below.

1 large potato or medium sweet potato

½ tablespoon cold pressed flaxseed oil

FILLING SUGGESTIONS:

1 tablespoon hummus, baba ghanoush or tzatziki

2 teaspoons homemade low-fat mayonnaise

1 teaspoon tahini or nut butter

Fresh herbs (basil, parsley or coriander)

¼ small avocado

1 teaspoon toasted seeds: pumpkin, sesame, sunflower or LSA

2 teaspoons leek or shallots, finely chopped

1 tablespoon natural yoghurt (LF: lactose-free yoghurt), mix with 2 teaspoons lemon

2 teaspoons salsa

½ teaspoon Dijon mustard

¼ cup (19 g/3/4 oz) steamed vegetables, small dices (carrot, corn, peas, broccoli, zucchini or capsicum)

¼ cup (19 g/¾ oz) cooked chicken pieces, salmon or tuna flakes, firm tofu or legumes (chickpeas, kidney beans or broad beans)

TOPPING SUGGESTION:

Low-fat cheddar cheese or feta (LF: vegan cheese)

Preheat oven to 200°C (400°F/Gas 6).

Thoroughly wash potato and wrap in foil. Bake for 60 minutes until potato is cooked through.

Slice the top off potato and scoop out its soft filling. Make sure the skin stays in tack. Mix together desired fillings, potato and flaxseed oil in a small bowl.

Scoop mixture back into potato jackets and sprinkle with cheese.

Place under the griller or pop back in the oven until cheese has melted.

Makes 1 potato jacket.

Tuna, cottage cheese & sesame melt

Ideal for a quick lunch or snack this tasty tuna melt is packed with healthy omega-3 fats, calcium and protein.

125 g (4½ oz) tin light tuna, drained
⅓ cup (83 g/ 3 oz) low-fat cottage cheese
(LF: vegan cheese)
1 tablespoon lemon juice
1 tablespoon thinly sliced shallots
2 slices crusty wholegrain bread
(GF: gluten-free bread)
1 teaspoon sesame seeds

In a small bowl gently combine tuna, cottage cheese, shallots and lemon juice, using a fork.

Lightly toast bread then top with tuna mixture.

Sprinkle with sesame seeds and place under a medium grill until heated through.

Makes 2.

Variation: for vegetarians replace tuna with small can of corn kernels.

Avocado, salmon & feta melt

This filling salmon melt is rich in monounsaturated and omega-3 fats as well as protein. Include the soft salmon bones for an extra calcium boost.

125 g (4½ oz) tin salmon, drained
¼ avocado, small dices
2 teaspoons crumbled low-fat feta
(LF: grated vegan cheese)
2 teaspoons lemon juice
2 slices crusty wholegrain bread
(GF: gluten-free bread)

Remove any large salmon bones then gently mash salmon and small softer bones together in a bowl.

Add avocado, feta and lemon juice, gently combine using a fork.

Lightly toast bread and top with salmon mixture.

Place under a medium grill until heated through.

Makes 2.

Variation: For vegetarians replace salmon with tomato pieces.

Tomato, basil & hummus bruschetta

This light and flavoursome bruschetta is topped with tomatoes which contain lycopene, a powerful antioxidant which helps fight free radical damage in the body. Hummus made from chickpeas and tahini is an excellent source of protein, dietary fibre, B vitamins and calcium.

¼ cup (63 g/2¼ oz) hummus (refer to recipe)
1 medium ripe roman tomato, small dices
2 teaspoons fresh basil, finely chopped
1 teaspoon balsamic vinegar
2 thick slices sourdough bread (GF: gluten-free bread)

In a small bowl gently combine basil, tomato and balsamic vinegar.

Lightly toast bread and spread with hummus.

Top with tomato mixture and serve.

Makes 2.

Baked rice balls

These delicious balls of goodness make an ideal snack or lunch on the run. Pack one in your kid's lunch box or pop one in a salad wrap.

3 shallots, finely chopped
1 clove garlic, crushed
2 ½ cups cooked Japanese rice
1 medium carrot, finely diced
2 celery sticks, finely diced
1 tablespoon tamari (wheat-free)
2 tablespoons sesame seeds or linseeds
1 tablespoon sunflower seeds
Olive oil spray

Preheat oven to 220°C (400°F/Gas 6). Line a baking tray with baking paper.

Lightly spray a small frying pan with olive oil and place over a medium heat. Lightly cook carrot, shallots, seeds, celery and garlic for a couple of minutes.

Place mixture in a bowl with cooled rice and tamari, and mix together. Form balls, about a heaped tablespoon each, then place on baking tray.

Lightly spray balls with olive oil and cook for 20 minutes until golden brown. Turn after 10 minutes.

Corn & spinach rice timbales

Like other dark green leafy vegetables, spinach is an excellent source of iron. These nutritious timbales make a well-balanced school lunch or dinner served with a salad.

1 onion, finely chopped

1 clove garlic, crushed

1 cup (63 g/21/4 oz) spinach, finely chopped

1 cup (160 g/51/2 oz) zucchini, grated

½ cup (100 g/31/2 oz) corn kernels

2 cups (370 g/13 oz) cooked brown rice

¼ cup (63 g/21/4 oz) crumbled low-fat feta (LF: grated vegan cheese)

Pinch sea salt

5 egg whites and 3 egg yolks

2 tablespoons pepitas (pumpkin seeds)

Preheat oven to 200°C (400°F/Gas 6). Lightly spray a 6-hole muffin tray with olive oil.

Lightly spray a frying pan with olive oil and place over a medium heat. Cook onion and garlic until tender.

In a large bowl grate zucchini then add vegetables from frying pan, spinach, corn, cooked rice, feta and sea salt.

In another smaller bowl whisk eggs together then add to larger bowl, combining well.

Scoop mixture into muffin holes and sprinkle with pepitas. Cook for 35-40 minutes, until golden brown and cooked through.

Sprinkle with pepitas and cook for 35-40 minutes, until golden brown and cooked through.

Tip: Soak brown rice in water for 30 minutes before cooking (for improved texture and reduced cooking time).

Vegetable bake with almond & sunflower crumble

This fabulous vegetable dish is a substantial meal on its own or a wonderful side dish to grilled salmon, chicken or beef. This dish is abundant in nutrients such as protein, beta-carotene, calcium, zinc and B vitamins.

4 potatoes or 1 large sweet potato, thinly sliced

2 cups (320 g/11¼ oz) thinly sliced carrots

2 cups (100 g/3½ oz) small broccoli florets

1 thinly sliced red capsicum

1 bunch fresh chives, finely chopped

¼ cup (30 g/1 oz) finely chopped leek or shallots

1 cup (250 g/9 oz) natural yoghurt (LF: lactose-free yoghurt)

¼ cup (63 ml/2¼ fl oz) low-fat milk (LF: rice, almond, soy or lactose-free milk)

4 eggs

CRUMBLE TOPPING:

1 ½ cups (120 g/4¼ oz) wholegrain breadcrumbs, approx 2 slices (GF: gluten-free bread crumbs)

2 tablespoons almonds flakes

1 tablespoon pepitas (pumpkin seeds)

¼ cup (30 g/1 oz) crumbled low-fat cheddar cheese (LF: vegan cheese)

Preheat oven to 200ºC (400ºF/Gas 6). Lightly spray an ovenproof casserole dish with olive oil.

Lightly steam potato, carrot and broccoli until tender but not too soft.

Layer potato, carrot, broccoli and capsicum into casserole dish.

In a bowl whisk yoghurt, milk and eggs together. Mix through chives and shallots and pour mixture over vegetables.

In another bowl combine topping ingredients. You can make your own breadcrumbs by processing bread in a blender. Sprinkle topping evenly over vegetables.

Bake for 35-40 minutes.

Broccoli & feta quiche with brown rice base

This lovely light quiche has a delightful yoghurt tang. The grainy brown rice base complements this protein-rich quiche by supplying added complex carbohydrates and dietary fibre. This quiche is also lovely made with a cous cous or quinoa base.

BASE:

2 ½ cups (463 g/16¼ oz) cooked brown rice

¼ cup (40 g/1½ oz) sesame seeds

FILLING:

½ cup (50 g/1¾ oz) small broccoli florets

1 tablespoon finely chopped shallots or leek

4 eggs, lightly beaten

1 cup (250 g/9 fl oz) natural yoghurt (LF: lactose-free yoghurt)

Pinch of sea salt

1 tablespoon finely chopped fresh basil or parsley

¼ cup (63 g/2¼ oz) crumbled low-fat feta (LF: grated vegan cheese)

2 tablespoons sunflower seeds

Preheat oven to 180°C (350°F/Gas 4). Lightly spray a quiche dish with olive oil.

Place base ingredients in a bowl and mix until well combined. Firmly press base into quiche dish.

Cut broccoli into small pieces, scatter over base and sprinkle with shallots.

In a bowl whisk together eggs, yoghurt, herbs and sea salt, then pour over broccoli.

Sprinkle with cheese and sunflower seeds, then bake for 50 minutes, or until firm and golden brown.

Tip: Soak brown rice in water for 30 minutes before cooking (for improved texture and reduced cooking time).

Variation: Use couscous or quinoa for the base instead of brown rice (follow grain cooking chart).

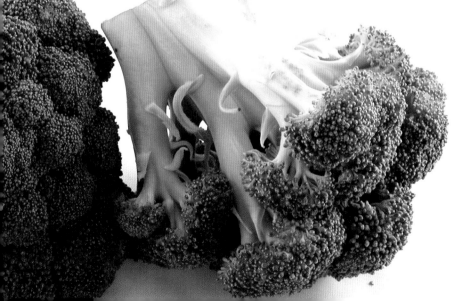

Mini capsicum & salmon quiches with kumera base

These tasty little quiches are bursting with flavour and nutrients. Salmon is an excellent source of omega-3 fats (include the soft bones for extra calcium). This light and crispy base is a healthy low-fat alternative to commercially prepared quiche bases which are high in saturated and trans fats. These mini quiches freeze well for school lunches.

BASE:

1½ cups (180 g/6¼ oz) wholemeal flour
(GF: gluten-free plain flour)

1 cup (260 g/9 oz) cold mashed kumera
(sweet potato)

QUICHE FILLING:

1 onion, finely chopped

4 eggs, lightly beaten

1 cup (250 ml/9 fl oz) natural yoghurt
(LF: lactose-free yoghurt)

¼ cup (30 g/1 oz) grated low-fat cheddar cheese
(LF: vegan cheese)

½ cup (80 g/2¾ oz) red capsicum, finely diced

1 tablespoon finely chopped fresh parsley

220 g (7 ¾ oz) tin salmon, drained with
large bones removed

2 tablespoons sesame seeds or linseeds

Preheat oven to 180°C (350°F/Gas 4). Lightly spray 8 individual quiche shells with olive oil.

Combine all base ingredients in a bowl and mix until well combined.

Knead base on a floured board, roll out and cut into squares to fit quiche holes. You can use an egg ring.

Place a circle of pastry in each hole and press into shape. Bring the pastry up the edges of the dish. Prick each base several times with a fork and bake for 8 minutes.

Lightly spray a frying pan with olive oil and place over a medium heat. Cook onion until tender.

In a bowl whisk eggs, natural yoghurt and cheese together. Stir through onion, capsicum and parsley.

Remove larger salmon bones and gently mash salmon with a fork. Add salmon to egg mixture and combine well.

Fill each quiche base with mixture.
Sprinkle with sesame seeds and bake for 35-40 minutes until firm and golden brown.

Makes 8 individual quiches.

Variation: Add a handful of your child's favourite diced vegies. Add some corn kernels. Replace salmon with cooked chicken, tofu or tuna.

Pumpkin & ricotta quiche with pecan base

This quiche is a real taste treat with creamy ricotta and pumpkin and a pecan spiked crust. This dish will provide your child with protein, omega-3 fats, beta-carotene and calcium. Sprinkle with pepitas to give an added zinc boost, needed for healthy immune function.

BASE:

½ cup (60 g/2 oz) wholemeal flour (GF: gluten-free plain flour)

¾ cup (75 g/2¾ oz) ground pecans or LSA (ground linseeds, sunflower seeds and almonds)

2 tablespoons water

2 tablespoons cold pressed virgin olive oil

1 ½ tablespoons lemon juice

FILLING:

1 clove garlic, crushed

1 small onion, finely chopped

4 eggs

½ cup (125 ml/4½ fl oz) low-fat milk (LF: rice, almond, soy or lactose-free milk)

1 teaspoon rosemary

1 cup (150 g/5¼ oz) small dices of pumpkin

1 cup (63 g/2¼ oz) finely chopped spinach (or grated zucchini)

¼ cup (63 g/2¼ oz) low-fat ricotta or grated cheese (LF: vegan cheese)

1 tablespoon pepitas (pumpkin seeds)

Preheat oven to 190°C (350°F/Gas 4). Lightly spray a quiche dish with olive oil.

In a bowl add base ingredients and mix with hands until mixture is a crumbly consistency.

Press mixture into quiche dish and press firmly, bringing base up the edges.

Bake for 10 minutes.

Lightly spray a frying pan with olive oil and place over medium heat. Cook onion and garlic until tender. Add pumpkin and partially cook.

In a small bowl whisk eggs, milk and rosemary together.

Cover base with vegetables from frying pan and spinach. Sprinkle with cheese.

Pour mixture into quiche dish and sprinkle with pepitas.

Bake for 40-45 minutes until set and golden brown. When cooked you should be able to bring a knife out of the centre cleanly.

Roast vegetable & hummus pies

These delicious pies are a feast for the eyes as well as the taste buds. Packed with lots of vegies and hummus, these pies provide an array of antioxidants along with dietary fibre, complex carbohydrates and protein.

BASE:

1 cup (120 g/4¼ oz) wholemeal flour (GF: gluten-free plain flour)

3 tablespoons cold pressed virgin olive oil

1 tablespoon water

1 egg

2 tablespoons LSA (ground linseeds, sunflower seeds and almonds)

FILLING:

1 cup (150 g/5¼ oz) diced beetroot

1 cup (150 g/5¼ oz) diced pumpkin or sweet potato

1 cup (150 g/5¼ oz) diced carrot

1 cup (150 g/5¼ oz) diced zucchini

1 cup (50 g/1¾ oz) small broccoli florets

2 cups (500 g/17¾ oz) thick hummus

¼ cup (63 g/2¼ oz) crumbled low-fat feta or goat's cheese (LF: grated vegan cheese)

Preheat oven to 200°C (400°F/Gas 6). Lightly spray 8 individual pie shells with olive oil.

Place flour and LSA together in a bowl. Add olive oil and water and combine with your hands until mixture resembles breadcrumbs.

Add egg and knead until a dough like consistency. Wrap dough in plastic wrap and refrigerate for 30 min.

Roll dough out on a floured board and divide into 4 pieces.

Press each base into pie shells and press firmly, bring up the edges. Prick each base several times with a fork. Bake bases for 8 minutes.

Line a baking tray with baking paper. Place beetroot, carrot and pumpkin pieces on tray and bake for 30 minutes.

Add zucchini and bake for another 10 minutes until pumpkin and beetroot are cooked through.

Lightly steam broccoli.

Spoon hummus into each pie base. Top with vegetables then sprinkle with cheese.

Place pies back in the oven for a few minutes, until cheese has melted and golden brown.

Makes 8 individual pies.

Wholemeal spaghetti & meatballs

Spaghetti and meatballs is a favourite with most kids. These tasty bite sized meatballs are high in protein, iron and zinc. Wholemeal spaghetti is a good source of complex carbohydrates, and tomatoes are a rich source of antioxidants.

½ cup (40 g/1½ oz) breadcrumbs (GF: gluten-free bread crumbs)

500 g (17¾ oz) lean minced beef

1 tablespoon tamari (wheat-free)

½ red onion, finely chopped

1 clove garlic, crushed

1 egg, lightly beaten

1 tablespoon tomato paste

1 tablespoon sesame seeds

1 teaspoon mixed Italian herbs

1 tablespoon finely chopped fresh parsley

250g (9 oz) wholemeal spaghetti (GF: gluten-free spaghetti)

3 cups (750 ml/26¼ fl oz) fresh tomato sauce (refer to recipe)

¼ cup (30 g/1 0z) grated parmesan cheese (LF: vegan cheese)

You can make your own breadcrumbs by placing bread in a food processor and blending until they're fine crumbs. Place bread crumbs in a large bowl.

In a food processor, blend onion, garlic, minced meat, herbs, tomato paste, tamari, sesame seeds and egg. Mix until well combined.

Add mixture to breadcrumbs and combine well.

Using floured hands shape mixture into 15 small balls (1 heaped tablespoon each).

Place meatballs on a plate, cover in cling wrap and refrigerate for 30 minutes.

Lightly spray a frying pan with olive oil and place over a medium heat. Cook meatballs for 2 minutes each side, until golden brown and cooked through. Return meatballs to frying pan and cover them with tomato sauce. Cook for a few minutes and reduce heat to a simmer.

Cook pasta in a large saucepan of boiling water, according to packet instructions, then drain.

Place spaghetti on each plate and top with meatballs and tomato sauce. Sprinkle with parmesan cheese. Serve with a green salad.

Serves 4.

Variation: Replace minced beef with lean minced lamb, chicken, canned tuna or salmon. For a vegetarian option, replace mince meat with mashed, cooked chickpeas or lentils.

Bean falafels in mini pita pockets

Your kids will love eating this scrumptious Middle Eastern inspired dish. Eaten with warm wholegrain pitas, these bean falafels provide a complete protein meal as well as supplying important nutrients such as iron and B vitamins. Delicious served with tabouli, baba ghanoush, tzatziki or mango chutney.

½ cup (93 g/3¼ oz) millet, rinse well

2 x 440 g (15 ½ oz) cans broad beans or butter beans, drained

1 clove garlic, crushed

½ teaspoon ground cumin

1 teaspoon ground coriander

2 tablespoons fresh parsley, finely chopped

1 teaspoon fresh ginger, minced

Extra wholemeal flour for dusting (GF: brown rice or gluten-free plain flour)

10 wholemeal pita pockets (GF: gluten-free pita pockets)

Salad filling: lettuce, tomato, alfalfa Tzatziki

Place a saucepan over medium heat and bring 1¼ cups (313 ml/11 fl oz) of water to boil. Add millet and reduce heat, leave to simmer covered for 15-20 minutes until millet becomes fluffy.

In a blender add beans, garlic, ginger and herbs, mix until well combined.

In a bowl combine millet and chickpea mixture.

Using floured hands, shape mixture into 10 small balls (2 heaped tablespoons each). Dust each patty lightly with flour and shake off any excess.

Lightly spray a frying pan with olive oil and place over a medium heat. Cook falafels for 2 minutes each side, until golden brown and cooked through. Makes 10 falafels.

Warm some mini pita pockets under the grill or in the oven.

Split pocket breads open and fill with lettuce, falafel, tomato, alfalfa, and top with tzatziki.

Serves 5.

Variation: If using dried legumes refer to legume cooking chart. You can also use quinoa or couscous instead of millet (refer to grain cooking chart).

Serving suggestion: Add falafels to a green salad and top with tzatziki.

Chickpea vegie burger

These tasty chickpea patties form a complete protein meal, supplying all the essential amino acids needed for children's growth and development. These patties also provide your child with dietary fibre, iron and B vitamins.

1 onion, finely chopped

1 clove garlic, crushed

½ teaspoon ground cumin

½ teaspoon ground coriander

½ cup (75 g/ 2½ oz) grated zucchini

½ cup (75 g/2½ oz) grated carrot

2 teaspoons tamari (wheat-free)

1 egg, lightly beaten

¼ cup (25 g/¾ oz) finely chopped fresh basil

2 x 440g (15½ oz) cans chickpeas, drain well

1 ½ cups (278 g/9¾ oz) cooked brown rice

Wholemeal flour, for dusting (GF: brown rice or gluten-free plain flour)

Wholegrain bread rolls (GF: gluten-free bread rolls)

Salad filling: lettuce, tomato, beetroot, pineapple and avocado

Preheat oven to 200°C (400°F/Gas 6). Line a baking tray with baking paper. Lightly spray a frying pan with olive oil, cook onion and garlic until tender.

Place all ingredients (except rice) in a blender, mix until combined.

Place chickpea mixture and rice in a large bowl, mix until well combined.

Using floured hands, shape mixture into 10 medium patties (1/4 cup each). Dust each patty lightly with flour and shake off any excess.

Place patties on a plate, cover with cling wrap and refrigerate for 30 minutes. This helps the ingredients to bind, preventing patties from crumbling.

Place patties on baking tray and cook for 30 minutes, turning after 20 minutes. You could also cook patties in a frying pan lightly sprayed with olive oil, 5-6 minutes each side.

Makes 8 medium patties.

Spread rolls with avocado. Place patties on wholegrain bread rolls, top with salad, add desired healthy sauce or mayonnaise.

Variation: If using dried chickpeas refer to legume cooking chart. You can use millet or quinoa instead of brown rice (refer to grain cooking chart).

Tip: Soak brown rice in water for 30 minutes before cooking (for improved texture and reduced cooking time).

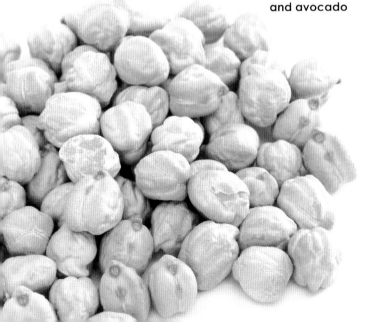

Lentil & millet patties

These lentil and millet patties make a well-balanced meal or snack. Lentils are nutrition powerhouses packed with protein, iron and zinc. Millet is a North African grain that is gluten-free and rich in magnesium and B vitamins.

¼ cup (30 g/1 oz) leek, finely chopped

1 clove garlic, crushed

2 x 440g (15½ oz) cans lentils, drained

1 egg, lightly beaten

1 cup (185 g/6½ oz) millet, rinse well

½ teaspoon finely grated ginger

1 teaspoon curry powder

2 teaspoons tamari (wheat-free)

1 tablespoon finely chopped fresh coriander

¼ cup (45 g/1½ oz) crushed walnuts

Extra wholemeal flour, for dusting (GF: brown rice or gluten-free plain flour)

Preheat oven to 200°C (400°F/Gas 6). Line a baking tray with baking paper.

Place a saucepan over medium heat and bring 2 ½ cups (625 ml/22 oz) of water to boil. Add millet and reduce heat, leave to simmer covered for 15-20 minutes until millet becomes fluffy.

Lightly spray a frying pan with olive oil and cook leek and garlic until tender.

Place all ingredients in a blender (except millet), mix until combined.

Place lentil mixture and millet in a large bowl, mix until well combined.

Using floured hands, shape mixture into 10 medium patties (1/4 cup each).

Dust each patty lightly with flour and shake off any excess.

Place patties on a plate, cover with cling wrap and refrigerate for 30 minutes. This helps the ingredients to bind, preventing patties from crumbling.

Place patties on baking tray and cook for 30 minutes, turning after 15 minutes. You could also cook patties in a frying pan lightly sprayed with olive oil, 5-6 minutes each side.

Makes 10 medium patties.

Variation: If using dried lentils refer to legume cooking chart.

Sesame crumbed tuna & zucchini patties

These flavoursome tuna patties with a hint of lemon are a great way to increase your child's fish intake. Tuna is an excellent source of essential omega-3 fats, important for the growth and development of the brain and nervous system. Tuna is also a rich source of protein plus minerals such as iodine, zinc and iron.

2 large potatoes, diced

500g (17¾ oz) can light tuna, drain well

¼ cup (30 g/1 oz) finely chopped shallots

2 tablespoons finely chopped fresh chives

1 clove garlic, crushed

2 tablespoons lemon juice

2 eggs

1 cup (150 g/5 ¼ oz) grated zucchini

Pinch sea salt

¼ cup (40 g/1½ oz) sesame seeds

¾ cup (60 g/2 oz) wholemeal breadcrumbs (GF: gluten-free breadcrumbs)

Extra wholemeal flour, for dusting(GF: brown rice or gluten-free plain flour)

Preheat oven to 200°C (400°F/Gas 6). Line a baking tray with baking paper.

Steam potato dices and mash (without milk).

Place potato, tuna, shallots, chives, garlic, lemon juice, 1 lightly beaten egg, zucchini and sea salt in a large bowl, combine well using a fork.

Using floured hands, shape mixture into 9 medium patties.

Dust each patty lightly with flour and shake off any excess.

In a small bowl place other egg and lightly whisk. Dip each patty in egg, until well covered.

In another bowl place breadcrumbs and sesame seeds, cover each patty in mixture.

Place patties on a plate, cover with cling wrap and refrigerate for 30 minutes. This helps the ingredients to bind and prevents crumbling.

Place patties on baking tray and cook for 30 minutes, turning after 15 minutes. You could also cook patties in a frying pan lightly sprayed with olive oil, 5-6 minutes each side.

Makes 9 medium patties.

Variation: For a vegetarian option replace tuna with a can of cannelloni beans (mashed).

Salmon, kumera & quinoa patties

Quinoa, an ancient South American grain, is quick to prepare and light and easy to digest. This gluten-free grain is very nutritious and known for its high protein content and lovely nutty flavour. These flavoursome salmon patties are a great way to increase your child's omega-3 fat intake.

¾ cup (150 g/5¼ oz) quinoa, rinse well

400g (14¼ oz) kumera (sweet potato), diced

½ onion, finely chopped

2 cloves garlic, crushed

440g (15½ oz) can pink salmon, drained with large bones removed

¾ cup (113 g/4 oz) grated carrot

2 tablespoons lemon juice

1 tablespoon finely chopped basil

1 egg, lightly beaten

Pinch sea salt

3 tablespoons wholemeal flour (GF: brown rice or gluten-free plain flour)

2 tablespoons salsa or tomato paste

Extra wholemeal flour, for dusting (GF: brown rice or gluten-free plain flour)

Preheat oven to 200°C (400°F/Gas 6). Line a baking tray with baking paper.

Rinse quinoa under cold running water for a couple of minutes to remove its bitter protective coating. Place a saucepan over medium heat and bring 1 ½ cups of water to boil. Add quinoa and reduce heat, leave to simmer covered for 15-20 minutes until tender.

Steam sweet potato dices until tender, then mash, do not add milk.

Lightly spray a frying pan with olive oil, cook onion and garlic until tender.

Place salmon in a large bowl, remove large bones then mash with a fork, including small soft bones. Add remaining ingredients and combine well.

Using floured hands, shape mixture into 10 medium patties (1/4 cup each).

Dust each patty lightly with flour and shake off any excess.

Place patties on a plate, cover with cling wrap and leave in the fridge for 30 minutes. This helps the ingredients to bind and prevent crumbling.

Place patties on baking tray and cook for 30 minutes, turning after 15 minutes. You could also cook patties in a frying pan lightly sprayed with olive oil, 5-6 minutes each side.

Makes 10 medium patties.

Variation: Replace salmon with tuna or chicken mince (make sure chicken is cooked through). For a vegetarian option replace salmon with chickpeas.

Tasty tortillas

Tortillas are a flat round unleavened bread made from either wheat or corn. These versatile Mexican breads can be used in a number of different ways to make delicious meals and snacks. Warmed tortillas make fantastic fajitas, toasted they make tasty quesadillas or wraps, and baked they make healthy low-fat crispy tacos or tortilla chips. Keep tortillas in the freezer until ready for use.

Healthy nachos

Kids love eating nachos with their hands, using corn chips as scoops. Corn chips however, are cooked in hydrogenated vegetable oils and contain unhealthy trans-fats. This healthy version, using tortilla chips, still has the same authentic taste without all the fat.

2 wheat tortillas (GF: 4 smaller corn tortillas)

¼ **teaspoon paprika**

¼ **iceberg lettuce, shredded**

Kidney bean mince (refer to recipe)

½ **cup (125 g/4½ oz) guacamole (refer to recipe)**

1 cup (250 g/9 oz) low-fat cottage cheese (LF: grated vegan cheese)

¼ **cup (30 g/1 oz) grated low-fat cheddar cheese (LF: vegan cheese)**

Preheat oven to 200°C (400°F/Gas 6). Line a baking tray with baking paper.

Cut tortillas into small triangles the size of corn chips. Sprinkle with a little paprika and place on a baking tray.

Bake for 4 minutes until crisp (careful they don't burn).

In 4 flat bowls lay iceberg lettuce around edges (make sure it's not too moist).

Place tortilla chips with edges sticking out around the lettuce.

Fill the centre with kidney bean mince, top with a heap tablespoon of cottage cheese and a tablespoon of guacamole. Then sprinkle a little low-fat grated cheese.

Makes 4.

Variation: Add ¼ cup (50 g/¾ oz) cooked corn kernels to bean mix. Add ¼ cup (38 g/1¼ oz) cooked pumpkin dices to bean mix.

Kidney bean tacos

Tacos are one of the most popular Mexican foods and a big hit with kids. Your kids will have fun packing their own taco shells with these tasty healthy fillings. Commercially made taco shells are usually cooked in hydrogenated vegetable oils and contain unhealthy trans-fats. These delicious crunchy taco shells made by baking tortillas are a low-fat healthy alternative. Use leftover kidney bean mix as wrap fillers.

4-6 wholewheat tortillas (GF: 6-8 smaller corn tortillas)

2 tomatoes, diced

½ shredded iceberg lettuce

½ cup (60 g/2¼ oz) low-fat grated cheddar or cottage cheese (LF: vegan cheese)

½ cup (125 g/4½ oz) guacamole or diced avocado

Salsa

KIDNEY BEAN MINCE:

1 medium onion, diced

2 cloves garlic, crushed

250 g (8¾ oz) lean minced meat – optional

440g (15½ oz) can red kidney beans, drained

½ red capsicum, diced

½ green capsicum, diced

2 teaspoons ground cumin

2 teaspoons ground paprika

¼ teaspoon chilli powder

400 g (14 oz/2 cups) can tomatoes, chopped

2 tablespoons tomato paste

1 cup (250 ml/9 fl oz) salt-reduced vegetable stock or water

Preheat oven to 180°C (350°C/Gas 4).

Lightly spray a frying pan with olive oil and place over a medium heat. Cook onion and garlic until tender.

Add mince and spices and cook for a further 5 minutes, breaking mince up.

Add kidney beans, capsicum, herbs, tomatoes, tomato paste and vegetable stock. Reduce heat and simmer for 20 minutes, stirring occasionally.

Hang each tortilla bread evenly over 3 rungs of oven rack. Bake for 8-10 minutes until they are crisp and hold their shape. Watch that they don't burn.

Place filling ingredients in separate bowls and serve with a plate of warm taco shells.

Take a taco shell, fill with 2 tablespoons of bean mince, diced tomato, lettuce, avocado, a sprinkling of cheese and a teaspoon of salsa.

Serves 4.

Variation: For a vegetarian option replace minced meat with more kidney beans or dices of firm tofu. If you are using dried kidney beans refer to legume cooking chart.

Toasted chicken, roast vegetable & feta quesadillas

Quesadillas are toasted tortillas filled with melted cheese and other tasty fillings. You can get creative using any combination of nutritious fillings you like. These quesadillas make a nice alternative to toasted sandwiches, great for weekend lunches and light dinners served with a salad.

2 corn tortillas

¼ cup (45 g/1½ oz) shredded cooked chicken breast

2 tablespoons crumbled low-fat feta (LF: vegan cheese)

Roast vegetables, thin slices (kumera, zucchini, eggplant, potato and capsicum)

Lightly spray a frying pan with olive oil and place over a medium heat. Place one tortilla in pan and cover with shredded chicken, sprinkle with cheese and top with roast vegetable slices.

Place other tortilla on top and cook until browned on one side. Flip and cook until other side is browned and cheese has melted.

Cut into 4 triangles and serve hot with a side salad.

Serves 1-2.

Variation: Replace chicken with a small can of salmon or tuna, sliced roast turkey, beef, or firm tofu. Add salsa, pesto, avocado, mango or beetroot chutney, or hummus.

Crispy almond & sesame chicken nuggets

These scrumptious chicken nuggets are packed with protein, needed for children's growth and development. Commercial chicken nuggets are usually made with poor quality chicken and high in unhealthy fats and chemical additives. These healthy nuggets are low in fat and contain nutrients such as iron, zinc and calcium. As a snack serve with a dipping sauce, or for a nutritious dinner serve with vegetables and mash. Pack leftovers for school lunches.

500 g (17¾ oz) chicken breast, cut into nuggets

1 cup (250 ml/9 fl oz) low-fat milk (LF: rice, almond, soy or lactose-free milk)

1 cup (120 g/4¼ oz) wholemeal flour (GF: gluten-free plain flour)

2 teaspoons mixed dried herbs (rosemary, oregano, garlic, basil or chives)

Pinch sea salt

¾ cup (45 g/1½ oz) natural corn flakes, crushed

½ cup (85 g/3 oz) almond flakes, crushed

2 tablespoons sesame seeds

Preheat oven to 190°C (375°F/Gas 5). Line a baking tray with baking paper.

You will need 3 separate bowls. In one bowl place milk. In a second bowl place flour, sea salt and herbs. In a third bowl place corn flakes, sesame seeds and almonds.

Coat each chicken piece in flour, coat in milk, then roll in almond and sesame mix until well coated.

Place nuggets on baking tray and cook for 15-20 minutes, until chicken is well cooked. Make sure chicken nuggets are not pink in the centre.

Oven baked crumbed fish

Crumbed fish bought from fish and chip shops or frozen varieties are usually deep fried in hydrogenated vegetable oils and contain harmful trans-fats. This healthy low-fat version with a delightful crispy crust is as tasty as it is good for you. Serve with homemade chips and a crispy green salad.

¾ cup (90 g/3¼ oz) wholemeal or spelt flour (GF: gluten-free plain flour)

3 tablespoons low-fat milk (LF: rice, almond or lactose-free milk)

2 eggs, lightly beaten

¾ cup (60 g/2 oz) wholemeal bread crumbs (GF: gluten-free bread crumbs)

¼ cup (40 g/11/2 oz) sesame seeds

¼ cup (23 g/¾ oz) parmesan, finely grated (LF: vegan cheese) – optional

500g (17 ¾ oz) fish fillets, boneless

Preheat oven to 200°C (400°F/Gas 6). Line a baking tray with baking paper.

You will need 3 dishes. Place flour in the first dish. Combine milk and egg in a second and combine breadcrumbs, sesame seeds and parmesan in a third.

Pat fish pieces dry with a paper towel. Coat fish with flour, dip into milk mixture, then dip into sesame and bread crumb mixture, making sure fish is well coated.

Place crumbed fish on a plate, cover with cling wrap and place in the fridge for 20 minutes.

Place on baking tray and cook for 25 minutes, until golden brown and cooked through. Turn after 15 minutes.

Nori rolls

These Japanese rolls are wrapped in toasted seaweed and filled with rice and other nutritious ingredients. Seaweed is a highly nutritious food, rich in protein, calcium, iron and iodine. Seaweed is also known to have immune boosting powers. These rolls are great for school lunches or cut up into smaller rolls and served with miso soup. Kids always have lots of fun trying to eat these rolls with chopsticks.

4 nori roll sheets

1 cup (185 g/6½ oz) cooked brown rice

2 tablespoons rice wine vinegar or lemon juice

1 egg

1 tablespoon milk

4 nori sheets

Avocado, long thin strips

Lettuce, finely shredded

Lebanese cucumber, long thin strips

Carrot, finely grated

Alfalfa sprouts

Creamy mayonnaise (refer to recipe) – optional

You will need a bamboo mat

Cook rice to packet instructions, stir in vinegar and allow rice to cool.

Deseed cucumber by cutting in half lengthways and scooping out the seeds. Cut into long thin strips.

Lightly spray a frying pan with olive oil and place over a medium heat. In a small bowl whisk an egg with 1 tablespoon of milk. Fry egg and then place on a chopping board and cut into thin strips.

Place nori sheet shiny side down on a bamboo mat.

Dip your hands in water and pat a ¼ cup rice over 2/3 of the nori sheet, leaving the end clear.

Lay some avocado, egg, lettuce, carrot, cucumber and alfalfa width ways along the centre of the rice. Add a little mayonnaise if desired. Holding the mat roll the nori over and over to the edge of the rice.

Dampen the remaining nori and roll it up. Using the mat pull the roll tightly to seal.

Makes 4 large nori rolls

Variations: Replace egg with cooked strips of chicken, salmon, tuna or tofu.

Rice paper rolls

Rice paper rolls can be made with any nutritious fillings you like. Let your kids create their own combinations. Great as a healthy snack or for school lunches.

10 large rice paper sheets

2-3 tablespoons sweet chilli sauce (or mango chutney)

250 g (8¾ oz) cooked chicken breast, shredded

50g dried mung bean or rice vermicelli noodles

1 carrot, cut into thin strips

½ red capsicum, cut into thin strips

Handful fresh mint, finely chopped

Handful fresh coriander, finely chopped

3 tablespoons crushed cashew nuts (raw and unsalted)

¼ lettuce, shredded

In a medium bowl soak vermicelli noodles, carrot and capsicum in boiling water for 10 minutes. Drain when noodles are soft and separated. Add sweet chilli sauce and mix until well coated.

Fill a shallow, wide dish with warm water. Cover a chopping board with a damp clean tea towel.

Dip rice paper sheets into the warm water for a few seconds, until they soften, then place on moist tea towel.

In the centre of the paper place some chicken, carrot, capsicum, vermicelli, lettuce, a sprinkling of herbs and cashew nuts. Don't add too much filling or you will not be able to roll it properly.

Flatten the filling down and fold in the two sides, roll it up tightly. Lay the seam side down on a plate and cover them with a damp tea towel. If they start to go brittle spray them with a little water.

Makes 10 rice paper rolls.

Tip: When you pack rice paper rolls in a lunch box, spray them with a little water so they don't go brittle and wrap them in cling wrap.

Variations: Replace chicken with cooked tuna, salmon, tofu, thin beef or lamb strips. Add avocado strips.

Tuna & corn pasta bake

This nutritious pasta bake makes a well-balanced meal, containing energy giving complex carbohydrates, protein, omega-3 fats and a good dose of calcium. Serve with a green salad or steamed vegetables.

**4 cups (622 g/2 ¾ oz) uncooked penne pasta
(GF: gluten-free pasta)**

½ cup (100 g/3½ oz) corn kernels (frozen)

440 g (15½ oz) tin tuna, drained

**1½ cups (375 ml/12¾ fl oz) low-fat milk (LF: rice,
almond, soy or lactose-free milk)**

**½ cup (125 g/4½ oz) low-fat cottage cheese
(LF: grated vegan cheese)**

¼ cup (13 g/½ oz) finely chopped parsley

2 cloves garlic, crushed

**3 tablespoons spelt or flour (GF: brown rice or
gluten-free plain flour)**

**⅓ cup (80 g/2¾ oz) grated low-fat cheddar cheese
(LF: vegan cheese)**

¼ cup (30 g/1 oz) finely sliced leek

Preheat oven to 200°C (400°F/Gas 6). Lightly spray a baking dish with olive oil.

In a large saucepan cook pasta according to packet instructions, drain and rinse. Add corn kernels to saucepan for the last 4 minutes of cooking.

In a bowl combine pasta, tuna flakes and corn.

In a small saucepan bring milk to nearly boiling point then reduce heat. Add cottage cheese, garlic and herbs, whisk until well combined. Add flour and stir until sauce thickens. Add in grated cheese and leek, continue stirring.

Pour half the pasta mix in baking dish and cover with half the cheese mixture and repeat.

Bake for 25-30 minutes until golden brown. Allow pasta to sit for 10 minutes, then cut into squares and serve.

Serves 4.

Variation: You can sprinkle breadcrumbs, seeds and a little cheese on top for a crusty topping.

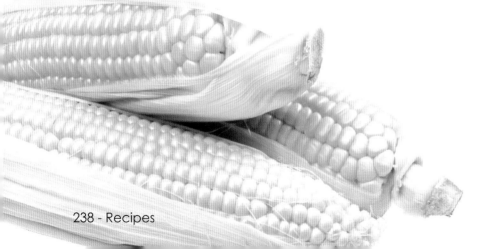

Vegie lasagna

This gluten-free vegetarian lasagna is packed full of antioxidant rich vegetables and topped with a delicious pesto sauce. Served with a crisp green salad this lasagna is even better the next day, so be sure to make enough for leftovers.

6 large rice lasagna sheets

¼ cup (63 g/2¼ oz) pesto

1 eggplant, thin slices

2 red capsicums, thin strips

1 large onion, finely chopped

2 cloves garlic, crushed

2 large zucchini's, small dices

400 g (14 oz/2 cups) can tomatoes

1 cup (250 ml/9 fl oz) tomato pasta sauce

3 large spinach leaves, finely chopped

440g (15½ oz) can lentils, drained

1 teaspoon dried Italian herbs

2 large sweet potatoes, diced

1 tablespoon low-fat milk (LF: rice, almond, soy or lactose-free milk)

1 tablespoon pepitas (pumpkin seeds)

Handful of grated cheddar cheese (LF: vegan cheese)

Preheat oven to 180°C (350°F/Gas 4). Lightly spray a lasagna dish with olive oil.

Steam sweet potato until tender, transfer to a bowl and mash with a little milk.

In a small bowl mix pesto and mash together.

Lightly spray a frying pan with olive oil and place over a medium heat. Lightly fry eggplant and capsicum strips and transfer to a plate.

Add onion, garlic and zucchini to frying pan and cook until soft. Add tomatoes, tomato sauce, spinach, lentils and herbs and cook for a further 10 minutes.

Layer lasagna in this order: tomato sauce, lasagna sheets, tomato sauce, eggplant, lasagna sheets, tomato sauce, capsicum, lasagna sheets, tomato sauce, and pesto mash.

Sprinkle with pepitas and cheese and bake for 60 minutes, until golden brown and cooked through. Cover with foil when browned.

Serves 4-6.

Variation: Add cooked lean minced beef or lamb, or tuna or salmon to tomato sauce.

Lamb & vegetable kebabs

These kebabs are a fun way to serve vegetables and iron-rich lamb to your kids. Perfect for BBQs and picnics served with a salad or rice.

500g (17¾ oz) cubes of lamb

1 tablespoon cold pressed virgin olive oil

1 clove garlic, crushed

2 tablespoons lemon juice

1 tablespoon tamari (wheat-free)

1 tablespoon grated fresh ginger

8 cherry tomatoes

2 thick slices pineapple, cut into large pieces

1 red capsicum, large pieces

2 steamed cobs of corn, cut each into 4 pieces

8 skewers, soak in water for an hour (stops them from burning and splitting)

Place meat cubes in a bowl and sprinkle with garlic, ginger, tamari, lemon juice and olive oil. Rub mixture into meat.

Leave meat covered to marinate in the fridge for a few hours or overnight.

Thread corn, meat, cherry tomatoes, pineapple and capsicum on skewers.

Baste with a little lemon juice.

Grill or BBQ kebabs for 12-15 minutes, turning every 3 minutes, until meat has cooked through.

Makes 8 kebabs.

Variation: Instead of lamb, use cubes of salmon, tuna or chicken. For a vegetarian option use firm tofu cubes.

Tandoori chicken skewers with turmeric rice

This aromatic Indian dish is a lovely way to introduce your children to an array of herbs and spices. Delicious served with colourful turmeric and currant rice and a spoonful of mango chutney.

4 x 200g chicken breast (or lamb or fish), cut into cubes

½ cup natural yoghurt (LF: lactose-free yoghurt)

2 tablespoon lemon juice

1 tablespoon finely grated fresh ginger

1 tablespoon garlic, minced

½ teaspoon turmeric

1 teaspoon cumin

1 teaspoon coriander

½ teaspoon chilli

½ teaspoon ground cardamon

1 teaspoon garam masala

1 teaspoon of cinnamon

OPTIONAL

Mango chutney (refer to recipe)

TURMERIC RICE:

1½ cups (278 g/9¾ oz) basmati rice, rinse well

2 cups (500 ml/18 fl oz) low-salt vegetable stock

½ teaspoon turmeric

2-3 tablespoons currants

2-3 tablespoons flaked almonds

skewers, soak in water for an hour (stops them from burning and splitting)

Thread chicken cubes on skewers. Combine yoghurt , lemon, garlic, ginger, and spices together in a bowl. Marinade chicken skewers in the mixture, in the fridge, covered, for a few hours or overnight.

To make rice, add rice, vegetable stock, cinnamon and turmeric to a saucepan and bring to boil. Reduce heat, cover and simmer for 12 minutes.

When rice is tender remove from heat and add currants and almonds, leave for 10 minutes covered.

Grill or BBQ skewers for 12-15 minutes, turning every 3 minutes, until chicken is cooked through.

Serves 4.

Rice and skewers taste delicious served with some mango chutney.

Variation: Instead of chicken cover salmon fillets with tandoori mixture and bake, uncovered. Cook in a 200°C oven for around 30-40 minutes, until cooked to your liking.

Mild lamb curry

This delicious, wholesome curry is a perfect way to introduce your child to spicy foods. Feel free to substitute any of the vegetables in this dish for your favourite seasonal vegetables. Serve with steamed rice and a spoonful of mango chutney.

1 kg (35 oz) lean lamb (or beef or chicken)

1 onion, chopped

1 clove garlic, minced

2 large carrots, large dices

1 cup (170 g/6 oz) potato, diced

4 celery sticks, thick slices

1 medium apple, grated

2 teaspoons mild curry powder

400g (14 oz) can tomatoes

2 cups (500 ml/17¾ oz) water

2 teaspoons raw organic honey

2 teaspoons lemon juice

1 tablespoon spelt flour (GF: brown rice or arrowroot flour)

1 cup (185 g/6½ oz) brown rice, rinse well

1 tablespoon sesame or sunflower seeds

Trim fat from meat and cut into cubes. Lightly spray frying pan with olive oil and place over a medium heat. Place onion, garlic and meat in frying pan and cook until lightly browned.

Add vegetables and apple to frying pan and cook for a couple of minutes. Add curry powder, tomato, water, honey and lemon juice. Combine well.

Cover and simmer for 45 minutes until meat and vegetables are cooked through, stirring occasionally and adding more water if becoming too dry.

Blend flour in a little water and add to curry, stirring until curry starts to thicken.

Cook brown rice according to packet instructions. Serve curry with rice and sprinkle with sesame seeds.

Serves 4.

Variation: You can add ½ cup (80 g/2¾ oz) of diced red capsicum or 2 slices of fresh pineapple (thickly diced).

Tip: Soak brown rice in water for 30 minutes before cooking (for improved texture and reduced cooking time).

Chickpea curry

This aromatic and delicately spiced curry is packed with protein, dietary fibre, B vitamins and iron. Serve with brown rice for a well-balanced, 'complete protein' meal.

1 large onion, chopped

2 cloves garlic, crushed

1 teaspoon ground turmeric

1 teaspoon ground paprika

1 teaspoon ground cumin

1 teaspoon ground coriander

2 x 440g (15½ oz) cans chickpeas, drained

1 cup (260 g/9 oz) mashed pumpkin

400 g (14 oz) can tomatoes

3 tablespoons 100% apple juice (no-added-sugar)

1 cup (150 g/5¼ oz) diced zucchini

Lightly spray a frying pan with olive oil and place over medium heat. Cook onion and garlic until tender.

Add chickpeas, tomatoes, zucchini, apple juice, herbs and spices, cook for 5 minutes. Reduce heat and simmer for 20 minutes, stirring occasionally.

Steam pumpkin and mash in a small bowl. Stir through curry until well combined and curry thickened.

Serve with steamed rice and warmed wholemeal pita bread.

Serves 4.

Variation: if using dried chickpeas refer to legume cooking chart.

Spicy pea & lentil dahl

This tasty Indian dish is a quick and nutritious meal. Lentils are an excellent source of protein, dietary fibre, B vitamins, iron and zinc. Dahl goes perfectly with warm pita bread.

1 teaspoon finely grated fresh ginger

1 onion, finely chopped

1 clove garlic, crushed

1 ¼ cups (234 g/8¼ oz) green lentils, rinse well

1 teaspoon ground turmeric

1 teaspoon garam masala

½ cup (80 g/2¾ oz) peas (fresh or frozen)

½ cup (100 g/3½ oz) corn kernels (frozen)

1 carrot, diced

3 tablespoons lemon juice

400 g (140 oz) can tomatoes

Lightly spray a large saucepan with olive oil and place over a medium heat. Add onion and garlic and cook until tender.

Add lentils, carrot, ginger, spices and 4 cups (1250 ml/43 ½ fl oz) of water, and then bring to the boil. Reduce heat and simmer covered for 30-45 minutes, until lentils are tender and water has been absorbed. If lentils are not cooked through you can add more water.

Just before lentils have finished cooking, add peas, corn, tomato and lemon juice, and cook for another 5 minutes.

Serves 4.

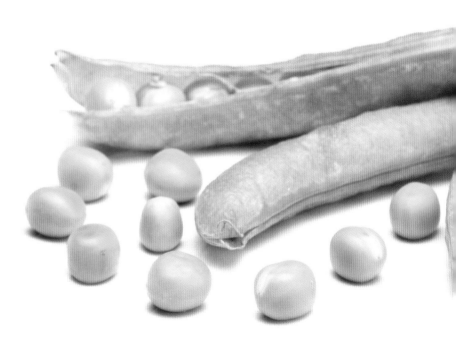

Vegetable & lima bean casserole

This hearty casserole is sure to warm those tummies on a cold winters night. You can use a variety of different seasonal vegetables for this dish. Delicious served with rice, millet, quinoa or mashed potato. Leftovers packed in a warm thermos make a nutritious school lunch.

1 onion, finely chopped

1 clove garlic, crushed

1 celery stalk, finely chopped

440g (15½ oz) can lima beans, drained

1 small carrot, thick slices

2 large potatoes, medium sized dices

1 small zucchini, thick slices

400 g (14 oz/2 cups) can tomato, diced

1 teaspoon dried oregano

Handful fresh parsley or basil, chopped

1 cup (250 ml/9 fl oz) salt-reduced vegetable stock or water

Preheat oven to 200°C (400°F/Gas 6). Lightly spray a casserole dish with olive oil.

Spray a frying pan with olive oil and place over a medium heat. Cook onion and garlic until tender.

Place all ingredients in casserole dish, stir until combined.

Cover and bake for 40 minutes or until vegetables are tender, stir occasionally. If casserole is a little dry you can add some extra fluid.

Serves 4.

Variation: Replace lima beans with lamb, beef or chicken cubes. If using dried lima beans refer to legume cooking chart.

Rosemary chicken & kumera risotto

This Italian classic is sure to be a favourite with the kids. Ideal any time of year, this tasty risotto is low in saturated fats and packed with protein and energy giving complex carbohydrates. Serve with a green salad or pack leftovers in a warm thermos for school lunches.

1 tablespoon cold pressed virgin olive oil

1 onion, finely chopped

1 clove garlic, crushed

Handful fresh rosemary, finely chopped

2 cups (440 g/15½ oz) aborio rice, rinse well

6 cups (1½ Litres/52½ fl oz) salt-reduced vegetable stock

1 medium kumera (sweet potato), peeled and chopped

1 medium zucchini, diced

300g (10½ oz) chicken breast, cubes

½ cup (46 g/1½ oz) grated low-fat parmesan cheese (LF: vegan cheese)

Cook chicken, sweet potato and zucchini in a frying pan over a medium heat. Transfer to a plate when chicken is well cooked and sweet potato is tender.

In a large saucepan add olive oil and place over a medium heat. Add onion, garlic and rosemary and cook until tender. Add rice and stir until rice is well coated.

Cook for a couple of minutes and then slowly add stock. Pour ½ cup of stock at a time, stirring until fully absorbed. Continue until all stock has been absorbed and rice is tender.

Add chicken, sweet potato and zucchini to rice, gently combine. Cook for another few minutes until chicken and vegetables have heated through.

Stir through cheese and leave covered for a few minutes before serving. Garnish with parmesan cheese.

Serves 4.

Lentil & vegie cottage pie

Winter wouldn't be the same without a hearty cottage pie. My version of this old time classic is a perfect way to sneak extra vegetables into your child's diet - add any combination of vegetables you like. Lentils in this pie can easily be replaced with minced beef, lamb or chicken.

1 clove garlic, crushed

½ tablespoon tamari (wheat-free)

500g (17¾ oz) cooked lentils (or minced lean beef, lamb or chicken)

2 tablespoons spelt flour (GF: brown rice or gluten-free plain flour)

1 small onion, finely chopped

2 ripe tomatoes, small dices

2 tablespoons chopped fresh parsley

4 large potatoes

¼ cup (63 ml/3 oz) low-fat milk (LF: rice, almond, soy or lactose-free milk)

1 cup (160 g/5½ oz) peas (fresh or frozen)

1 cup (170 g/6 oz) small dices of carrot

1 cup (200 g/7 oz) corn kernels

¼ cup (30 g/1 oz) grated low-fat cheddar cheese (LF: vegan cheese)

Preheat oven to 190°C (375°F/Gas 5). Lightly spray 6 individual oven proof bowls with olive oil.

Lightly spray a frying pan with olive oil and place over a medium heat. Cook onion, garlic and minced meat until mince is lightly browned.

Add corn, carrot, tomato and flour, cook for 5 minutes, stirring until well combined.

Add lentils, peas, tamari and parsley and simmer for another 3 minutes. Add a little water if too dry.

Steam or boil potatoes until soft, transfer to a bowl, add milk and peas, and mash until a smooth consistency.

Spoon meat mixture into individual heat proof bowls and top with potato mash.

Sprinkle cheese on top and bake for 15 minutes until tops are golden.

Makes 6 individual pies.

Variation: Use a wholemeal base (see quiche recipe). Use sweet potato instead of potato and peas for mash topping. Make one large cottage pie in a casserole dish. If you are using minced meat or chicken brown it first in the frying pan with the onion and garlic.

Individual pizzas

Why order a pizza dripping with saturated fats and low on nutritious toppings when you can make your own healthy pizza at home. If you don't have time to make the base yourself use flat breads such as pita breads, Lebanese bread or tortillas. You can even use wholemeal muffins for mini pizzas. Your kids will love making their own pizza creations. Here is a delicious, light and crispy wholemeal base for you to try along with some tasty topping suggestions.

WHOLEMEAL PIZZA BASE:
2 cups (240 g/8½ oz) wholemeal flour (GF: gluten-free plain flour)

1 teaspoon baking powder (GF: gluten-free baking powder)

¼ cup (63 ml/2¼ fl oz) cold pressed virgin olive oil

2/3 cup (167 ml/5¾ fl oz) water

BASE SPREADS:
Tomato paste, hummus, sun dried tomato or basil pesto

VEGETABLES:
Roast vegetables (pumpkin, kumera or potato), spinach, mushrooms, lightly steamed broccoli florets, corn, zucchini, capsicum, onion (sauté first), pitted olives finely sliced

FRUIT:
Pineapple, tomatoes or fig slices

PROTEIN:
Cooked strips of lamb, chicken or tofu, salmon or tuna, or a small can of legumes

HERBS, SPICES & SEEDS:
Crushed garlic, fresh basil or coriander, oregano, sesame seeds, pepitas or sunflower seeds

SPRINKLE WITH LOW-FAT CHEESE:
Grated cheddar, mozzarella, parmesan or crumbled feta, ricotta or cottage cheese (LF: vegan cheese). You can also use spoonfuls of natural yoghurt instead of cheese (it melts and sets just like cheese).

Preheat oven to 200°C (400°F/Gas 6). Line baking trays with baking paper.

In a bowl combine flour and baking powder. Add oil and water, combine with your hands until mixture resembles a soft dough.

Roll dough out onto a well-floured board, divide into 4, and then roll into 4 round bases.

Place bases on trays, prick with a fork several times and bake for 15 minutes.

Cover pizza base with desired spread.

Top with a selection of vegetables, fruit and protein.

Sprinkle with desired herbs and top with cheese.

Cook for 20 minutes, until golden brown and topping is bubbling.

You can serve topped with a handful of baby spinach or a spoonful of chutney or natural yoghurt.

Makes 4 small pizzas.

Variation: Use ½ teaspoon of xanthan gum if using brown rice flour for the base.

Dessert

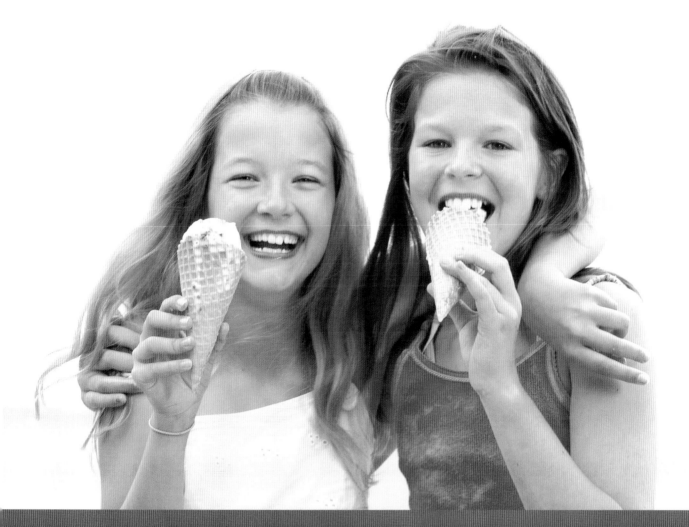

Made with 100% all natural ingredients these delicious desserts are packed with fresh fruit, wholegrain cereals and calcium-rich yoghurt. You can feel guilt-free knowing you're giving your child something that's good for their health.

Ice blocks

These refreshing ice blocks are a healthy alternative to commercially made icy poles that are full of sugar and artificial colours and flavourings.

Raspberry & watermelon ice block:
Both raspberry and watermelon are packed with antioxidants, vitamin C and dietary fibre.

¼ of a watermelon (remove seeds) • 2 cups (267 g/9¼ oz) raspberries (frozen or fresh)

Place watermelon and raspberries in a blender and mix until well combined. Pour into ice block moulds and freeze.

Yoghurt topped fruit ice block:
This ice block is a good way to increase your child's yoghurt intake. Yoghurt contains beneficial live bacteria which helps strengthen the immune system and improve digestion. Yoghurt is also an excellent source of protein and calcium.

1 cup (250 g/9 oz) fruit yoghurt (LF: lactose-free yoghurt) • 2 cups (250 m/9 fl oz) 100% fruit juice (tropical, apple, orange or mango)

Fill ¼ of each ice block mould with yoghurt. Place in the freezer until it starts to set. Fill the rest of the moulds with fruit juice then place back in the freezer to set.

Orange & mango ice block: Oranges
and mangoes are both rich in vitamin C, beta-carotene and dietary fibre.

8 oranges (freshly squeezed) • 1 large mango • 1 cup (250 ml/9 fl oz) apple juice (100% with no added sugar)

Place oranges, mango and apple juice in a blender and mix until well combined. Pour into ice block moulds and place in the freezer to set.

Yoghurt ice blocks: These yoghurt ice blocks
are an excellent way to increase your child's protein and calcium intake for the day.

1 cup (250 g/9 oz) vanilla or fruit yoghurt (LF: lactose-free or soy yoghurt) • 1 cup (150 g/5¼ oz) desired fruit (mango, berries or banana) • ¾ cup (167 ml/5¾ fl oz) low-fat milk (LF: rice, almond, soy or lactose-free milk)

Place yoghurt, fruit and milk in a blender and mix until well combined. Pour into ice block moulds and freeze.

Carob coated banana ice creams:
Your kids are going to love these creamy banana ice creams with a crunchy carob coating. Carob is a great source of calcium and is a caffeine-free alternative to chocolate.

2 large bananas, cut into thirds • 125g (4½ oz) carob buds, unsweetened (LF: soy carob) • 3 paddle pop sticks, cut in half • crushed nuts or desiccated coconut

Push a paddle pop stick up the centre of each banana piece. Melt carob in a water bath over a medium heat. When carob is melted keep bowl in the water bath on low heat. Dip banana pieces into carob mixture, coating the whole banana. Place in the freezer to set. Variation: Once dipped in carob, roll each banana in crushed nuts or desiccated coconut.

Fruit jelly

Commonly used in Asian desserts agar-agar is a type of seaweed that acts like a vegetarian gelatin. Commercial jellies are made with gelatin made from cow's bones and contain lots of sugars and artificial colourings and flavourings. This jelly makes a delicious healthy summer dessert served with fresh fruit, homemade ice cream or yoghurt.

1 cup (150 g/4¼ oz) diced fresh fruit (mango, pineapple, berries or peach).

2 tablespoons agar-agar powder or 6 tablespoons of flakes

3 ¼ cups (813 ml/28½ fl oz) fruit juice (freshly squeezed or 100% no added sugar)

Very lightly spray 6 jelly moulds with olive oil so jellies come out cleanly when set. Quarter fill each mould with diced fruit.

In a small bowl dissolve agar-agar powder in ¼ cup (63 ml/2¼ fl oz) of juice, stir well. In a small saucepan over a medium heat add fruit juice and agar-agar, stir until well combined.

Remove from heat and allow to cool slightly then pour into jelly moulds. Place in the fridge to set. When set turn out onto a plate and top with fresh fruit. Serves 6.

Creamy mango jelly

This delicious creamy jelly is a taste of the tropics in every mouthful. Made with juicy mango pieces this jelly is rich in vitamin C, beta-carotene and antioxidants.

1 cup (150 g/5¼ oz) diced mango

2 tablespoons agar-agar powder or 6 tablespoons of flakes

3¼ cups (813 ml/28½ fl oz) almond milk

2 tablespoons raw organic honey

Lightly spray 6 jelly moulds with olive oil so jellies come out cleanly when set. Quarter fill each mould with diced mango.

In a small bowl dissolve agar-agar powder in ¼ cup (63 ml/2¼ fl oz) of milk and stir well. In a small saucepan over a medium heat add milk and agar-agar and stir until well combined. Remove from heat and stir in honey.

Allow to cool slightly and then pour into jelly moulds. Place in the fridge to set. When set turn out onto a plate and top with fresh fruit. Serves 6.

Raspberry baked rice pudding

This old time classic with a raspberry twist will be a sure winner with the kids. This dessert is an excellent source of energy giving complex carbohydrates, protein and calcium. Raspberries give this dessert an extra vitamin C and antioxidant boost.

2 cups cooked jasmine or basmati rice

2 ½ cups (625 ml/21¾ fl oz) low-fat milk (LF: almond, soy or lactose-free milk)

3 tablespoons raw organic honey

1 large ripe banana, small dices

2 eggs

1 vanilla bean

1 cup (150 g/5 ¼ oz) raspberries (fresh or frozen)

1 teaspoon cinnamon

2 tablespoons almond flakes

Preheat oven to 180°C (350°F/Gas 4). Lightly spray an ovenproof baking dish with olive oil.

Using a sharp knife slice vanilla bean in half, lengthways. Scrape out the vanilla seeds with the tip of the knife.

Place eggs, milk, honey and vanilla seeds in a blender and mix until well combined.

Place rice, banana and raspberries in baking dish and cover with milk mixture.

Bake in moderate oven for 15 min. Take out of oven and gently stir until rice and raspberries are evenly mixed through pudding. Sprinkle with cinnamon and almond flakes and return to oven for 30-35 minutes, until pudding is set. Cover with foil if pudding is becoming too brown.

Let stand for 5 minutes before serving. Serve warm or cold.

Serves 4-6.

Variation: Replace raspberries with sultanas and diced apple, or mango, peaches or pear.

Apricot creamy rice

This delicious creamy rice is packed with energy giving complex carbohydrates, protein and calcium. Get creative and use any combination of fruits, nuts and seeds you like.

½ cup (110 g/3 ¾ oz) aborio rice, rinse well

3 cups (750 ml/26 fl oz) low-fat milk (LF: almond, soy or lactose-free milk)

1 tablespoon raw organic honey

½ teaspoon cinnamon

1 teaspoon vanilla essence

8 sun-dried apricot halves

2 tablespoons almond flakes

Cut apricots into strips. Place apricots in a bowl of boiling water and cover. Leave for 30 minutes.

Pour milk in a saucepan and add rice, vanilla and cinnamon. Bring to the boil, then leave to simmer with lid on for 25 minutes, until rice is soft and creamy. Add apricots at the end and heat through.

Take off the heat and stir in honey.
Serve topped with almonds.

Serves 4.

Variation: Replace apricots with fresh berries, mango, banana or sultanas. Sprinkle with sesame or sunflower seeds or grated carob.

Ice cream

Made from fresh fruit and other nutritious ingredients these delicious low-fat ice creams will satisfy the cravings of any ice cream loving kid. These ice creams are a healthy alternative to commercial ice creams that are high in sugar, saturated fats and artificial additives. Try some different toppings such as fresh fruit, shaved carob, fruit puree sauce or toasted nuts.

Strawberry yoghurt ice cream: This creamy ice cream will supply your kids with protein, calcium and vitamin C. Yoghurt is rich in beneficial live bacteria, important for boosting your child's immunity and digestive health.

1 cup (250 g/9 oz) strawberry yoghurt (LF: lactose-free strawberry yoghurt) • 1 cup (250 ml/9 fl oz) low-fat milk (LF: rice, almond, soy or lactose-free milk) • 2 tablespoon raw organic honey • ½ cup (75 g/2¾ oz) finely diced strawberries

Whisk yoghurt, milk and honey together in a bowl. Pour into a shallow dish and place in the freezer for 2 hours. Gently stir strawberries through ice cream and return to the freezer to set. Before serving remove from the freezer and allow ice cream to soften. Makes ½ litre.

Banana ice cream: Bananas have a creaminess and natural sweetness that make them ideal for making ice cream. Bananas are one of the best sources of potassium, an essential mineral for maintaining blood pressure and heart function.

3 organic eggs yolks • ¼ cup raw organic honey • ½ teaspoon vanilla essence or seeds • 2 ripe bananas • 2 tablespoon arrowroot or corn flour • 2 cups (500 ml/17¾ fl oz) low-fat milk (LF: rice, almond, soy or lactose-free milk)

Place eggs, honey, vanilla and bananas into a blender, mix until smooth and well combined. Heat milk in a saucepan over a medium heat until milk is just about to boil. In a small bowl mix flour and a little water to make a smooth paste. Add banana mixture to milk and stir over low heat. Add flour paste and stir until mixture thickens. Pour mixture into a shallow dish and place in the freezer until set. Stir with a fork after 2 hours. Before serving remove from the freezer and allow ice cream to soften. Makes ½ litre.

Fresh fruit soft serve ice cream: This ice cream is an excellent way to increase you child's fruit intake for the day. Use any combination of fruit you like.

¼ cup (63 ml/2 ¼ fl oz) apple or orange juice (freshly squeezed or 100% no added sugar) • ¾ cup (113 g/4 oz) blueberries or diced mango (frozen) • 1 frozen banana

Place sliced fruit in the freezer until partially frozen. Place fruit and juice in a blender and mix until thick and creamy. Transfer ice cream to an airtight container and place back in the freezer for an hour and then serve.

Vanilla & carob chip ice cream: This healthy version of choc chip ice cream will be a sure winner with the kids. You can replace the carob chips with roasted almonds or hazelnuts for an added boost of healthy fats.

3 organic eggs yolks • ¼ cup raw organic honey • 1 teaspoon vanilla essence or seeds • 2 cups (500 ml/17¾ fl oz) low-fat milk (LF: rice, almond, soy or lactose-free milk) • 2 tablespoons arrowroot or corn flour • ½ cup carob chips, unsweetened (LF: soy carob)

In a small bowl whisk together egg yolks, honey and vanilla. Heat milk in a saucepan over a medium heat, until milk is just about to boil. In a small bowl add flour and a little water to make a smooth paste. Add egg mixture to milk and stir until well combined. Add flour paste and stir until mixture thickens. Pour mixture into a shallow dish and place in the freezer for 2 hours. Gently stir through carob chips and return to the freezer until set. If you can only find larger carob buds, place them in a plastic bag and crush them into smaller pieces. Before serving remove from the freezer and allow ice cream to soften. Makes ½ litre.

Peach & blueberry crumble

This scrumptious winter dessert is a great way of increasing your child's fruit and fibre intake. Get creative and use any combination of seasonal fruit you like. Delicious served with homemade custard and ice cream, or a spoonful of yoghurt.

8 peach halves, diced (tinned in natural juice)

1 cup (150 g/5¼ oz) blueberries

1 teaspoon cinnamon

1 cup (100 g/13½ oz) rolled oats (GF: flaked millet or quinoa)

½ cup (80 g/2¾ oz) coconut flakes

½ cup (86 g/3 oz) almond flakes

1 tablespoon light olive oil

2 tablespoons raw organic honey

Preheat oven to 190°C (375°F/Gas 5). Lightly spray individual ovenproof dishes with olive oil.

Combine fruit together in a bowl and spoon some mixed fruit into each dish.

In a separate bowl mix oats, almonds, coconut flakes, flour and cinnamon. Whisk oil and honey together in a small bowl. Using your fingers mix honey and oil into oat mixture, until mixture has a crumbed consistency.

Top fruit with crumble and bake for 30-40 minutes, until golden brown. Serve hot with custard.

Serves 4.

Variations: Use different fruit combinations such as peach, pear and mango.

Vanilla custard

This smooth, velvety custard is free from artificial additives and sugars found in commercial varieties. Quick and easy to make this custard is perfect poured over fruit crumbles and warm muffins.

3 cups (750 ml/26¼ fl oz) low-fat milk (LF: almond, soy or lactose-free milk)

1 vanilla bean

2 tablespoons corn flour or arrowroot

2 organic egg yolks

2 tablespoons raw organic honey

Using a sharp knife slice vanilla bean in half, lengthways. Using the tip of the knife scrape out vanilla seeds and place in a small bowl.

In a small saucepan over a medium heat slowly bring milk to boil.

In a bowl mix flour with 2 tablespoons of warm milk, until a smooth paste forms.

Whisk in egg yolks, vanilla seeds and honey. Add hot milk and whisk until well combined.

Tip back into saucepan and bring to the boil, stirring slowly. Reduce heat and simmer, stirring slowly, until custard has thickened enough to coat the back of a spoon.

Serves 4.

Variation: Add one small ripe banana and blend until smooth. Add slices of banana, mango, peach, pear or berries. Add ¼ teaspoon of carob powder. Add a pinch of spice (cinnamon, cardamom or star anise).

Tip: Do not discard the vanilla pod, store them in a jar and use them to add flavour to sauces.

Carob coated strawberries

These decadent, easy-to-prepare carob coated strawberries are a sure way to impress. Strawberries are rich in antioxidants and vitamin C, both important for healthy immune function. Serve as an after dinner treat or at your child's next party.

2 punnets of large strawberries

1 bag of carob buds, unsweetened (LF: soy carob buds)

¼ cup (40 g/1½ oz) shredded coconut - optional

¼ cup (43 g/1½ oz) crushed almonds - optional

Wash strawberries and pat dry with a paper towel.

Toast coconut in a small saucepan over a medium heat and transfer to a small bowl. Toast almonds in saucepan and transfer to another small bowl.

Melt carob in a small bowl, in a water bath, over a medium heat. When the carob has melted keep the bowl in water bath on a low heat.

Dip each strawberry in carob, covering ¾ of the strawberry all the way around. Place on a flat tray covered in baking paper.

Once all strawberries are coated in carob sprinkle some with coconut and almonds and leave some plain. If coconut and almonds are not sticking pat gently until strawberries are well coated. Place in the fridge to set.

Serves 4-6.

Tip: Keep any left over carob in the fridge to grate over desserts.

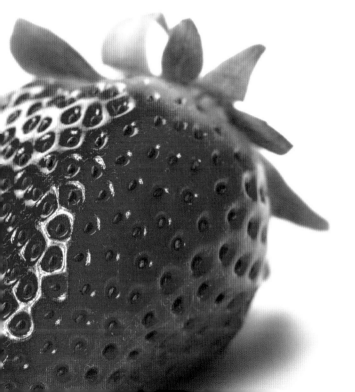

Beverages

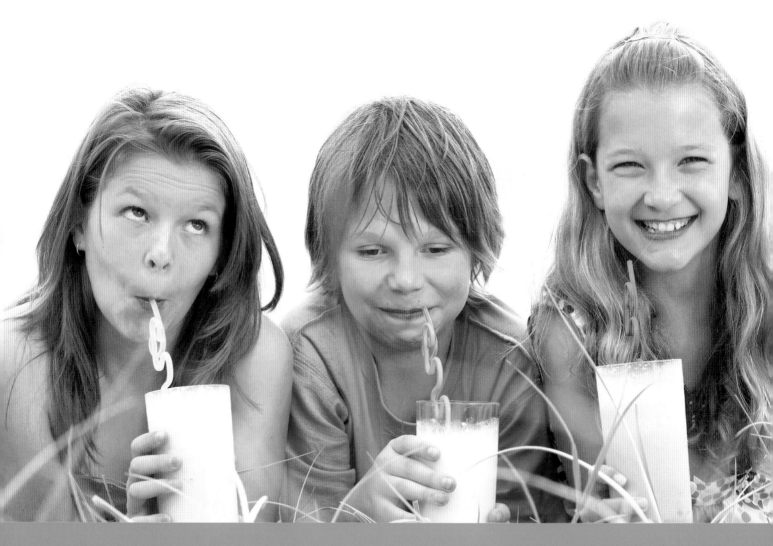

All these delicious drinks are healthy alternatives to soft drinks, flavoured milks and cordials that are full of sugars, artificial additives and caffeine. Sugary drinks, especially soft drinks, can have devastating effects on children's teeth and general health. Serve these drinks with peace of mind that you're doing something good for your child's health.

Delicious smoothies

These nutritious smoothies provide the perfect opportunity to increase your child's fruit intake. Naturally sweetened with fresh fruit and packed with protein-rich milk and yoghurt, these smoothies make an ideal breakfast on the go or afternoon snack.

Berry & yoghurt smoothie: This nutritious smoothie is packed with berries and yoghurt which both help to strengthen the immune system. Berries are an excellent source of antioxidants that help protect the body against free radical damage.

1 ripe banana • 1 cup (150 g/5¼ oz) mixed berries (strawberry, blueberry and raspberry) • 3 tablespoons vanilla yoghurt (LF: lactose-free yoghurt) • 1 cup (250 ml/9 fl oz) low-fat milk (LF: rice, almond, soy or lactose-free milk) • 1 teaspoon raw organic honey

Place banana, berries, yoghurt, milk and honey in a blender and mix until smooth and well combined. For a thicker smoothie use frozen fruit or add a handful of ice. Keep over ripe bananas in the fridge for smoothies. If you would like a thinner smoothie add extra milk. Serves 2. **Variation:** Add 2 teaspoons of LSA for extra omega-3 fats, calcium and protein. Add 1 tablespoon of muesli for added complex carbohydrates and fibre.

Carob & banana smoothie: This calcium rich carob smoothie is a healthy alternative to chocolate milk shakes.

2 ripe bananas • 1 cup (250 ml/9 fl oz) low-fat milk (LF: rice, soy or lactose-free milk) • ½ cup (125 ml/4½ fl oz) iced water • ¼ teaspoon carob powder • 1-2 teaspoons raw organic honey

Place all ingredients in a blender, mix until smooth and well combined. For a thicker smoothie use frozen bananas or add more ice. Keep over ripe bananas in the fridge for smoothies. If you would like a thinner smoothie add extra milk. Serves 2. **Variation:** Add 2 teaspoons of LSA for extra omga-3 fats, calcium and protein.

Strawberry & vanilla smoothie: This delicious light and refreshing smoothie will provide your child with protein, calcium, vitamin C and antioxidants.

½ cup (75 g/2½ oz) diced strawberries • 1 cup (250 ml/9 fl oz) low-fat vanilla rice milk • ½ cup (125 g/4½ fl oz) vanilla yoghurt (LF: lactose-free yoghurt) • 3 ice cubes • 1 teaspoon raw organic honey

Add strawberries, milk, yoghurt, honey and ice cubes to a blender, mix until well combined. For a thicker smoothie use frozen strawberries or add more ice. If you would like a thinner smoothie add extra milk. Serves 1. **Variation:** Add 2 teaspoons of LSA for extra omega-3 fats, calcium and protein. Add 1 tablespoon of muesli for added complex carbohydrates and fibre.

Mango smoothie: This sweet tropical smoothie is rich in vitamin C, beta-carotene, protein and calcium.

1 cup (150 g/5¼ oz) diced mango • ½ cup (125 g/4½ oz) vanilla yoghurt (LF: lactose-free yoghurt) • ½ cup (125 ml/4½ fl oz) low-fat milk (LF: rice, almond, soy or lactose-free milk) • 6 ice cubes • ¼ cup (63 ml/2¼ fl oz) orange juice, freshly squeezed

Place mango, yoghurt, milk, ice cubes and orange juice into a blender and mix until well combined. For a thicker smoothie use frozen fruit or add more ice. If you would like a thinner smoothie add extra orange juice. Serves 2. **Variation:** Add 2 teaspoons of LSA for extra omega-3 fats, calcium and protein. Add 1 tablespoon of muesli for added complex carbohydrates and fibre. For added sweetness add 1 teaspoon of honey.

Fruit crushes

These icy treats are a perfect way to cool down on a hot summer's day. Packed with fruit rich in vitamin C, these drinks are an excellent way to serve extra fruit to your children.

Tropical fruit crush

2 thick slices fresh pineapple • 1 passionfruit • 1 mango • ½ cup (125 ml/4½ fl oz) freshly squeezed orange juice • 6 ice cubes

Place pineapple, passionfruit, mango, orange juice and ice into a blender. Mix until well combined. Add more ice if needed. Makes 2 glasses. **Variation:** Add a handful of fresh mint.

Watermelon & strawberry fruit crush

4 thick slices of watermelon (remove seeds) • 6 strawberries • 6 ice cubes • ½ cup (125 ml/4½ fl oz) 100% apple juice

Place watermelon, strawberries, ice and apple juice in a blender and mix until well combined. Add more ice if needed. Makes 2 glasses.

Fizzy drinks

This refreshing drink is a healthy alternative to sugary, chemical laden soft drinks. Use any combination of fruit juice you like. Tropical, pineapple and mixed berry juices work well.

Fruit juice (freshly squeezed or 100% no added sugar) • natural sparkling mineral water

Fill ¼ of a glass with fruit juice then fill the glass with mineral water. Add ice then serve.

Party punch

This refreshing tropical punch is a must at kid's parties. A healthy alternative to soft drink, this colourful punch looks and tastes great.

1 punnet frozen strawberries • 2 passionfruit • 2 cups (500 ml/18 fl oz) iced water • 2 cups (500 ml/18 fl oz) 100% pineapple juice • 2 cups (500 ml/18 fl oz) 100% orange juice • 2 cups (500 ml/18 fl oz) 100% apple juice • 3 cups (750 ml/27 fl oz) sparkling mineral water • 1 orange, thinly sliced • 1 cup halved grapes • 1 tray of ice cubes

Place strawberries, passion fruit and iced water in a blender and process until well mixed. Add mix to a large punch bowl, add pineapple, orange and apple juice, blend with a hand mixer. Stir through mineral water, orange slices and grapes and add ice. Serve with a ladle and small punch cups. Serves 12.

Juices

These delicious fresh fruit and vegetable juices are a fantastic way of supplying your kids with an abundance of vitamins such as vitamin C, A and beta-carotene.

Carrot, celery, apple & beetroot juice

2 large carrots • 1 medium beetroot • 3 apples • 3 celery sticks

Peel carrots, beetroot and apples (unless organic). Place ingredients in juicer, then serve with some ice cubes. Serves 2.

Pineapple, orange, banana & spirulina juice

½ small pineapple • 2 oranges • 1 ripe banana • 1 teaspoon spirulina • 3 ice cubes

Juice pineapple and oranges. Pour into blender with banana and spirulina and a few ice cubes and process. Serves 2.

Berry yoghurt drink

1½ cups (225 g/7 ¾ oz) raspberries • 125g (4oz) blueberries • 1 cup (250 ml/9 fl oz) unsweetened cranberry juice • 1 banana • 3 tablespoons natural yoghurt (LF: lactose-free yoghurt)

Place all ingredients in blender and process until a smooth consistency. Serves 2-3.

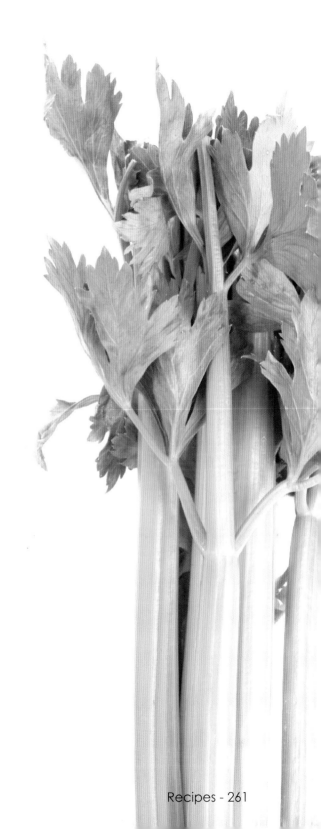

Healthy party food

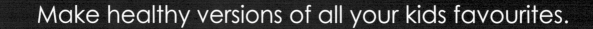

Make healthy versions of all your kids favourites.

Unfortunately most food served at kids parties are laden with sugar, salt and fat. They are commonly made from poor quality ingredients and contain a large cocktail of artificial additives. If you don't feel right about giving these foods to your kids and all their friends, try serving a healthy party spread. By serving nutritious food at your kid's next party you can feel guilt-free knowing they are eating something good for them. Healthy party food doesn't have to be tasteless and boring. You can make up healthy versions of all your kid's party favourites.

The trick to serving a popular party spread is to make the food look bright, fun and appealing. Cut sandwiches and fruit into shapes. Use brightly coloured themed tablecloths, plates and cups. Make bite sized finger foods such as pizzas, quiches and hamburgers. Kids love food served on toothpicks or on skewers with some tasty dipping sauces.

These days a lot of children follow special diets as food intolerances, allergies and diabetes is common. Make sure you check if any of your guests have special dietary requirements. On the invites have a section at the bottom for any dietary requirements, so you can adjust your party menu accordingly. Due to an increasing number of children with peanut allergies, err on the side of caution and don't serve food that contains nuts

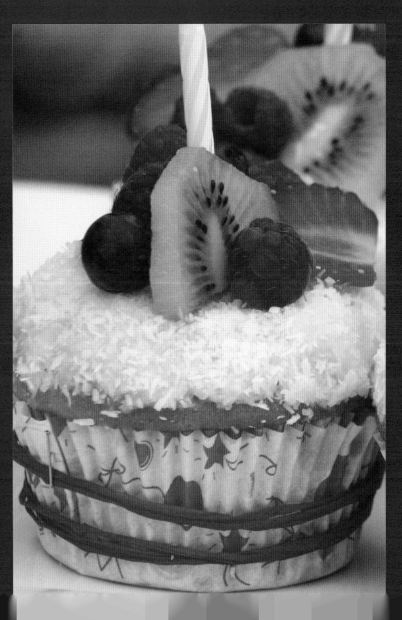

Healthy party food ideas

Here are some tasty ideas to help you create a healthy birthday feast that your kids will love.

Savoury Food:

Here are some delicious savoury suggestions that are healthy alternatives to junk food party favourites.

• Mini hamburgers: Using long Turkish bread, cut into small bread rolls with a round scone cutter. Separate each roll into two halves and fill with mini patties (lean meat, chicken, legume, salmon or tuna), lettuce and tomato sauce.

• Mini quiches: Using any of the quiche recipes in this book make small individual sized quiches.

• Mini pizzas: Using wholemeal muffin halves, pita bread or small homemade bases make tasty individual sized pizzas with a variety of healthy toppings.

• Mini sandwich swirls: Choose from different types of flat bread (mountain or tortillas). Place flat bread in a moderate oven for a couple of minutes until soft. Cover with desired spreads (avocado, hummus, baba ghanoush, beetroot dip, chutneys, homemade mayonnaise etc), and top with desired fillings (thin slices of salad, roast vegetables, cheese, chicken, turkey, lean meat, salmon or tuna). Do not over do it with the filling or your rolls will not stay together. Roll up and cut into inch wide swirls. You can hold them together with a tooth pick if they keep unravelling.

• Dips served with rice crackers, toasted flat breads, turkish bread pieces and raw vegie sticks.

• Potato and sweet potato wedges with dipping sauce.

• Mini meatballs or bean falafels on toothpicks with dipping sauce.

• Crispy sesame chicken nuggets with dipping sauce (replace almonds in this recipe with breadcrumbs).

• Kebab skewers (lamb, beef, fish, chicken or vegetable) with dipping sauces.

• Tandoori chicken skewers with dipping sauce.

• Nachos and kidney bean tacos made with baked tortillas.

• If you're having a BBQ, serve good quality sausages made with lean meat or chicken; make up homemade patties (lean meat, chicken, fish or legume); cook up pieces of fish or lean cuts of meat or kebabs; make up any of the delicious salads from this book; toad in the hole (egg in bread hole); and buy wholegrain bread and rolls.

Sweet treats:

These healthy treats won't send your party guests on a sugar high. Naturally sweetened with fruit and honey these foods are highly nutritious and don't have the high fat content of commercial cakes and other baked goods. Due to the increased number of children with peanut allergies these days, leave out the nuts from the following recipes. If any of your guests are gluten or lactose intolerant you can change the following recipes accordingly.

• Fruit shapes on skewers with dipping yoghurt: Thread fruit shapes and melon balls on skewers or place a toothpick through each of them. Kids love dipping them in flavoured yoghurt (make sure it contains no artificial sweeteners).

• Carob goodies: Carob coated strawberries, carob coconut roughs, carob chip oatmeal cookies or apple and beetroot carob brownies.

• Apricot sesame bars (drizzle with carob) and crunchy muesli bars.

• Decorative cupcakes. Choose from any of the delicious muffin recipes in this book. Make in colourful paper muffin cups and top with different flavoured coconut icing (carob, passionfruit and vanilla). Decorate cakes with slices of fruit, coconut, carob buds or grated carob shavings.

• Honey popcorn mix: In a large bowl place 6 cups (180 g/6 oz) puffed corn cereal, ½ cup (45 g/1½ oz) rice bran, ½ cup (26 g/1 oz)) coconut flakes, ¼ cup (40 g/1½ oz) pepitas, ¼ cup (40 g/1½ oz) sunflower seeds and 1 tablespoon sesame seeds. Heat ⅓ cup (83 ml/3 fl oz) raw organic honey in a small saucepan. Pour honey over mixture and combine until well coated. Preheat oven to 180°C. Line a slice tray with baking paper, spread with mixture and bake for 15 minutes, tossing occasionally. Cool mixture and serve or store in a airtight container in the fridge.

• Birthday cake suggestions: Use any of the muffin recipes from this book and bake in a round cake tin or deep slice tray. Bake for an extra 10 minutes until cake is golden brown and cooked through. Top with coconut icing and decorate.

Cool treats:

Instead of serving ice creams packed with sugar and artificial colourings and flavourings, serve these nutritious fruit packed cool treats.

• Fruit and yoghurt ice blocks.

• Watermelon ice blocks: Cut thick slices of watermelon into rectangles, place a paddle pop stick down the centre of each and place in the freezer until ready to serve.

• Carob coated banana ice creams.

• Homemade ice cream in cones.

Refreshing Drinks:

For party drinks steer clear of soft drinks laden with sugar and chemicals. Try these refreshing fruity drinks.

• Party punch.

• Healthy fizzy fruit drinks.

• Milk shakes: Add desired ingredients to low-fat milk (LF: rice, almond, soy or lactose-free milk). Add strawberries, banana, blueberries or mango. Add carob powder for a chocolate like milkshake. Give extra sweetness with organic raw honey, vanilla essence, homemade ice cream or flavoured yoghurt. Don't forget the coloured swirly straws.

Goodie bags for younger children:

For younger children's parties, where the guests take home a party bag of goodies, avoid filling them with lollies and junk food. Instead fill them with stickers, balloons, swirly straws, pencil and rubber sets, mini toys (yo-yo, games, figurines), fun key rings, puzzles, dress up jewellery, hair clips and bands, and collector cards. Give each child a slice of cake or cupcake to take home.

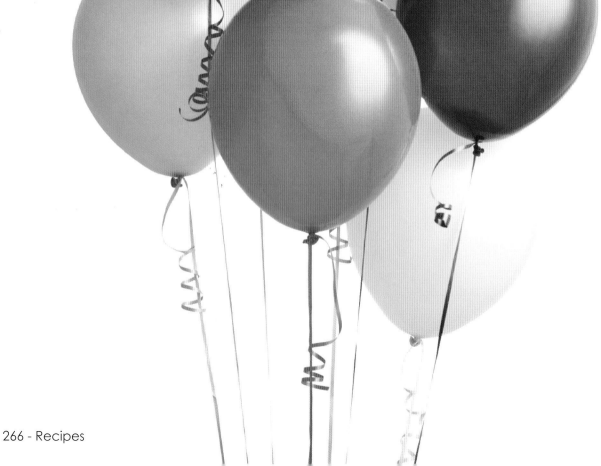

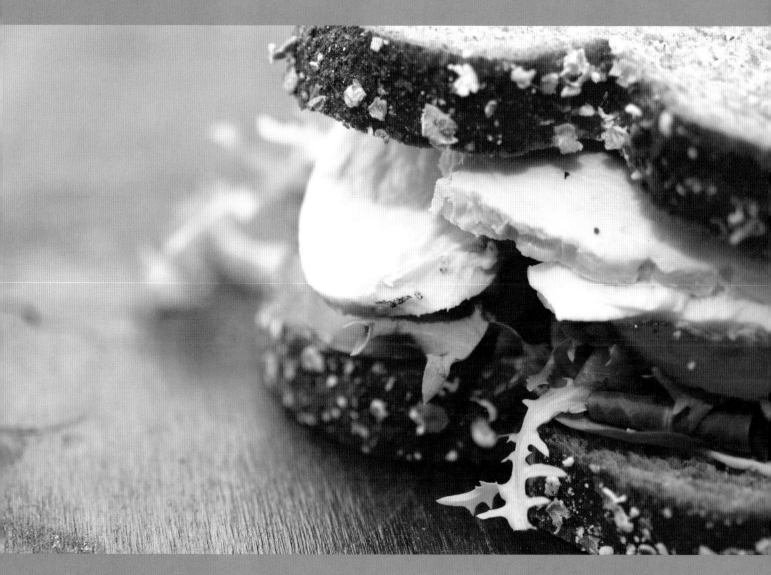

Sandwiches
& lunch box ideas

As a parent it can be difficult to keep coming up with interesting and nutritious school lunches. The following section is packed with healthy sandwich and lunch box suggestions for you to try. No more trading sandwiches at school or bringing lunches home uneaten.

Lunch box ideas

1. Use a variety of breads:
Make sandwiches and wraps with different types of breads (preferably wholegrain or wholemeal): rolls or flat breads (lavash, Lebanese bread, mountain bread, pita pockets or tortillas). Try breads made from different types of grains including: sourdough, oat, rye (pumpernickel), spelt, corn, barley, rice, fruit bread, sunflower and pumpkin seed, or multi-grain.

2. Roast vegetable slices:
Oven roast or grill a selection of thinly sliced vegetables such as pumpkin, zucchini, eggplant, potato, sweet potato and beetroot. Keep them in the fridge to use for school sandwiches and wraps. These vegies wont make sandwiches soggy.

3. Avoid soggy sandwiches:
Pack a pita pocket and a small container filled with grated and diced salad (carrot, beetroot, cucumber, avocado, pineapple, tomato, cheese and roast vegies). Get your kids to fill the pita pocket with salad at lunchtime - no more soggy sandwiches. Pack a small can of tuna or salmon with a fork along with pita pocket and salad (tabouli). When making sandwiches for school lunches make sure you dry the lettuce. Make sure you drain any juice from beetroot and pat dry with a paper towel so it's not messy.

4. Healthy butter alternatives:
Use avocado, hummus or baba ghanoush as a healthy alternative to butter on sandwiches.

5. Yoghurt:
Low-fat yoghurts are a nutritious addition to your child's lunch, high in protein and calcium. Pack yoghurts next to an ice pack or a frozen drink.

6. Always pack a piece of fruit:
Always pack a piece of fruit in your child's lunch box. Pack an apple, orange, mandarin, banana, kiwi fruit (with a spoon), strawberries, handful of grapes, slices of watermelon or a fruit salad.

7. No added salt:
Don't add salt to your kid's sandwiches or wraps.

8. Liven up sandwiches & wraps with spreads & chutneys:
Use spreads such as hummus, baba ghanoush, healthy mayonnaise, avocado spread, nut butters, tahini, mild mustards, and mango or beetroot chutneys to liven up sandwiches and wraps.

9. Pack a salad:
Pack a separate container or cool thermos full of salad. Don't forget to pack a fork. Have a mix of cherry tomatoes, cubes of low-fat cheese, seeds (sunflower or pepitas), lettuce, corn kernels, carrot, cucumber and some form of protein (dices of cooked chicken, turkey, salmon or tuna, a boiled egg, or a small can of legumes). Go to the salad section in this book for some great salad ideas. Pack a wholemeal roll or pita pocket in your kid's lunch box so they can fill it with salad.

10. Pack winter soups, casseroles, curries & pasta dishes:
In winter pack soups and leftover casseroles, curries and pasta dishes in a hot thermos with a crusty bread roll. Fill thermos with hot water first to heat it up, empty, then fill with hot food.

11. Always pack a bottle of water:
Always pack a 600 ml bottle full of water with your child's lunch. Freeze it so it stays nice and cool throughout the day.

12. Other drink ideas:
Other drinks which are healthy options to pack in lunch boxes include small juices (no added sugar) or a small drink bottle with a mix of 1/4 juice diluted with water. Fruit smoothies, carob or vanilla rice drinks are also healthy drink choices. Freeze drinks overnight and pack in lunchbox to keep lunch cool and bacteria free.

Sandwich, wrap & pita filling suggestions

- Salmon or tuna mixed with healthy mayonnaise and lettuce.

- Turkey, roast vegies, baby spinach and chutney.

- Lean roast beef, low-fat cheddar cheese, lettuce and chutney.

- Chicken, avocado, shredded lettuce and tomato.

- Tuna patty, baba ghanoush and low-fat cheese.

- Tabouli, hummus and falafel ball or patty.

- Chickpea patty with salad (lettuce, tomato, cucumber, beetroot).

- Boiled egg mixed with healthy mayonnaise and shredded lettuce.

- Shredded chicken/tuna or salmon with coleslaw.

- Low-fat cottage cheese mixed with corn kernels and salad.

- Nut butter with sliced banana and a little honey.

- Low-fat cream cheese with grated carrot, cucumber and shredded lettuce.

- Hummus and salad or roast veges.

- Thin frittata slices with salad (lettuce, tomato, cucumber, beetroot).

Other lunch ideas

- Soups, curries or casseroles in a thermos with a wholemeal roll or pumpkin muffin.

- Individual mini frittatas.

- Rice timbales.

- Patties (chickpea, lentil, tuna or salmon) with a dipping sauce and salad.

- Crispy almond and sesame chicken nuggets with dipping sauce (baba ghanoush or tomato sauce).

- Puffed rice or corn cakes with low-fat cheese (cottage, cheddar, cream), avocado, hummus, slices of chicken, turkey, salmon or tuna, or tahini with banana.

- Mini quiches or vegetable hummus pies with a salad.

- Nori rolls or rice paper rolls with sweet chilli dipping sauce.

Lunch box snack ideas

- Pancakes with a spread of jam (no-added sugar), low-fat ricotta cheese, date or prune puree, or organic raw honey. Pack a small container of sliced fruit to wrap pancakes around (sliced strawberries, blueberries or banana).

- ½ cooked corn cob.

- Small container of corn kernels mixed with cottage cheese and some celery stick dippers.

- Fresh fruit salad. Squeeze lemon juice on apple pieces to prevent them going brown.

- Small container of grapes, cherries or berries.

- Small can of fruit in natural juice.

- Raw carrot, celery sticks or apple slices with a tub of hummus, baba ghanoush, avocado dip or low-fat cottage cheese.

- Low-fat cheese stick.

- Boiled egg in its shell.

- A whole orange (peel in a spiral), mandarin, apple or banana.

- Crisp bread with low-fat cream cheese or avocado.

- Carob covered rice or buckwheat cakes.

- Tub of low-fat flavoured yoghurt.

- Small container of yoghurt mixed with LSA and fresh berries.

- Tub of yoghurt topped with muesli.

- Small tub of Bircher muesli.

- Fruit tapioca pudding.

- Carob coconut roughs.

- Healthy muesli bars from this book.

- Any of the healthy cookies from this book.

- Apricot protein balls.

- Date wholemeal scone.

- Pumpkin muffins spread with some avocado, hummus or cream cheese.

- Whole kiwi fruit are fun for kids to scoop out with a spoon.

- Any of the healthy muffins or cakes from this book.

Trail mix

Combine a mix of the following in a small plastic bag:

Raw, unsalted seeds (sunflower or pepitas)
Sun-dried fruit (apricots, pear, peaches, mango, apple, banana, sultanas, dates, figs or goji berries)
Unsweetened carob buds
Yoghurt coated sultanas
Carob coconut roughs
Apricot protein balls

Savory crackers & dip mix

Combine a mix of the following in a small plastic bag:

Plain rice crackers (no MSG or added preservatives)
Cheese and sesame crackers
Baked pretzels (low-sodium)
Plain air popped popcorn
Mini rice or corn cakes

Pack a small container of dip:

Guacamole
Beetroot & cumin dip
Low-fat cottage cheese
Hummus
Baba ghanoush

Cooking grains & legumes

If the grain or legume packet has cooking instructions follow them, otherwise here are some cooking charts to follow. Consider these charts as a general guide as some varieties of grains and legumes require a few minutes more or less.

Basic cooking directions for grains

1. Rinse grains thoroughly to remove any dirt or pesticide residue. Some grains, like quinoa, need to be rinsed well to remove their bitter natural coating.

2. Place grain in a large saucepan and cover with water. Bring to boil over a high heat. Turn heat down to low and simmer for the recommended cooking time. (Buckwheat is the exception to these basic directions. Because the grain is so porous and absorbs water quickly, it's best to bring the water to a boil first and then add grain.)

3. If the grain needs more cooking time and all the water has been absorbed, add ¼ cup of water, cover and continue cooking. When grains are tender, turn off the heat and allow the grains to rest 5 to 10 minutes, fluff with a fork and then serve.

Cooking tip: For improved texture and reduced cooking time, soak brown rice in water for 30 minutes before cooking.

Grain cooking chart

Grain (1 cup dry)	water (cups)	cooking time (minutes)	cups yield (cups)
Amaranth	2	25-30	2 ½
Barley, pearled	3	45-50	3 ½
Barley, whole hulled	3	90	3 ½
Barley, flakes	2	30-40	2 ½
Buckwheat, whole	2	15-20	2 ½
Cornmeal (fine grind)	4	8-10	2 ½
Cornmeal (polenta, coarse)	4	20-25	2 ½
Kamut	3	120	2 ½
Millet, hulled	3	25	3 ½
Oats, whole	3	30-60	3 ½
Oats, rolled	2	5-15	2
Quinoa	2	20	2 ¾
Rice, brown basmati	2½	35-40	3
Rice, white basmati	1 ¾	15	3 ½
Rice, brown, long grain	2 ½	45-50	3
Rice, brown, short grain	2-2 ½	45-50	3
Rice, brown, quick	1 ¼	10	2
Rice, wild	3	50-60	4
Rice, arborio	2 ½	30	2 ½
Rye, whole	3-4	60	3
Rye, flakes	2	10-15	3
Spelt	3-4	40-50	2 ½
Wheat, whole	3	120	2 ½
Wheat, couscous	1	5	2
Wheat, cracked	2	20-25	2 ¼
Wheat, bulgur	2	15	2 ½

Basic cooking directions for legumes

1. Legumes cook quicker and their digestibility is improved by soaking them first. Cover legumes in water for eight hours or overnight (for longer-cooking legumes), changing the water a couple of times. Split peas and lentils do not need to be soaked.

2. Drain legumes and discard the water. Place legumes in a large saucepan, add water, and bring to the boil over a high heat. Reduce heat and simmer, cover and cook for the recommended time. Foaming can be reduced by adding a teaspoon of olive oil.

3. When legumes are tender, drain and serve.

Cooking tip: Many people are concerned with the reputation that legumes have for causing flatulence. Soaking and cooking the legumes thoroughly helps to break down the complex sugars (oligosaccharides), which challenge our digestive systems and can cause flatulence. Adding a kombu (seaweed) strip to the saucepan while cooking will also improve their digestibility.

Legume (1 cup dry)	water (cups)	cooking time (minutes)	cups yield (cups)
Adzuki	4	50-60	3
Black beans	4	60-90	2 ¼
Black-eyed peas	3	60	2
Cannellini (white kidney beans)	3	45-60	2 ½
Fava beans (broad beans)	3	40-60	1 ²/₃
Garbanzos (chick peas)	4	120-180	2
Green split peas	4	45-60	2
Yellow split peas	4	60-90	2
Green peas, whole	6	60-120	2
Kidney beans	3	60	2 ¼
Lentils, brown	2 ¼	30-45	2 ¼
Lentils, green	2	30-45	2
Lentils, red	3	20-30	2-2 ½
Lima beans, large	4	45-60	2
Mung beans	2	45-60	2
Navy beans	3	60-90	2 ²/₃
Pinto beans	3	90-120	2 ²/₃
Soybeans	4	180-240	3

References

Introduction

1. Magarey AM, Daniels LA & Boulton TJC. Prevalence of overweight and obesity in Australian children and adolescents: Reassessment of 1985 and 1995 data against new standard international definitions. The Medical Journal of Australia 2001; 174:561-4.
2. Wake M, Lazarus R, Hasketh R & Waters E. Are Australian Children getting fatter? Journal of Paediatrics and child health 1999; 35-47.
3. Booth ML, Wake M, Armstrong T, Chey T, Hesketh K, Mathur S. The epidemiology of overweight and obesity amoung Australian children and adolescents, 1995-1997. Australian and New Zealand Journal of Public Health 2001; 25:162-9.
4. NSW Health. NSW Schools Physical Activity and Nutrition Survey (SPANS) 2004: Summary Report. NSW Centre for overweight and obesity. 2006 April; iv.
5. ibid, iv.
6. Kraakv & Pelletier DL. The influence of commercialism on the food purchasing behaviour of children and teenage youth. Family Economic and Nutrition Review 1998; 11:15-23.
7. Byrd-Bredbenner C & Grasso D. Health, medicine, and food messages in television commercials during 1992 and 1998. Journal of School Health 2000; 70:61-5.
8. Pincus G. Food advertisements and nutrition. Paper presented at conference: Children and Advertising a fair game? Sydney, July 1994.
9. Campbell K & Crawford D. Family food environments as determinants of preschool-aged children's eating behaviours: Implications for obesity prevention policy - a review. Australian Journal of Nutrition and Dietetics 2001; 58:19-25.

Chapter 1: Back to basics

Going organic

1. UK Food Commission. Additives do cause temper tantrums. The Food Magazine 25th October 2002; http://www.foodcomm.org.uk/parentsjury/add_2.htm
2. Food Standards Australia New Zealand. Food Additives List (February 2007) http://www.foodstandards.gov.au/newsroom/publications/choosingtherightstuff/foodadditive/salphaup1679.cfm
3. Baker BP, Benbrook CM, Groth III E & Benbrook KL. Pesticide residues in conventional, IPM-grown and organic foods: Insights from three U.S. data sets. Food Additives and Contaminants 2002; 19(5): 427-446.
4. Batelle Memorial Institute. Background Report on Fertilizer use, Contaminants and Regulations. Washington, DC: National Program Chemicals Division, US Environmental Protection Agency 1999; 27–51.
5. Aehnelt E & Hahn J. Animal fertility: A possibility for biological quality assay of fodder and feeds. Biodynamics 1978; 25: 36–47.
6. Vogtmann H. From healthy soil to healthy food: An analysis of the quality of food produced under contrasting agricultural systems. Nutrition and Health 1988; 6: 21–35.
7. Plochberger K. Feeding experiments: A criterion for quality estimation of biologically and conventionally produced foods. Agriculture, Ecosystems and Environment 1989; 27: 419–428.
8. Velimirov A, Plochberger K, Huspeka UW & Schott W. The influence of biologically and conventionally cultivated food on the fertility of rats. Biological Agriculture and Horticulture 1992; 8: 325–337.
9. Worthington V. Nutritional Quality of Organic Versus Conventional Fruits, Vegetables, and Grains. The Journal of Alternative and Complementary Medicine 2001; 7(2): 161.
10. Worthington V. Effect of Agricultural Methods on Nutritional Quality: A Comparison of Organic with Conventional Crops. Alternative Therapies 1998; 4: 58-69.
11. ibid.
12. ibid.
13. Asami DK, Hong YJ, Barrett DM & Mitchell AE. Comparison of the Total Phenolic and Ascorbic Acid Content of Freeze-Dried and Air-Dried Marionberry, Strawberry, and Corn Grown Using Conventional, Organic, and Sustainable Agricultural Practices. Journal of Agricultural and Food Chemistry 2003; 51 (5): 1237-1241.
14. Grinder-Pedersen L, Rasmussen SE, Bügel S, Jørgensen LV, Dragsted LO, Gundersen V & Sandström B. Effect Of Diets Based On Foods From Conventional Versus Organic Production On Intake And Excretion Of Flavonoids And Markers Of Antioxidative Defense In Humans. Journal of Agricultural and Food Chemistry 2003; 51 (19): 5671-5676.
15. Greenpeace. Monsanto Ordered to Make Secret Study Public. 20 June 2005 http://eu.greenpeace.org/issues/news.html#050620=5Fa

Healthy cooking

1. Vallejo F, Tomas-Barberan FA, Garcia-Viguera C, et al. Phenolic compound contents in edible parts of broccoli inflorescences after domestic cooking. Journal of the Science of food and Agriculture 2003; 83(14): 1511-1516.
2. ibid.
3. NHMRC. Dietary Guidelines for children and adolescents in Australia. Endorsed 10 April 2003. National Health and Medical Research Council. Chapter 3.1: 74.
4. Gil MI, Ferreres F & Tomas-Barberan FA. Effects of post harvest storage and processing on the antioxidant constituents (Flavanoids and vitamin C) of fresh cut spinach. Journal of Agriculture and Food Chemistry 1999; 47(6): 2213-7.
5. Anderson KE, Kadlubar FF, Kulldorff M, Harnack L, Gross M, Lang NP, Barber C, Rothman N & Sinha R. Dietary intake of Heterocyclic Amines and Benzo(a)pryrene: Associations with pancreatic cancer. Cancer Epidemiology Biomarkers and Prevention 2005; 14: 2261-2265.

Phytochemicals

1. Talalay P & Fahey JW. Phytochemicals from plants protect against cancer by modulationg carcinogen metabolism. Supplement: AICR's 11th Annual Research Conference on Diet, Nutrition and Cancer. Journal of Nutrition 2001; 131: 3027S-3033S.
2. Giovannucci E. Tomatoes, tomato-based products, lycopene, and cancer: Review of the epidemiologic literature. Journal of the National cancer Institute 1999; 91(4): 317-331.
3. Hamilton CA. Low density lipoprotein and oxidized low-density lipoprotein: their role in the development of atherosclerosis. Pharmacology Therapeutics 1997; 74: 55-72.
4. Tapiero H, Townsend DM & Tew KD. The role of carotenoids in the prevention of human pathologies. Biomedical Pharmacotherapy 2004; 58: 100–10.
5. Giovannucci E. Tomatoes, tomato-based products, lycopene, and cancer: Review of the epidemiologic literature. Journal of the National cancer Institute 1999; 91(4): 317-331.
6. Krinsky NI. Carotenoids as antioxidants. Nutrition 2001; 17(10): 815-17.
7. Sies H & Stahl W. Lycopene: Antioxidant and biological effects and its bioavailability in the human body. Proceedings for the Society of Experimental Biology and Medicine 1998; 218: 121-124.
8. Stahl W & Sies H. Lycopene: a biologically important carotenoid for humans? Archives of Biochemistry and Biophysics 1996; 336: 1-9.
9. Gerster H. The potential role of lycopene for human health. Journal of the American College of Nutrition 1997; 16: 109-126.
10. Gerster, H. The potential role of lycopene for human health. Journal of the American College of Nutrition 1997; 16: 109-126.
11. Gabrielska J & Oszmianski JC. Antioxidant activity of anthocyanin glycoside derivatives evaluated by the inhibition of liposome oxidation. Journal of Biosciences 2005; 60(5-6): 399-407.

Fibre

1. NHMRC, Dietary Guidelines for children and adolescents in Australia. Endorsed 10 April 2003. National Health and Medical Research Council. Chapter 3.2; 86.
2. Komaroff AL. Constipation, fibre and colon cancer. Journal Watch 14 July 1998.
3. Brown L, Rosner B, Willett WW & Sacks FM. Cholesterol-lowering effects of dietary fiber: a meta-analysis. American Journal of Clinical Nutrition 1999; 69: 30-42.
4. UN Food and Agriculture Organisation. Carbohydrates in human nutrition: report of a joint FAO-WHO expert consultation. Rome, 1998.
5. Brown I, Warhurst M, Arcot J, Playne M, Illman RJ & Topping DL. Fecal numbers of bifidobacteria are higher in pigs fed Bifidobacterium longum with a high amylose cornstarch than with a low amylose cornstarch. The Journal of Nutrition 1997; 127: 1822-1827.
6. Leake LL. Analyzing Resistant Starch. Laboratory. Food Technology July 2006; 67.
7. Archer SY, Meng S, Shei A & Hodin RA. P21 WAF1 is required for bytyrate-mediated growth inhibition of human colon cancer cells. Cell Biology 1998; 95 (12): 6791-6796.
8. Toden S, Bird AR, Topping DL & Conlon MA. Resistant starch prevents colonic DNA damage induced by high dietary cooked red meat or casein in rats. Cancer Biology and Therapy 2006.
9. Barlow J. Legumes found to contain starch carrying a fiber-like punch. Nutrition 2001; 217: 333-5802.
10. Leake LL. Analyzing Resistant Starch. Laboratory. Food Technology 2006; July: 67.
11. Cummings JH, Macfarlane G & Englyst HN. Prebiotic digestion and fermentation. American Journal of Clinical Nutrition 2001; 73(2): 415S-420S.
12. Australian Government. National Health and Medical Research Council. Nutrient reference values for Australia and New Zealand: including recommended dietary intakes. Australia 2006; 47.

Glycaemic Index

1. Brand-Miller JC, Pawlak DB & McMillan J. Glycaemic index and obesity. American Journal of Clinical Nutrition July 2002; 76(1): 281S-285S.
2. ibid.
3. Ludwig DS, Majzoulb JA, Al-Zahrani A, Dallal GE, Blanco I & Roberts SB. High glycaemic index foods, overeating, and obesity. Pediatrics 1999; 103(3): e26.
4. Roberts B. High gycaemic index foods, hunger and obesity: is there a connection? Nutrition Review 2000; 58: 163-9.

5. Lui S, Willet WC, Stampfer MJ, Hu FB, Franz M, Sampson L, Hennekens CH & Manson JE. A prospective study of dietary glycaemic load, carbohydrate intake and risk of coronary heart disease in US women. *American Journal of Clinical Nutrition* 2000; 71(6): 1455-61.

6. Roberts B. High gycaemic index foods, hunger and obesity: is there a connection? *Nutrition Review* 2000; 58:163-9.

7. Lustig RH. Childhood obesity: behavioral aberration or biochemical drive? Reinterpreting the First Law of Thermodynamics. *Nature Clinical Practice Endocrinology & Metabolism* 2006; 2: 447-458.

8. Holt S & Brand Miller J. Particle size, satiety and the glycaemic response. *European Journal of Clinical Nutrition* 1994; 48 :496-502.

9. Astrup A, Ryan L, Grunwals G, Storgaard M, Saris W, Melanson E, et al. The role of dietary fat in body fatness: evidence from a preliminary meta-analysis of ad libitum low-fat dietary intervention studies. *British Journal of Nutrition* 2000; 83: 25S-32S.

10. Ludwig DS. Dietary glycaemic index and obesity. *Journal of Nutrition* 2000; 130: 280S-3S.

11. NHMRC, Dietary Guidelines for children and adolescents in Australia. Endorsed 10 April 2003. National Health and Medical Research Council. Chpt.3.2; 89.

12. David Mendosa. Revised International Table of Glycaemic Index (GI) and Glycaemic Load (GL) Values—2002. http://www.mendosa.com/gilists.htm (Last modified 01/03/2006).

Chapter 2: Essential nutrients

Protein

1. USDA. United States department of agriculture. Agricultural Research Service. Nutrient Data Laboratory. Food composition database. http://nal.usda.gov/fnic/cgi-bln/nut_search.pl (Last modified 16/04/2008).

2. Australian Government. National Health and Medical Research Council. Nutrient reference values for Australia and New Zealand: including recommended dietary intakes. Australia 2006; 30.

Fats

1. Kris-Etherton PM, Pearson TA, Wan Y, Hargrove RL, Moriarty K, Fishell V & Etherton TD. High–monounsaturated fatty acid diets lower both plasma cholesterol and triacylglycerol concentrations. *American Journal of Clinical Nutrition* 1999; 70(6): 1009-1015.

2. Rasmussen OW, Thomsen C, Hansen KW, Vesterlund M, Winther E & Hermansen K. Effects on blood pressure, glucose, and lipid levels of a high-monounsaturated fat diet compared with a high-carbohydrate diet in NIDDM subjects. *Diabetes Care* 1993; 16(12): 1565-1571.

3. ibid.

4. Garg A. High-monounsaturated-fat diets for patients with diabetes mellitus: a meta-analysis. *American Journal of Clinical Nutrition* 1998; 67: 577S-582S.

5. ibid.

6. Kris-Etherton PM, Taylor DS, Yu-Poth S, Huth P, Moriarty K, Fishell V, et al. Polyunsaturated fatty acids in the food chain in the United States. *American Journal of Clinical Nutrition* 2000; 71S.

7. Simopoulos AP. The importance of the ratio of omega-6/omega-3 essential fatty acids. *Biomedical Pharmacotherapy* 2002; 56(8): 365-79.

8. Simopoulos AP. Omega-3 fatty acids in health and disease and in growth and development. *American Journal of Clinical Nutrition* 1991; 54: 438–63.

9. Simopoulos AP, Kifer RR & Martin RE. Health effects of polyunsaturated fatty acids in seafood. Orlando, FL: Academic Press, 1986.

10. Galli C & Simopoulos AP. Dietary 3 and 6 fatty acids. Biological effects and nutritional essentiality. New York: Plenum Press, 1989.

11. Galli C, Simopoulos AP & Tremoli E. Fatty acids and lipids: biological aspects. *World Review of Nutrition and Dietetics* 1994; 75: 1–197.

12. Salem N Jr, Simopoulos AP, Galli C, Lagarde M & Knapp HR. Fatty acids and lipids from cell biology to human disease. *Lipids* 1996; 31: S1–326.

13. Raheja BS, Sadikot SM, Phatak RB & Rao MB. Significance of the n-6/n-3 ratio for insulin action in diabetes. *Annals of the New York Academy of Sciences* 1993; 683: 258–71.

14. Connor WE, Prince MJ, Ullmann D, et al. The hypotriglyceridemic effect of fish oil in adult-onset diabetes without adverse glucose control. *Annals of the New York Academy of Sciences* 1993; 683: 337–40.

15. Burr ML, Fehily AM, Gilbert JF, et al. Effect of changes in fat, fish and fibre intakes on death and myocardial reinfarction: diet and reinfarction trial (DART). *Lancet* 1989; 2: 757–61.

16. De Lorgeril M, Renaud S, Mamelle N, et al. Mediterranean -linolenic acid–rich diet in secondary prevention of coronary heart disease. *Lancet* 1994; 343: 1454–9.

17. Morris MC, Sacks F & Rosner B. Fish oil to reduce blood pressure: a meta-analysis. *Annals of Internal Medicine* 1994; 120: 10.

18. Appel LJ, Miller ER, Seidler AJ & Whelton PK. Does supplementation of diet with "fish oil" reduce blood pressure? A meta-analysis of controlled clinical trials. *Archives of Internal Medicine* 1993; 153: 1429–38.

19. Kremer JM. Effects of modulation of inflammatory and immune parameters in patients with rheumatic and inflammatory disease receiving dietary supplementation of n-3 and n-6 fatty acids. *Lipids* 1996; 31: 243S–7S.

20. Din JN, Newby DE & Flapan AD. Clinical review Science, medicine, and the future: Omega 3 fatty acids and cardiovascular disease—fishing for a natural treatment. *British Medical Journal* 2004; 328: 30-35.

21. Connor WE, Neuringer M & Reisbick S. Essential fatty acids: the importance of n-3 fatty acids in the retina and brain. *Nutrition Review* 1992; 50: 21–9.

22. Starling S. Study links nutrition and children's behaviour. *Functional Foods & Nutraceuticals* 2005; July.

23. Painter FM. Fish Oil Monograph. *Alternative Medicine Review* 2000; 5(6): 576-580.

24. ibid.

25. Lands WEM. Biochemistry and physiology of eicosanoid precursors in cell membranes. *European Heart Journal*; 3: 22D-25D.

26. Weiss LA, Barrett-Connor E & Von MD. Ratio of n-6 to n-3 fatty acids and bone mineral density in older adults: the Rancho Bernardo Study. American Journal of Clinical Nutrition 2005; 81(4): 934-938.
27. Simopoulos AP. The importance of the ratio of omega-6/omega-3 essential fatty acids. Biomedical Pharmacotherapy 2002; 56(8): 365-79.
28. Simopopoulos AP, Leaf A & Salem Jnr N. Workshop statement on the essentiality of and recommended dietary intakes for omega-6 and omega-3 fatty acids. Prostaglandins, leucotrienes and essential fatty acids 2000; 63: 119-21.

Calcium

1. Halioua I & Anderson JJ. Lifetime calcium intake and physical activity habits: interdependent and combined effects on the radial bone of healthy premenopausal caucasian women. American Journal of Clinical Nutrition 1989; 49: 534–41.
2. Matkovic V, Jelic T, Wardlaw GM, Ilich JZ, Goel PK, Wright JK et al. Timing of peak bone mass in Caucasian females and its implications for the prevention of osteoporosis. Journal of Clinical Investigation 1994; 93: 799–808.
3. Nieves JW, Golden AL, Sirs E, Kelsey JL & Lindsay R. Teenage and current calcium intake are related to bone mineral density of the hip and forearm in women aged 30–39 years. American Journal of Epidemiology 1995; 141: 342–51.
4. Sandler RB, Slemenda CW, LaPorte RE, Cauley JA, Schramm MM, Barresi ML et al. Postmenopausal bone density and milk consumption in childhood and adolescence. American Journal of Clinical Nutrition 1985; 42: 270–4.
5. Oregon State University. Linus Pauling Institute. Micronutrient research for optimum health. http://lpi.oregonstate.edu/infocenter/minerals/calcium (Last modified 01/06/2006).
6. National Health and Medical Research Council. Nutrient reference values for Australia and New Zealand: including recommended dietary intakes. Australian Government 2006; 157.

Iron

1. National Health and Medical Research Council. Dietary Guidelines for children and adolescents in Australia. Endorsed 10 April 2003. Australian Government; Chapter 3.3: 104-105.
2. Walter T, Kovalsky SJ & Stekel A. Effect of a mild iron deficiency on infant mental development scores. Journal of Paediatrics 1983; 102: 519-22.
3. Lozoff B, Brittenham GM, Wolf AW, McClish DK, Kuhnert PM, Jimenez E, et al. Iron deficiency anaemia and iron therapy effects on infant development: test performance. Paediatrics 1987; 79: 981-95.
4. De Andraca I, Walter T, Castillo M, Pino P, Rivera P & Cobo C. Iron deficiency anemia and its effects upon psychological development at preschool age: a longitudinally study. Nestle Foundation annual report 1990; 53-62.
5. Lozoff B, Jimenez E & Wolf AW. Long-term developmental outcome of infants with iron deficiency. New England Journal of Medicine 1991; 325(10): 687-94.
6. Ballot D, Baynes RD, Bothwell TH, Gillooly M, MacFarlane BJ, MacPhail AP, et al. The effects of fruit juices and fruits on the absorption of iron from a rice meal. British Journal of Nutrition 1987; 57: 331–43.
7. Oregon State University. Linus Pauling Institute. Micronutrient research for optimum health. http://lpi.oregonstate.edu/infocenter/minerals/iron (Last modified 01/06/2006).
8. National Health and Medical Research Council. Nutrient reference values for Australia and New Zealand: including recommended dietary intakes. Australian Government 2006; 188.

Zinc

1. Hambidge M. Human zinc deficiency. Journal of Nutrition 2000; 130(5): 1344S-1349S.
2. Ibid.
3. Oregon State University. Linus Pauling Institute. Micronutrient research for optimum health. http://lpi.oregonstate.edu/infocenter/minerals/zinc (Last modified 01/06/2006).
4. National Health and Medical Research Council. Nutrient reference values for Australia and New Zealand: including recommended dietary intakes. Australian Government 2006; 236.

Vitamin C

1. Carr AC & Frei B. Toward a new recommended dietary allowance for vitamin C based on antioxidant and health effects in humans. American Journal of Clinical Nutrition 1999; 69(6): 1086-1107
2. Enstrom JE. Counterpoint: vitamin C and mortality. Nutrition Today 1993; 28: 28-32.
3. Oregon State University. Linus Pauling Institute. Micronutrient research for optimum health. http://lpi.oregonstate.edu/infocenter/vitamins/vitamin C (Last modified 01/06/2006).
4. Australian Government. National Health and Medical Research Council. Nutrient reference values for Australia and New Zealand: including recommended dietary intakes. Australia 2006; 120.

Vitamin A & beta-carotene

1. Field CJ, Johnson IR & Schley PD. Nutrients and their role in host resistance to infection. Journal of Leukocyte Biology 2002; 71(1): 16-32.
2. Ross AC. Vitamin A and retinoids. Nutrition in Health and Disease 1999; 9: 305-327.
3. Oregon State University. Linus Pauling Institute. Micronutrient research for optimum health. http://lpi.oregonstate.edu/infocenter/vitamins/vitamin A (Last modified 01/06/06).
4. National Health and Medical Research Council. Nutrient reference values for Australia and New Zealand: including recommended dietary intakes. Australian Government 2006; 60.

Vitamin E

1. Rimm EB, Stampfer MJ, Ascherio A, Giovannucci E, Colditz GA & Willett WC. Vitamin E consumption and the risk of coronary heart disease in men. New England Journal of Medicine 1993; 328(20): 1450-1456.
2. Stampfer MJ, Hennekens CH, Manson JE, Colditz GA, Rosner B & Willett WC. Vitamin E consumption and the risk of coronary disease in women. New England Journal of Medicine 1993; 328(20): 1444-1449.
3. Yu W, Sanders BG & Kline K. RRR-alpha-tocopheryl succinate-induced apoptosis of human breast cancer cells involves Bax translocation to mitochondria. Cancer Research 2003; 63(10): 2483-2491.
4. You H, Yu W, Munoz-Medellin D, Brown PH, Sanders BG & Kline K. Role of extracellular signal-regulated kinase pathway in RRR-alpha-tocopheryl succinate-induced differentiation of human MDA-MB-435 breast cancer cells. Mol Carcinog. 2002; 33(4): 228-236.
5. Oregon State University. Linus Pauling Institute. Micronutrient research for optimum health. http://lpi.oregonstate.edu/infocenter/vitamins/vitamin E (Last modified 01/06/06).
6. National Health and Medical Research Council. Nutrient reference values for Australia and New Zealand: including recommended dietary intakes. Australian Government 2006; 141.

B vitamins

1. Fenech M, Aitken C & Rinaldi J. Folate, vitamin B12, homocysteine status and DNA damage in young Australian adults. Carcinogenesis 1998; 19(7): 1163-71.
2. Fenech M & Rinaldi J. A comparison of lymphocyte micronuclei and plasma micronutrients in vegetarians and non-vegetarians. Carcinogenesis 1995; 16(2): 223-30.
3. Li D, Sinclair AJ, Mann NJ, Turner A & Ball MJ. Selected micro-nutrient intake and status in men with differing meat intakes, vegetarians and vegans. Asia Pacific Journal of Clinical Nutrition 2000; 9: 18-23.
4. Law MR & Morris JK. By how much fruit and vegetable consumption reduce the risk of ischaemic heart disease? European Journal Clinical Nutrition 1998; 52: 549-56.
5. Verhoef P, Stampfer MJ & Rimm EB. Folate and coronary heart disease. Current Opinion in Lipiology 1998; 9: 17-22.
6. National Health and Medical Research Council. Nutrient reference values for Australia and New Zealand: including recommended dietary intakes. Australian Government 2006; 93.

Chapter 3: The five food groups

Wholegrain cereals

1. European Cancer Prevention organization consensus Panel on Cereals and Cancer. Consensus statement on cereals, fibre and colorectal and breast cancers. European Journal of Cancer Prevention 1998; 7(2): 1S-2S.
2. ibid.
3. Herbert J, Hurley T, Olendzki B, Teas J, Ma Y & Hampl J. Nutritional and socioeconomic factors in relation to prostate cancer mortality: a cross national study. Journal of the National Cancer Institute 1998; 90: 1637–47.
4. World Cancer Research Fund and American Institute for Cancer Research. Food, Nutrition and the prevention of cancer: a global perspective. Washington, DC, American Institute for cancer research, 1997.
5. European Cancer Prevention organization consensus Panel on Cereals and Cancer. Consensus statement on cereals, fibre and colorectal and breast cancers. European Journal of Cancer Prevention 1998; 7(2): 1S-2S.
6. National Heart Foundation. Dietary fibre: a policy statement prepared by the diet and heart Disease Advisory Committee for the National Heart Foundation. Canberra, 1997.
7. Jacobs D, Pereira M, Slavin J & Marquart L. Defining the impact of whole-grain intake on chronic disease. Cereal foods World 2000; 45: 51-3.
8. Kushi L, Meyer K & Jacobs D. Cereals, legumes, and chronic disease risk reduction: evidence from epidemiological studies. American Journal of Clinical Nutrition 1999; 70: 451S-458S.
9. Munoz de Chavez M & Chavez A. Diet that Prevents cancer: recommendations from the American Institute for cancer Research. International Journal of Cancer 1998; 11: 85-9.
10. Truswell A. Cereal grains and coronary heart disease. European Journal of Clinical Nutrition 2002; 56: 1-14.

11. Liu S, Manson J, Stampfer M, Hui F, Giovannucci E, Colditz G, et al. A prospective study of wholegrain intake and risk of type-2 diabetes mellitus in US women. American Journal of Public Health 2000; 90: 1409-15.
12. Rolls B & Hill J. Carbohydrates and weight management. Washington, DC: ILSI Press, 1998.
13. Franklin J & Caterson I. Setting the record straight: the role of carbohydrates in weight control. Sydney: Grains research and development corporation and BRI Australia, 1999.
14. Yao M & Roberts S. Dietary energy density and weight regulation. Nutrition Review 2001; 59: 247-58.
15. National Health and Medical Research Council. Dietary Guidelines for children and adolescents in Australia. Endorsed 10 April 2003; 88.

Fruit

1. Ness AR & Powles JW. Fruit and vegetable, and Cardiovascular disease: a review. International Journal of Epidemiology 1997; 26: 1-13.
2. Law MR & Morris JK. By how much fruit and vegetable consumption reduce the risk of ischaemic heart disease? European Journal of Clinical Nutrition 1998; 52: 549-56.
3. Ascherio A, Hennekens C, Willett WC, Sacks F, Rosner B, Manson J, et al. Prospective study of nutritional factors, blood pressure and hypertension among US women. Hypertension 1996; 27: 1065–72.
4. Moore TJ, Vollmer WM, Appel LJ, Sacks FM, Svetkey LP, Vogt TM, et al. Effects of dietary patterns on ambulatory blood pressure: results from the Dietary Approaches to Stop Hypertension (DASH) trial. Hypertension 1999; 34: 472–7.
5. Ness AR & Powles JW. Fruit and vegetable, and Cardiovascular disease: a review. International Journal of Epidemiology 1997; 26: 1-13.
6. Gillman MW, Cupples LA, Gagnon D, Posher BM, Eilison RC, Castelli WP & Wolf PA. Protective effects of fruit and vegetables on development of stroke in men. Journal of American Medical Association 1995; 273: 113-17.
7. Rolls B & Hill J. Carbohydrates and weight management. Washington, DC: ILSI Press, 1998.
8. Franklin J & Caterson I. Setting the record straight-the role of carbohydrates in weight control. Sydney: Grains research and development corporation and BRI Australia, 1999.
9. Yao M & Roberts S. Dietary energy density and weight regulation. Nutrition Review 2001; 59: 247-58.
10. Platel K & Srinivasan K. Plant foods in the management of diabetes mellitus: vegetables as potential hypoglycaemic agents. Nahrung 1997; 41: 68–74.
11. Williams DE, Wareham DJ, Cox BD, Byrne CD, Hales CN & Day NE. Frequent salad vegetable consumption is associated with a reduction in the risk of diabetes mellitus. Journal of Clinical Epidemiology 1999; 52: 329–37.
12. World Cancer Research Fund and American Institute for cancer research: vegetables and fruits. Food nutrition and the prevention of cancer: a global perspective. Washington, US, American Institute for Cancer research 1997; 436-46.
13. Terry P, Giovannucci E, Michels KB, Bergkvist L, Hansen H, Holmberg L & Wolk A. Fruit, Vegetables, Dietary Fiber, and Risk of Colorectal Cancer. Journal of the National Cancer Institute 2001; 93(7): 525-533.
14. Susan A Lanham-New. Fruit and vegetables: the unexpected natural answer to the question of osteoporosis prevention? American Journal of Clinical Nutrition June 2006; 83(6): 1254-1255.
15. National Health and Medical Research Council. Dietary Guidelines for children and adolescents in Australia. Endorsed 10 April 2003; 68.
16. Dennison B, Rockwell HL & Baker SL. Excess fruit juice consumption by preschool aged children is associated with short stature and obesity. Pediatrics 1997; 99(1): 15-22.
17. O'Sullivan EA & Curzon MEJ. A comparison of acidic dietary factors in children with and without dental erosion. Journal of Dentistry for Children 2000; 67: 187-92.
18. Seow K. Biological mechanism of early childhood caries. Community Dentistry and Oral Epidemiology 1998; 26(1): 8S-27S.

Vegetables & Legumes

1. Ness AR & Powles JW. Fruit and vegetable, and Cardiovascular disease: a review. International Journal of Epidemiology 1997; 26: 1-13.
2. Law MR & Morris JK. By how much fruit and vegetable consumption reduce the risk of ischaemic heart disease? European Journal of Clinical Nutrition 1998; 52: 549-56.
3. Ness AR & Powles JW. Fruit and vegetable, and Cardiovascular disease: a review. International Journal of Epidemiology 1997; 26: 1-13.
4. Gillman MW, Cupples LA, Gagnon D, Posher BM, Eilison RC, Castelli WP & Wolf PA. Protective effects of fruit and vegetables on development of stroke in men. Journal of American Medical Association 1995; 273: 113-17.
5. Steinmetz KA & Potter JD. Vegetables, Fruit and Cancer prevention: a review. Journal of American Dietetic Association 1996; 96: 1027-39.
6. World Cancer Research Fund and American Institute for cancer research: vegetables and fruits. Food nutrition and the prevention of cancer: a global perspective. Washington, US, American Institute for Cancer research 1997; 436-46.
7. Platel K & Srinivasan K. Plant foods in the management of diabetes mellitus: vegetables as potential hypoglycaemic agents. Nabrung 1997, 41: 68-74.
8. Williams DE, Waneham DJ, Cox BD, Byrne CD, Hales CN & Day NE. Frequent salad and vegetable consumption is associated with a reduction in the risk or diabetes mellitus. Journal of Clinical Epidemiology 1999; 52: 329-37.
9. World Cancer Research Fund. Food, nutrition and the prevention of cancer: a global perspective. American Institute for cancer research. Washington, DC, 1997.
10. Duane WC. Effects of legume consumption on serum cholesterol, biliary lipids, and sterol metabolism in humans. Journal of Lipid Research 1997; 38: 1120-1128.
11. Rolls B & Hill J. Carbohydrates and weight management. Washington, DC: ILSI Press, 1998.
12. Franklin J & Caterson I. Setting the record straight-the role of carbohydrates in weight control. Sydney: Grains research and development corporation and BRI Australia, 1999.
13. Yao M & Roberts S. Dietary energy density and weight regulation. Nutrition Review 2001; 59: 247-58.

14. Lanham-New SA. Fruit and vegetables: the unexpected natural answer to the question of osteoporosis prevention? American Journal of Clinical Nutrition 2006; 83(6): 1254-1255.
15. National Health and Medical Research Council. Dietary Guidelines for children and adolescents in Australia. Endorsed 10 April 2003; Chapter 3.3; 61.
16. NSW Health. NSW Schools Physical Activity and Nutrition Survey (SPANS) 2004: Summary Report. NSW Centre for overweight and obesity. 2006 April.

Dairy foods

1. Heaney RP. Nutrition and risk for osteoporosis. Osteoporosis 1996; 483–509.
2. Peacock M. Calcium absorption efficiency and calcium requirements in children and adolescents. American Journal of Clinical Nutrition 1991; 54: 261S–265S.
3. Renner E. Dairy calcium, bone metabolism and prevention of osteoporosis. Journal of Dairy Research 1994; 77: 3489-505.
4. New SA, Bolton-Smith C, Grubb D & Reid D. Nutritional influences on bone mineral density; a cross sectional study in premenopausal women. American Journal of Clinical Nutrition 1997; 65: 1831-9.
5. Teegarden D, Lylke RM, Proulx W, Johnston C & Weaver C. Previous milk consumption is associated with greater bone density in young women. American Journal of Clinical Nutrition 1999; 69: 1014-17.
6. National Health and Medical Research Council. Dietary Guidelines for children and adolescents in Australia. Endorsed 10 April 2003; Chapter 3.3: 130.

Meat, poultry, fish

1. Mu Li, Creswell J Eastman, Kay V Waite, Gary Ma, Margaret R Zacharin, et al. Are Australian children iodine deficient? Results of the Australian National Iodine Nutrition Study. The Medical Journal of Australia 2006; 184(4): 165-169.
2. Fitzpatrick M, Mitchell K. Soy Formulas and the effects of isoflavones on the thyroid. New Zealand Medical Journal 2000; 113: 24-26.
3. Department of Health and Family Services. The Australian Guide to Healthy Eating: background information for nutrition educators. Canberra, 1998.

Chapter 4: Extra foods

Refined sugars

1. NSW Health. NSW Schools Physical Activity and Nutrition Survey (SPANS) 2004: Summary Report. NSW Centre for overweight and obesity, 2006; 16.
2. Girardi NL. Blunted Catecholamine Responses after Glucose Ingestion in Children with Attention Deficit Disorder. Pediatrics Research 1995; 38: 539-542.
3. Molteni R, et al. A High-fat, refined sugar diet reduces hippocampal brain-derived neurotrophic factor, neuronal plasticity, and learning. Neuroscience 2002; 112(4): 803-814.
4. Vaccaro O, Ruth KJ & Stamler J. Relationship of post load plasma glucose to mortality with 19 year follow-up. Diabetes Care 1992; 10: 328-334.
5. Schmidt AM, et al. Activation of receptor for advanced glycation end products: a mechanism for chronic vascular dysfunction in diabetic vasculopathy and atherosclerosis. Circulation Research 1999; 84(5): 489-97.
6. Scanto S & Yudkin J. The effect of dietary sucrose on blood lipids, serum insulin, platelet adhesiveness and body weight in human volunteers. Postgraduate Medicine Journal 1969; 45: 602-607.
7. Australian Bureau of Statistics. National Nutrition Survey: selected highlights, Australia, 1995. Canberra, 1997.
8. Lewis GF & Steiner G. Acute Effects of Insulin in the Control of VLDL Production in Humans. Implications for The insulin-resistant State. Diabetes Care 1996; 19(4): 390-3.
9. Sanchez A, et al. Role of Sugars in Human Neutrophilic Phagocytosis, American Journal of Clinical Nutrition 1973; 261: 1180-1184.
10. Ringsdorf W, Cheraskin E & Ramsay R. Sucrose, Neutrophilic Phagocytosis and Resistance to Disease. Dental Survey 1976; 52(12): 46-48.
11. Lemann J. Evidence that Glucose Ingestion Inhibits Net Renal Tubular Reabsorption of Calcium and Magnesium. Journal of Clinical Nutrition 1976; 70: 236-245.
12. Tjäderhane L, Larmas M. A High Sucrose Diet Decreases the Mechanical Strength of Bones in Growing Rats. Journal of Nutrition 1998; 128: 1807-1810.
13. U.S. Department of Agriculture (USDA). Database for the Added Sugars, Content of Selected Foods Release 1. Prepared by Nutrient Data Laboratory, Beltsville Human Nutrition Research Center (BHNRC). http://www.nal.usda.gov/fnic/foodcomp/Data/add_sug/addsug01.pdf (last modified Feb 2006).

Artificial sweeteners

1. Roberts HJ. American Board of Internal Medicine statement of HJ Roberts MD, concerning the use of products containing aspartame (nutrasweet) by persons with diabetes and hypoglycemia. West Palm Beach, August 9, 1994.
2. Soffritti M, et al. Aspartame induces lymphomas and leukaemias in rats. European Journal of Oncology 2005; 10(2): 107-116.
3. Soffritti M, et al. First experimental demonstration of the multipotenial carcinogenic effects of aspartame administered in the feed to Sprague-Dawley rats. Environmental Health Perspectives 2006; 114(3): 379-385.
4. The Food Commission. Aspartame: the litmus test for the FSA and EFSA. Food Magazine May 2006. http://www.foodcomm.org.uk/latest_aspartame_may_06.htm The Food Commission.
5. Roberts HJ. Sweet'ner dearest: Bittersweet vignettes about aspartame (nutrasweet). Sunshine Sentinel Press, West Palm Beach, Florida.

6. Lam M, Riedy C, Coldwell S, Milgrom P & Craig R. Children's acceptance of Xylitol-based foods. Community Dentistry and Oral Epidemiology 2000; 28(2): 97-101.
7. Gales MA & Nguyen TM. Sorbitol compared with Xylitol in prevention of dental caries. The Annals of Pharmacotherapy 2000; 34(1): 98-100.

Soft drink

1. Harnack L, Stang J & Story R. Soft drink consumption among US children and adolescents: nutritional consequences. Journal of the American Dental Association 1999; 99(4): 436-41.
2. NSW Health. NSW Schools Physical Activity and Nutrition Survey (SPANS) 2004: Summary Report. NSW Centre for overweight and obesity. 2006; 15.
3. Jacobson MF. Liquid Candy: how soft drinks are harming Americans health. Washington DC: Center for Sciences in the Public interest, 1998.
4. Whyshak G. Teenaged girls, carbonated beverages consumption, and bone fractures. Archives of Pediatrics and Adolescent Medicine 2000; 154: 610-13.
5. Crowley S, Antioch K, Carter R, Waters A-M, Conway L & Mathers C. Dietary Conditions for Children and Adolescents in Australia Incorporating the Infant Feeding Guidelines for Health Workers. National Health and Medical Research Council 2003 (Endorsed 10 April).
6. The American Dental Association. Diet and tooth decay. Journal of the American Dental Association 2002; 133 (4): 527.
7. Australian Dental Association. Dental health trends of young children. National Dental http://www.ada.org.au (Last modified June 2007).
8. Gibson S & Williams S. Dental caries in pre-school children: association with social class, tooth brushing habit and consumption of sugars and sugar containing foods. Caries Resource 1999; 33: 101–13.
9. Sank L. Dental nutrition. Nutrition Issues 1999; 19: 1-2.
10. Murry R & Drummond B. Are the risks to dental health with frequent use of carbohydrate foods and beverages? Australian Journal of Nutrition Dietetics 1996; 53(4): 47S.

Caffeine

1. Smith PF, Smith A, Miners J, McNeil J & Proudfoot A. Report from the Expert working Group on the safety Aspects of Dietary caffeine. Canberra: Australia New Zealand Food Authority, 2000.
2. Barrett-Connor e, Chang JC & Edelstein SL. Coffee-associated osteoporosis offset by daily milk consumption. Journal of the American Medical Association 1994; 271: 280-83.

Salt

1. Food Standards Agency. The National Diet and Nutrition Survey of Young People aged 4 to 18 years. HMSO June 2000, London.
2. Kurtz TW, Al-Bander H & Morris RC. 'Salt-sensitive' essential hypertension in man. Is the sodium ion alone important? New England Journal of Medicine 1987; 317: 1043-8.
3. Siani A, Guglielmucci F, Farinaro E & Strazzullo P. Increasing evidence for the roles of salt and salt-sensitivity in hypertension. Nutrition, Metabolism and Cardiovascular Diseases 1999; 2: 93-100.
4. NSW Health. NSW Schools Physical Activity and Nutrition Survey (SPANS) 2004: Summary Report. NSW Centre for overweight and obesity. 2006; 20.
5. Weaver CM, Proulx WR & Heaney RP. Choices for achieving adequate dietary calcium with a vegetarian diet. American Journal of Clinical Nutrition 1999; 70: 435S-85S.
6. Heaney RP. Bone mass, nutrition, and other lifestyle factors. Nutrition Review 1996; 54: 3S-10S.
7. Nutritional Health and Medical Research Council. Dietary guidelines for children and adolescents. Canberra: Australian Government Publishing Service, 1995.
8. Mu Li, Creswell J Eastman, Kay V Waite, Gary Ma, Margaret R Zacharin, Duncan J Topliss, et al. Are Australian children iodine deficient? Results of the Australian National Iodine Nutrition Study. The Medical Journal of Australia 2006; 184 (4): 165-169.
9. Eastman CJ. Where has all our iodine gone? Medical Journal of Australia 1999; 171: 455-456.
10. United States Department of Agriculture. USDA National Nutrient Database for Standard Reference, Release 18 Content of Selected Sodium Foods http://www.nal.usda.gov/fnic/foodcomp/Data/SR18/nutrlist/sr18a307.pdf (Last modified 16/04/2008).

Saturated & trans-fats

1. Beresford SA, Johnson KC, Ritenbaugh C, et al. Low-fat dietary pattern and risk of colorectal cancer: the Women's Health Initiative Randomized Controlled Dietary Modification Trial. Journal of the American Medical Association 2006; 295: 643-54.
2. Howard BV, Manson JE, Stefanick ML, et al. Low-fat dietary pattern and weight change over 7 years: the Women's Health Initiative Dietary Modification Trial. Journal of the American Medical Association 2006; 295: 39-49.
3. Howard BV, Van Horn L, Hsia J, et al. Low-fat dietary pattern and risk of cardiovascular disease: the Women's Health Initiative Randomized Controlled Dietary Modification Trial. Journal of the American Medical Association 2006; 295: 655-66.
4. Prentice RL, Caan B, Chlebowski RT, et al. Low-fat dietary pattern and risk of invasive breast cancer: the Women's Health Initiative Randomized Controlled Dietary Modification Trial. Journal of the American Medical Association 2006; 295: 629-42.
5. Suskind RM & Lewinter-Suskind Leds. Textbook of Pediatric Nutrition, 2nd ed. New York: Raven Press, 1993.
6. Magarey A, Nichols J & Boulton TJC. Food intake at age 8: energy, macro-and micro nutrients. Australian Paediatrics Journal 1987; 23: 173-8.
7. Jenner DA & Miller MR. Intakes of selected nutrients in year 7 Western Australian children: comparison between weekdays and weekend days and relationships with socio-economic status. Australian Journal of Nutrition and Dietetics 1991; 48: 50-5.

8. NSW Health. NSW Schools Physical Activity and Nutrition Survey (SPANS) 2004: Summary Report. NSW Centre for overweight and obesity, iv.
9. ibid, 20.
10. National Heart Foundation of Australia. A review of the relationship between dietary fat and cardiovascular disease. Australian Journal of Nutrition and Dietetics 1999; 56(4): 5S–22S.
11. Keys A. Seven Countries: A multivariate analysis of death and coronary heart disease. Cambridge, MA: Harvard University Press, 1980.
12. Penny M Kris-Etherton, Thomas A Pearson, Ying Wan, et al. High–monounsaturated fatty acid diets lower both plasma cholesterol and triacylglycerol concentrations. American Journal of Clinical Nutrition 1999; 70(6): 1009-1015.
13. Zhang J. et. Dietary fat intake is associated with psychosocial and cognitive functioning of school aged children in the United States. Journal of Nutrition 2005; 135(8): 1967-73.
14. Willett WC & Ascherio A. Trans fatty acids: Are the effects only marginal? American Journal of Public Health 1994; 84: 722-724.
15. Ascherio A, Stampfer MJ & Willett WC. Trans fatty acids and coronary heart disease. Departments of Nutrition and Epidemiology, Harvard School of Public Health. The Channing Laboratory, Department of Medicine, Brigham and Women's Hospital, Nov 15, 1999: 1-21.
16. Willett WC & Ascherio A. Trans fatty acids: Are the effects only marginal? American Journal of Public Health 1994; 84: 722-724.
17. Sun Q, Ma J, Campos H, Hankinson S, Manson J, Stampfer M. et al. A Prospective Study of Trans Fatty Acids in Erythrocytes and Risk of Coronary Heart Disease. Circulation April 10, 2007.
18. Salmeron J, Hu FB, Manson JE, Stampfer MJ, Colditz GA, Rimm EB, Willett W. Dietary fat intake and risk of type 2 diabetes in women. American Journal of Clinical Nutrition 2001; 73 (6): 1019-26.
19. US Department of Health and Human Services. US Food and Drug Administration consumer Magazine. Sept-Oct 2003; Pub No. FDA05-1329C. http://www.fda.gov/FDAC/features/2003/503_fats.html (Last modified Sept 2005).
20. Ibid.
21. National Health and Medical Research Council. Dietary Guidelines for children and adolescents in Australia. Endorsed 10 April 2003.

Chapter 5: Super foods

Berries

1. Wu X, Beecher GR, Holden JM, Haytowitz DB, Gebhardt SE & Prior RL. Lipophilic and hydrophilic antioxidant capacities of common foods in the United States. Journal of Agriculture Food Chemistry 2004; 52(12): 4026-37.
2. Bagchi D, Sen CK, Bagchi M & Atalay M. Anti-Angiogenic, Antioxidant, and Anti-Carcinogenic Properties of a Novel Anthocyanin-Rich Berry Extract Formula. Biochemistry 2004; 69(1): 75-80.
3. Schmidt BM, Howell AB, McEniry B, Knight CT, Seigler D, Erdman JW Jr & Lila MA. Effective separation of potent antiproliferation and antiadhesion components from wild blueberry (Vaccinium angustifolium Ait) fruits. Journal of Agriculture Food Chemistry 2004; 52(21): 6433-42.
4. Wu X. News release, American Chemical Society. Journal of Agricultural and Food Chemistry Nov 2004; http://pubs3.acs.org/journals/jafcau/promo/most_accessed/2004.html.
5. Halvorsen BL, Holte K, Myhrstad MC, Barikmo I, Hvattum E, et al. A Systematic Screening of Total Antioxidants in Dietary Plants. Journal of Nutrition 2002; 132: 461-471.
6. Wu X, Beecher GR, Holden JM, Haytowitz DB, Gebhardt SE & Prior RL. Lipophilic and hydrophilic antioxidant capacities of common foods in the United States. Journal of Agriculture Food Chemistry 2004; 52(12): 4026-37.
7. Wu X. News release, American Chemical Society. Journal of Agricultural and Food Chemistry Nov 2004; http://pubs3.acs.org/journals/jafcau/promo/most_accessed/2004.html.

Fish

1. Richardson AJ & Montgomery P. The Oxford-Durham study: a randomized, controlled trial of dietary supplementation with fatty acids in children with developmental coordination disorder. Pediatrics 2005; 1115: 1360-1366.
2. ibid.
3. ibid.
4. AJ Richardson & BK Puri. A randomized double-blind, placebo-controlled study of the effects of supplementation with highly unsaturated fatty acids on ADHD-related symptoms in children with specific learning difficulties. Progress in Neuro-Psychopharmacology and Biological Psychiatry 2002; 26(2): 233-9.
5. AJ Richardson. Long-chain polyunsaturated fatty acids in childhood developmental and psychiatric disorders. Lipids 2004; 39(12): 1215-22.
6. L Stevens, et al. EFA supplementation in children with inattention, hyperactivity, and other disruptive behaviors. Lipids 2003; 38(10): 007-21.
7. AJ Richardson. Clinical trials of fatty acid treatment in ADHD, dyslexia, dyspraxia and the autistic spectrum. Prostaglandins, Leukotrienes and Essential Fatty Acids 2004; 70(4): 383-90.
8. Horrocks LA & Yeo YK, Health Benefits of Docosahexaenoic acid (DHA). Pharmocological Research 1999; 40(3).

Garlic

1. Josling P. Preventing the common cold with a garlic supplement: two double-blind placebo-controlled survey. Advances in Therapy 200; 18(4): 189-93.

Yoghurt

1. Gill HS & Guarner F. Probiotics and human health: a clinical perspective. Postgraduate Medical Journal 2004; 80: 516-526.
2. Roberfroid M. Prebiotics and probiotics: are they functional foods? American Journal of Clinical Nutrition June 2000; 7(6): 1682S-1687S.

Chapter 6: Building healthy bones

1. Peacock M. Calcium Absorption Efficiency and Calcium Requirements in Children and Adolescents. American Journal of Nutrition 1991; 54: 261S-265S.
2. Anderson JJB and Rondano P. Peak Bone Mass Development of Females: Can Young Adult Women. Journal of the American College of Nutrition 1996; 15(6): 570-574.
3. ibid.
4. Peacock M. Calcium Absorption Efficiency and Calcium Requirements in Children and Adolescents. American Journal of Nutrition 1991; 54: 261S-265S.
5. Australian Bureau of Statistics, Musculoskeletal Conditions in Australia: A Snapshot, 2004-05. Released 28 Sept 2006; 4823.0.55.001.
6. Peacock M. Calcium Absorption Efficiency and Calcium Requirements in Children and Adolescents. American Journal of Nutrition 1991; 54: 261S-265S.
7. Pipes PL and CM. Trahms. Nutrition in Infancy and Childhood (5th ed.) 1993; Toronto: Mosby.
8. Dodiuk-Gad RP, Rozen GS, Rennert G, Rennert HS, and Ish-Shalom S. Sustained effect of short-term calcium supplementation on bone mass in adolescent girls with low calcium intake. American Journal of Clinical Nutrition 2005; 81(1): 168-174.
9. Matkovic V, Goel PK, Badenhop-Stevens NE, Landoll JD, et al. Calcium supplementation and bone mineral density in females from childhood to young adulthood: a randomized controlled trial. American Journal of Clinical Nutrition 2005; 81(1): 175-188.
10. Queensland Government. Healthy Kids Queensland Survey 2006 Summary Report. Queensland Health 2007; http://www.health.qld.gov.au/ph/documents/hpu/32848.pdf.
11. Lemann J. Evidence that Glucose Ingestion Inhibits Net Renal Tubular Reabsorption of Calcium and Magnesium. Journal of Clinical Nutrition 1976; 70: 236-245.
12. Tjäderhane L, Larmas M. A High Sucrose Diet Decreases the Mechanical Strength of Bones in Growing Rats. Journal of Nutrition 1998; 128: 1807-1810.
13. Thom J, Morris J, Bishop A, & Blacklock. The influence of refined carbohydrate on urinary calcium excretion. British Journal of Urology 1978; 50: 459-464.
14. Smith PF, Smith A, Miners J, McNeil J & Proudfoot A. Report from the Expert working Group on the safety Aspects of Dietary caffeine. Canberra: Australia New Zealand Food Authority 2000.
15. Barrett-Connor e, Chang JC & Edelstein SL. Coffee-associated osteoporosis offset by daily milk consumption. Journal of the American Medical Association 1994; 271: 280-83.
16. Shrapnel W & Truswell S. Vitamin D deficiency in Australia and New Zealand: what are the dietary options? Nutrition & Dietetics: The Journal of the Dietitians Association of Australia Dec 2006.
17. ibid.
18. ibid.
19. Whyshak G. Teenaged girls, carbonated beverages consumption, and bone fractures. Archives of Pediatrics and Adolescent Medicine 2000; 154: 610-13.
20. Licata A, et al. Acute effects of dietary protein on calcium metabolism in patients with osteoporosis. Journal of Gerontology 1981; 36: 14-19.
21. Tucker KL, Hannan MT & Kiel DP. The acid-base hypothesis: diet and bone in the Framingham Osteoporosis Study. European Journal of Clinical Nutrition 2001; 40: 231-237.
22. Buclin T, et al. Diet Acids and Alkalis Influence Calcium Retention in Bone. Osteoporosis International 2001; 12: 493-499.
23. Gur A, et al. The Role of Trace Minerals in the pathogenesis of postmenopausal osteoporosis and a new effect of calcitonin. Journal of Bone and Mineral Metabolism 2002: 20; 39-43.
24. Gaby, Alan R. Every Woman's Essential Guide to Preventing and Reversing Osteoporosis Prima Health 1990.
25. Australian Institute of Health and Welfare. Arthritis and musculoskeletal conditions in Australia. Canberra, 2005; PHE67.

Chapter 7: Vegetarian kids

1. Burr ML & Butland BK. Heart disease in British vegetarians. American Journal of Clinical Nutrition 1988; 48: 830-2.
2. Pronczuk A, Kipervarg Y & Hayes KC. Vegetarians have higher plasma alpha-tocopherol relative to cholesterol than do non-vegetarians. Journal of American College Nutrition 1992; 11: 50-5.
3. Prasad K, Reddy S, Saunders TAB. Plasma ubiquinone (Q10) concentrations in female vegetarians and omnivores. Proceedings of the Nutrition Society 1993; 52: 332A.
4. Haines AP, Chakraharti R, Fisher D, Meade TW, North WR & Stirling Y. Haemostatic variables in vegetarians and non vegetarians. Thrombosis Research 1980; 19: 139-48.
5. Sanders TAB & Key TJA. Blood pressure, plasma rennin activity and aldosterone concentrations in vegans and omnivore controls. Human Nutrition-Applied Nutrition 1987; 41: 101-8.

6. Margetts BM, Beilin LJ, Vandongen R & Armstrong Bk. Vegetarian diet in mild hypertension: a randomized controlled trial. British Medical Journal 1986; 293: 129-33.
7. American Dietetic Association. Position paper on vegetarian diets. Journal of American Dietitians Association 2003; 103: 748-765.
8. National Health and Medical Research Council. Dietary Guidelines for children and adolescents in Australia. Endorsed 10 April 2003; 113.

Chapter 8: Allergies & intolerances

1. Savalano DA, Abou El Anouar A, Smith DE, et al. Lactose malabsorption from yoghurt, pasteurized yoghurt, sweet acidophilus milk and cultured milk in lactase-deficient individuals. American Journal of Clinical Nutrition 1984; 40: 1219-23.
2. Pelletierx, Laure-Boussuge S & Danazzolo Y. Hydrogen excretion upon ingestion of dairy products in lactose-intolerant male subjects: importance of the live flora. European Journal of Clinical Nutrition 2001; 55: 509-12.

Chapter 9: Kids with special needs

Childhood obesity

1. Magarey AM, Daniels LA & Boulton TJC. Prevalence of overweight and obesity in Australian children and adolescents: reassessment of 1985 and 1995 data against new standard international definitions. Medical Journal of Australia 2001; 174: 561-4.
2. Wake M, Lazarus R, Hasketh R & Waters E. Are Australian Children getting fatter? Journal of Paediatrics and Child Health 1999; 35-47.
3. Booth ML, Wake M, Armstrong T, Chey T, Hesketh & Mathur S. The epidemiology of overweight and obesity among Australian children and adolescents, 1995-1997. Australian and New Zealand Journal of Public Health 2001; 25: 162-9.
4. NSW Health. NSW Schools Physical Activity and Nutrition Survey (SPANS) 2004: Summary Report. NSW Centre for overweight and obesity. 2006; 20.
5. ibid, iv.
6. Chagnon YC, Rankinen T, Snyder EE, et al. The human obesity gene map: the 2002 update. Obesity Research 2003; 11: 313-367.
7. Dollman J, Olds T, Norton K & Stuart D. The evaluation of fitness and fatness in 10-11 year old Australian children: Changes in distributional characteristics between 1985 and 1997. Pediatric Exercise Science 1999; 11: 108-21.
8. Law M. Dietary fat and adult diseases and the implications for childhood nutrition: an epidemiological approach. American Journal of Clinical Nutrition 2000; 72: 1291S-1296S.
9. Must A & Strauss R. Risks and consequences of childhood and adolescent obesity. International Journal of Obesity 1999; 22: 206-214.
10. Woutersen R, Appel M, Van Gardenen-Hoetmer A & Wijnands M. Dietary fat and carcinogenesis. Mutation Research 1999; 443(1-2): 111-127.
11. Siani A, Guglielmucci F, Farinaro E & Strazzullo P. Increasing evidence for the roles of salt and salt-sensitivity in hypertension. Nutrition, Metabolism and Cardiovascular Diseases 1999; 2: 93-100.
12. Kral VE, Rolls BJ. Energy density and portion size: their independent and combined effects on energy intake. Physiology and Behaviour 2004; 82: 131-138.
13. Dietz WH. Childhood weight affects adult morbidity and mortality. Journal of Nutrition 1998; 128: 5411-14S.
14. Power C, Lake JK & Cole TJ. Measurements of long-term health risks of child and adolescent fatness. International Journal of Obesity related Metabolic Disorders 1997; 21: 507-26.
15. National Health and Medical Research Council. Dietary Guidelines for children and adolescents in Australia. Endorsed 10 April 2003; Chapter 2: 27.
16. Department of Health and Human Services. Physical activity and health: a report of the Surgeon General. Atlanta, GA: DHHS, Centers for Disease Control and Prevention and National Center for Chronic Disease Prevention and Health Promotion, 1996.
17. NSW Health, op cit, 20.
18. Goran MI. Metabolic precursors and effects of obesity in children: a decade of progress, 1990-1999. American Journal of Clinical Nutrition 2001; 73: 158-71.
19. National Health and Medical Research Council, op cit. Chapter B, 252.
20. Lustig RH. Childhood obesity: behavioral aberration or biochemical drive? Reinterpreting the First Law of Thermodynamics. Nature Clinical Practice Endocrinology & Metabolism 2006; 2: 447-458.
21. Brand-Miller JC, Pawlak DB & McMillan J. Glycaemic index and obesity. American Journal of Clinical Nutrition 2002; 76(1): 281S-285S.
22. Dietz WH & Gortmaker SL. Do we fatten our children at the TV set? Television viewing and obesity in children and adolescents. Pediatrics 1985; 75: 807-12.
23. Garaulet M, Martinez A, Victoria F, Perez-Llama SF, Ortega R & Zamora S. Differences in dietary intake and activity level between normal-weight and overweight or obese adolescents. Journal of Pediatric Gastroenterology 2000; 30: 253-8.
24. NSW Health. NSW Schools Physical Activity and Nutrition Survey (SPANS) 2004: Summary Report. NSW Centre for overweight and obesity. April 2006; 5.
25. obid, iv.
26. Garg A. High-monounsaturated-fat diets for patients with diabetes mellitus: a meta-analysis. American Journal of Clinical Nutrition 1998; 67: 577S-582S.

Children with diabetes

1. Fagot-Campagna A. Emergence of type-2 diabetes mellitus in children: the epidemiological evidence. Journal of Pediatric Endocrinology and Metabolism 2000; 13(6): 1395S-402S.
2. Ehtisham S, Barrett TG & Shaw NJ. Type-2 diabetes mellitus in UK children: an emerging problem. Diabetic Medicine 2000; 17: 867-871.

3. Baur LA. Child and adolescent obesity in the 21st century: an Australian perspective. Asian Pacific Journal of Clinical Nutrition 2002; 11(3): 524S-528S.
4. McMahon SK, Haynes A, Ratnam N, Grant MT, Carne CL, et al. Increase in type-2 diabetes in children and adolescents in Western Australia. Medical Journal of Australia 2004; 180(9): 459-461.
5. Montonen J, Knekt P, Jarvinen R, Aromaa A & Reunanen A. Whole-grain and fiber intake and the incidence of type-2 diabetes. American Journal of Clinical Nutrition 2003; 77(3): 622-629.
6. Liu S, Manson J, Stampfer M, Hui F, Giovannucci E, Colditz G, et al. A prospective study of wholegrain intake and risk of type-2 diabetes mellitus in US women. American Journal of Public Health 2000; 90: 1409-15.
7. Salmeron J, Ascherio A, Rimm E & Colditz G. Dietary Fiber, glycaemic load and risk of NIDDM in men. Diabetes Care 1997; 20: 545-50.
8. Salmeron J, Manson J, Stampfer M, Colditz G, Wing A & Willett W. Dietary fiber, glycaemic load, and risk of non-insulin-dependant diabetes mellitus in women. Journal of the American Medical Association 1997; 277: 472-7.
9. Kris-Etherton PM, Pearson TA, Wan Y, Hargrove RL, Moriarty K, Fishell V & Etherton TD. High–monounsaturated fatty acid diets lower both plasma cholesterol and triacylglycerol concentrations. American Journal of Clinical Nutrition 1999; 70(6): 1009-1015.
10. Rasmussen OW, Thomsen C, Hansen KW, Vesterlund M, Winther E & Hermansen K. Effects on blood pressure, glucose, and lipid levels of a high-monounsaturated fat diet compared with a high-carbohydrate diet in NIDDM subjects. Diabetes Care 1993; 16(12): 1565-1571.
11. Garg A. High-monounsaturated-fat diets for patients with diabetes mellitus: a meta-analysis. American Journal of Clinical Nutrition 1998; 67: 577S-582S.
12. Raheja BS, Sadikot SM, Phatak RB, & Rao MB. Significance of the n-6/n-3 ratio for insulin action in diabetes. Annals of the New York Academy of Science 1993; 683: 258–71.
13. Connor WE, Prince MJ, Ullmann D, et al. The hypotriglyceridemic effect of fish oil in adult-onset diabetes without adverse glucose control. Annals of the New York Academy of Science 1993; 683: 337–40.
14. Burr ML, Fehily AM, Gilbert JF, et al. Effect of changes in fat, fish and fibre intakes on death and myocardial reinfarction: diet and reinfarction trial (DART). Lancet 1989; 2: 757–61.
15. De Lorgeril M, Renaud S, Mamelle N, et al. Mediterranean linolenic acid–rich diet in secondary prevention of coronary heart disease. Lancet 1994; 343: 1454–9.

Kids with ADHD

1. Kidd PM. Attention deficit/hyperactivity disorder (ADHD) in children: rational for its integrative management. Alternative Medicine Review Oct 2000; 5(5): 402-28.
2. Jacobson MF, Schardt MS. Diet, ADHD and behaviour: a quarter-century review. Washington DC: Centre for Science in the public interest, 1999.
3. Uhling T, Merkenschlager A, Brandmaier R & Egger J. Topographic mapping of brain electrical activity in children with food induced attention deficit hyperkinetic disorder. European Journal of Pediatrics 1997; 156(7): 557-61.
4. Bateman B, Warner JO, Hutchinson E, Dean T, Rowlandson P, Gant C, et al. The effects of a double blind, placebo controlled, artificial food colourings and benzoate preservative challenge on hyperactivity, in a general population sample of preschool children. Archives of Disease in Childhood 2004; 89(6): 506-11.
5. Swanson JM & Kinsbourne M. Food dyes impair performance of hyperactive children on a laboratory learning test. Science 1980; 207(4438): 1485-7.
6. Row KS & Row KJ. Synthetic food colouring and behaviour: a dose response effect in a double blind, placebo-controlled repeated-measured study. Journal of Pediatrics 1994; 125(5-Pt 1): 691-8.
7. Dengate S & Ruben A. Controlled trial of cumulative behavioural effects of a common bread preservative. Journal of Paediatrics and Child Health 2002; 38(4): 373-6.
8. Food standards ANZ. Food additives. http://www.foodstandards.gov.au/newsroom/publications/shoppersguide/index.cfm (Last modified Sept 2002).
9. Row KS & Briggs DR. Food additives and behaviour. The Medical Journal of Australia 1994; 161581-582.
10. Rapp DJ. Does diet effect hyperactivity? Journal of Learning Disabilities 1978; 11(6): 56-62.
11. Girardi NL. Blunted Catecholamine Responses after Glucose Ingestion in Children with Attention Deficit Disorder. Pediatrics Research 1995; 38: 539-542.
12. Stevens LJ, Zentall SS, Deck JL, Abate ML, Watkins BA, Lipp SR & Burgess JR. Essential fatty acid metabolism in boys with attention-deficit hyperactivity disorder. American Journal of Clinical Nutrition 1995; 62(4): 761-8.
13. Bourre JM, Bonneil M, Chaudiere J, Clement M, Bumont O, Durand G, Lafont H, Nalbone G, Pascal G & Piciotti M. Structural and functional importance of dietary polyunsaturated fatty acids in the nervous system. Advances in Experimental Medicine and Biology 1992; 318: 211-29.
14. Burgess JR, et al. Long Chain polyunsaturated fatty acids in children with attention deficit hyperactivity disorder. American Journal of Clinical Nutrition 2000; 71(1): 327S-30S.
15. Bekaroglu M, Aslan Y, Gedik Y, Deger O, Mocan H, Erduran E & Karahan C. Relationships between serum free fatty acids and zinc, and attention deficit hyperactivity disorder: a research note. The Journal of Child Psychology and Psychiatry 1996; 37(2): 225-7.

Recipes
Breakfast

1. Pollit E. Does breakfast make a difference in school? Journal of American Dietitians Association 1995; 95: 1134.
2. Pollit E, Leibel RL & Greenfield D. Brief fasting, stress and cognition in children. American Journal of Clinical Nutrition 1981; 34: 1526.

Index

A

ADHD   80, 101, 139, 140
Allergies   36, 48, 50, 52, 116, 117
Allergies, milk   117-119
Allergies, egg   120
Allergies, peanut   121
Alpha-linolenic acid (ALA)   38
Almond, coconut & peach muffins   199
Almond cream   174
Amino acids   34, 75, 79, 111-113
Anaemia   44, 123
Anaphylaxis   116, 118, 127
Antibiotics   13, 74, 102
Antioxidants   12, 13, 15, 19, 20, 32, 79,100, 110
Anxiety   80, 88, 140
Apple & cranberry sauce   174
Apple & beetroot carob brownies   205
Apple & zucchini carrot loaf   204
Apple, sultana & cinnamon muffins   201
Apricot creamy rice   253
Apricot protein balls   213
Apricot seed bar   209
Artificial additives   12, 85, 139, 140
Artificial sweeteners   70, 78, 84, 85
Aspartame   84
Asthma   36, 38, 52, 63
Avocado spread   167
Avocado, salmon & feta melt   217

B

Baba ghanoush   162
Baked beans   154
Baked potato jackets   216
Baked rice balls   218
Baked sweet potato wedges   165
Banana & berry breakfast smoothie   152
Banana & walnut muffins   203
Banana ice cream   284
B vitamins   54, 57, 60, 64, 68, 73, 75, 79, 88, 104
B12   54, 68, 70, 73-75
Bean tuna salad   179
Bean falafels in mini pita pockets   226
Beetroot & cumin dip   163
Beetroot chutney   170
Beetroot, pumpkin & goats cheese salad   180
Behavioural function   38
Behavioural problems   80, 101, 139, 140
Berries   20, 48, 49, 60-62, 72, 83, 100, 103
Berry & yoghurt smoothie   259
Berry Bircher muesli   149

Berry yoghurt drink   261
Beta-carotene   19, 50, 60, 64, 108
Blood pressure   8, 9, 37, 38, 90, 110, 116, 131, 133
Blood sugar levels   20, 22, 23, 26, 27, 32, 34, 37, 46, 58, 60, 65, 80, 135, 136-138
Blueberry buttermilk pancakes   158
Blueberry wholemeal muffins   200
Brain function & development   9, 20, 27, 32, 38, 44, 46, 48, 54, 74, 84, 90, 91, 101, 114, 139, 140
Broccoli & feta quiche with brown rice base   221
Bone density   38, 68, 106-108, 113
Bone health   41, 48, 61, 65, 68, 69, 85, 88, 90, 106-108, 111, 113, 114, 123
Bowel bacteria   21, 22, 23, 50, 54, 70, 104, 127
Breakfast   148
Breakfast cups   155
Breakfast eggs   156
Breakfast frittata   157
Buckwheat tabouli   182

C

Caffeine   41, 78, 85, 88, 102, 107
Carbohydrates   18, 26, 27, 32, 33, 46, 54, 64, 79
Cardiovascular   8, 16, 19, 20, 27, 38, 48, 58, 74, 130, 131, 138
Calcium   128
Carob   83, 88
Carob & banana smoothie   259
Carob & raspberry muffins   202
Carob chip oatmeal cookies   211
Carob coated banana ice creams   250
Carob coated strawberries   257
Carob coconut roughs   214
Carrot, apple & capsicum coleslaw   184
Carrot, celery, apple & beetroot juice   261
Carrot, orange & tomato soup   192
Carotenoids   16, 19, 50, 65
Calcium   13, 32, 41-43, 48, 49, 55, 56, 60, 63, 64, 68-72, 74, 79, 80, 85, 88, 90, 94, 106-108, 113, 114, 118, 123, 127, 128
Cancer   9, 13, 16, 19, 20, 22, 23, 36, 37, 38, 48, 50, 52, 57, 58, 61, 65, 79, 100
Cashew & tumeric rice salad   178
Cavities, dental   9, 17, 86
Char grilled beef & vegetable quinoa salad   187
Cheese & sesame crackers   166
Chicken curry   243
Chicken salad with wholegrain dressing & baked crotons   186
Chickpea, pineapple & tomato couscous salad   183

Chickpea vegie burger   227
Cholesterol   8, 22, 27, 36, 37, 54, 58, 65, 80, 94, 95, 110, 113, 133, 136, 138
Chromium   13, 79
Chronic disease   13, 19, 27, 38, 56, 57, 61, 65
Citrus dressing   172
Coeliac   122, 123, 126
Colds   9
Colon health   21-23
Constipation   9, 22, 24, 104
Cooking grains   271, 272
Cooking legumes   273
Cordial   17, 80, 83, 87
Corn & spinach timbales   219
Creamy mango jelly   251
Creamy mayonnaise   169
Crispy almond & sesame chicken nuggets   234
Crunchy nut muesli bar   208
Crunchy toasted muesli   151

D

Date or prune spread   167
Date spread   167
Date wholemeal scones   206
Depression   36, 38, 91, 101, 131
Diabetes   8, 9, 22, 23, 26, 27, 32, 36-38, 57, 58, 61, 65, 136-138, 110, 130, 131, 133, 135
Diarrhoea   50, 88, 104
Digestive enzymes   18, 33
Digestive health   21, 23, 50, 54
Docosahexaenoic acid (DHA)   38, 101
Dried fruit   22, 27, 28, 44, 62, 63, 72
Dysbiosis   104

E

Earth cookies   212
Ecoli   142
Eczema   36
Eggs   13, 14, 34, 42, 44, 46, 53, 54, 73, 75, 76, 110, 111, 113, 114, 116, 120, 138, 140, 142
Eicosapentaenoic acid   38
Energy drinks   88, 107
Enzymes   18, 66, 79
E series, food additives   139
Essential fatty acids (EFAs)   36, 37, 93, 113, 140
Exercise   44, 108, 131, 133, 136
Eye health   20, 36, 50

F

Fermented foods   104
Flavanoids   19, 20, 60, 61
Fibre, dietary   8, 21-25, 27, 28, 32, 33, 57 60, 63,
    64, 79, 80 110, 113, 125, 131, 132, 134, 137
Fig & date energy bars   210
Fish   16, 28, 34, 37-39, 43, 44, 46, 50, 53, 54, 67, 72-75
Fizzy drinks   260
Folic acid (folate)   48, 54, 123
Free radicals   19, 52, 100
Fresh fruit soft serve ice cream   254
Fructose   30, 32, 33, 60, 79, 81
Fruit crushes   260
Fruit jelly   251
Fruit juice   17, 24, 63, 83, 85, 87, 134

G

Garlic   64, 65, 67, 72, 92, 102, 103
Genetically modified (GM) food   12, 14
Glucose   22, 23, 27, 26, 30, 32-34, 44, 79, 81,
    135, 137
Gluten-intolerance   122, 123
Glycaemic Index   26, 28, 29, 30, 78, 81, 131,
    132, 134, 137, 138
Green pea & potato soup   195
Guacamole   162
Gum health   9, 50

H

Haem-iron   44, 45
Hay fever   52
Healthy nachos   231
Heart disease   9, 19, 20, 22, 26, 27, 36, 37, 52,
    54, 57, 58, 61, 65
Heavy metals   12
Herbal tea   88
Herbicides   12
High blood pressure   8, 9, 90, 110, 131
Honey   30-33, 79, 81, 83, 84, 88
Hummus   161
Hydrogenation   16, 36, 38, 95, 96, 98
Hyperactivity   80, 88, 140, 139
Hypertension   38, 57, 61, 90

I

Ice blocks   250
Ice creams   254
Immune health   9, 13, 14, 19, 21, 22, 23, 34, 38,
    44, 46, 48, 50, 52, 70, 73, 80, 88, 100, 102,
    104, 113, 114, 116, 122, 127
Individual pizza   248
Insoluble fibre   22-24, 60, 64
Insulin resistance   36, 135, 136

Insulin   8, 22, 27, 26, 32, 41, 46, 80, 131, 133,
    135, 136
Iodine   74, 75, 90, 91
Iron   13, 40, 44, 45, 48, 50, 57, 60, 64, 73, 75, 79,
    88, 110, 111, 114, 123
Iron deficiency   44
IQ   74, 90, 91, 101, 148

K

Kidney bean tacos   232
Kidney health   136
Kidney stones   85, 108

L

Lacto-ovo vegetarian   110, 113
Lactose   79, 81, 117-119, 123, 127
Lactose-free foods   112, 119, 122, 128
Lactose-intolerance   43, 70, 71, 122, 123, 127, 128
Lamb & vegetable kebabs   240
Learning difficulties   9
Legumes   14, 18-24, 27, 28, 33, 32, 34, 38, 44,
    46, 54, 64-67, 71, 73, 75, 76,
Lentil & millet patties   228
Lentil & vegie cottage pie   247
Lentil soup   189
Lentil rice salad with minted yoghurt   176
Linoleic acid   38
Listeria   142
Liver health   8, 32, 54, 130, 131
Liver disease   8
LSA   34, 39, 42, 71, 72, 76
Lunch box ideas   268, 270
Lycopene   19, 65

M

Magnesium   13, 42, 57, 60, 64, 68, 79, 88, 107,
    106, 108
Mango chutney   171
Mango smoothie   259
Mercury   12, 74
Mild lamb curry   242
Minestrone soup   191
Mini capsicum & salmon quiches with kumera
base   222
Mixed grain natural muesli   150
Monounsaturated fats   16, 36, 37, 39, 76, 93,
    94, 98, 138
Muesli bars, commercial   32, 39, 80, 81, 83, 104
Muscle health   32, 34, 41, 44, 52, 54, 89, 111,
    114, 135, 143

N

Nerve function   41, 52
Nervous system   12, 44, 54, 74, 38, 84, 88, 89,
    113, 136
Niacin (B3)   54, 73, 75
Nitrates   74
Non-haem iron   44, 45, 48
Non-sustainable farming   13
Nori rolls   236

O

Obesity   8, 9, 10, 26, 32, 33, 36, 58, 61, 63, 79,
    85, 94, 110, 130, 131-136
Olive oil   16, 36, 37, 39, 53, 67, 74, 76
Omega-3 fats   9, 37-39, 57, 73, 74, 76, 93, 95,
    101, 103
Omega-6 fats   37, 38, 39
Orange & mango ice blocks   250
Orange & mango sauce   174
Organic food   12-14, 24, 70, 74, 110, 140
Osteoporosis   9, 38, 41, 57, 61, 65, 68, 80, 85,
    88, 90, 106-108, 123
Oven baked crumbed fish   235

P

Party food, healthy   264-266
Party punch   260
Peach & blueberry crumble   255
Pear & carob chip muffins   198
Perfect porridge   153
Pesticides   12, 140
Pesto sauce   169
Phosphoric acid   85, 87, 107
Phosphorus   42 , 57, 60, 64, 68, 88, 106-108
Phytochemicals   13, 15, 16, 19, 20, 37, 56-58,
    60, 61, 64, 65, 79, 100
Pineapple, orange, banana & spirulina juice   261
Polyunsaturated fats   36, 37, 39, 74, 76, 93-95,
    98, 110, 134, 138
Potato salad with egg & fresh herbs   181
Potassium   13, 60, 63, 64, 79
Poultry   13, 16, 34, 54, 73-75
Prebiotic   23, 22
Preservatives   12, 69, 139, 140
Probiotic   104, 83
Processed foods   18, 32, 79, 78, 89, 91, 96, 118,
    119, 121, 124, 128, 130-132, 134, 139, 140
Protein   9, 13, 14, 18, 27, 28, 32, 34, 35,42, 44,
    46, 54, 57, 64, 68, 70, 71, 73, 75, 76
Protein complementation   34, 75, 112
Pumpkin & leek soup   190
Pumpkin & ricotta quiche with pecan base   223
Pyridoxine (B6)   54

R

Raspberry baked rice pudding   252
Raspberry sauce   174
Raw vegetable dippers   164
Recommended Daily Intake (RDI)
    Protein   35
    Calcium   43
    Iron   45
    Zinc   47
    Vitamin C   49
    Vitamin B12   54
Red blood cells   44, 50, 52, 54, 73, 114, 113
Red meat   16, 73-75
Reproductive system 12, 73, 114
Resistant starch   21, 23, 24, 58, 64, 137
Ribroflavin (B2)   54, 75
Rice paper rolls   237
Rickets   106, 107
Roast vegetable & hummus pies   224
Roast vegetable salad with tahini dressing   177
Raspberry & watermelon ice block   280
Rosemary chicken & kumera risotto   246

S

Salmon & pesto pasta salad   185
Salmon, kumera & quinoa patties   230
Salmonella   142
Salt   8, 59, 69, 78, 89, 90-92
Sandwich, wrap & pita filling suggestions   269
Saturated fats   8, 16, 36, 39, 69, 74, 78, 80, 83, 92, 92-98, 110, 130, 133, 134, 138, 140
Savoury spicy pumpkin & corn muffins   207
Seaweed   34, 38, 67, 91, 103
Selenium   58, 64
Sesame crumbed tuna & zucchini patties   229
Skin health   20, 34, 36, 44, 48, 50, 52, 54
Sodium   41, 63, 69, 73, 81, 89, 90-92
Soft drinks   8, 12, 17, 32, 33, 41, 78, 80, 84, 85, 87, 88, 107, 134, 136
Soluble fibre   22-24, 60, 64
Soy food   14, 41-43, 70, 71, 101, 103, 110, 112, 113, 118, 119, 121, 124, 125, 127, 128
Spicy pea & lentil dahl   244
Sprouts   18
Staphylococcus   142
Stevia   84
Strawberry & vanilla smoothie   259
Strawberry yoghurt ice cream   254
Sustainable farming   13
Sugar, refined   17, 27, 33, 32, 63, 62, 68, 70, 72, 78-81, 83-89, 118, 128, 131-134, 136, 138, 140
Sugars, total   81, 82
Sugar cravings   26, 34, 79
Sulfur dioxide   63
Sweet dessert dressings   174

T

Tahini   34, 38, 39, 42-44, 62, 71-73, 76, 83, 92, 103, 110, 111, 113, 114, 140
Tahini dressing   172
Tandoori chicken skewers with tumeric rice   241
Tasty toast toppings   159
Tasty tortillas   231
Tea   83, 88, 106, 107
Teeth   9, 41, 48, 62, 68, 86, 87
Thiamine (B1)   54, 73, 75
Thyroid function   74, 90, 91
Toasted banana cream   174
Toasted chicken, roast vegetable & feta quesadilas   233
Toasted flat bread chips   165
Tomato, basil & hummus brushetta   218
Tomato sauce   168
Tooth decay   9, 80, 84, 86, 87, 79
Tooth erosion   8, 63, 86, 87
Trail mix   270
Trans-fats   16, 36, 38, 93-98, 78, 80
Tropical fruit crush   260
Tuna & corn pasta bake   238
Tuna, cottage cheese & sesame melt   217
Tzatziki   164

U

Unsaturated fats   27, 36, 37, 39, 74, 76, 138

V

Vanilla & carob chip ice cream   254
Vanilla coconut icing   197
Vanilla custard   256
Vegan   110, 113, 114, 118, 127
Vegetable & lima bean casserole   245
Vegetable bake with almond & sunflower crumble   220
Vegetable miso soup   194
Vegetable oil   14, 16, 37, 38, 63, 74, 93
Vegetable stock   193
Vegetarian diets   45, 64, 108, 109, 110-114
Vegie lasagna   239
Vinaigrette herb dressing   173
Vitamin A   19, 40, 50, 51, 66, 68, 107, 108
Vitamin B2   120
Vitamin B12   110, 111, 113, 120, 123
Vitamin C   9, 18, 20, 45, 48, 49, 56, 63, 66, 80, 103, 107, 108, 114
Vitamin D   41, 42, 68, 70, 106-108, 114, 118, 128
Vitamin E   37, 52, 53, 57, 103
Vitamin K   104, 118, 123

W

Water   17
Watermelon & strawberry fruit crush   260
Wholegrain cereals   19, 24, 33, 34, 38, 45, 54, 57-59, 71, 75
Wholegrain mustard dressing   173
Wholemeal spaghetti & meatballs   225

X

Xylitol   84, 136, 137

Y

Yoghurt   27, 28, 34, 39, 42, 54, 62, 66, 69, 72, 76, 80, 81, 83, 93, 94, 98, 102, 104, 106, 108, 110, 112, 113, 118, 119, 124, 127, 128, 134, 142
Yoghurt ice blocks   250
Yoghurt topped fruit ice blocks   250

Z

Zinc   9, 13, 40, 46, 47, 57, 64, 68, 73-76, 80, 102, 103, 111, 113, 123, 140